The
PLANNED PARENTHOOD®
WOMEN'S
HEALTH
ENCYCLOPEDIA

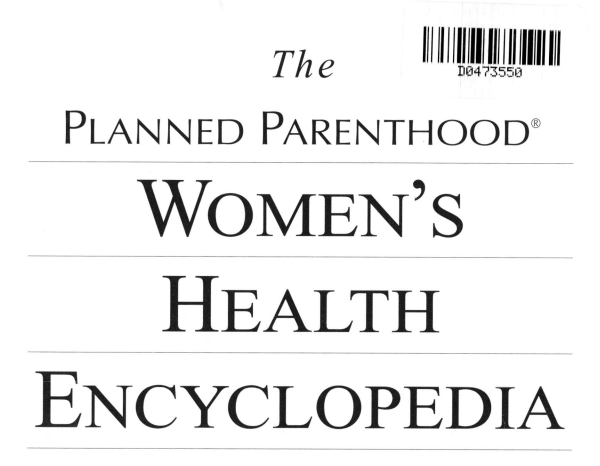

Crown Trade Paperbacks

New York

Published by Crown Trade Paperbacks, 201 East 50th Street, New York, New York 10022. Member of the Crown Publishing Group.

Random House, Inc. New York, Toronto, London, Sydney, Auckland
http://www.randomhouse.com/

CROWN TRADE PAPERBACKS and colophon are trademarks of Crown Publishers, Inc.

Printed in the United States of America

Design by Jerry O'Brien

Library of Congress Cataloging-in-Publication Data

The planned parenthood women's health encyclopedia
        p.   cm.
    Includes index.
    1. Women—Health and hygiene.   I. Planned Parenthood Federation
of America
    RA778.P655 1996
    613'.04244 — dc20   96-29188
                                                        CIP

ISBN 0–517–88823–8

10 9 8 7 6 5 4 3 2 1

First Edition

CONTENTS

ACKNOWLEDGMENTS

Books of this magnitude are created with the input and assistance of many dedicated people. We especially want to thank the following individuals for their special contributions:

The Planned Parenthood Federation of America Staff:

Michael Burnhill, M.D., Vice President for Medical Affairs

Wendy Lund, Vice President for Marketing

Barbara Snow, Vice President for Communications

Kate Thomsen, M.D., M.P.H., Associate Medical Director

Particular thanks go to Jon Knowles, Director of Sexual Health Information, for serving as editor and for working tirelessly on this project.

Medical Reviewers:

Schales Atkinson, M.D., Clinical Professor, Gynecology and Obstetrics, University of Oklahoma College of Medicine, Oklahoma City, Oklahoma

Jerry Edwards, M.D., Medical Director, Planned Parenthood of Houston and Southeast Texas, Inc., Houston, Texas

Judith E. Freedman, C.S.W., Private Practice, New York, New York

Donald Greydanus, M.D., Professor, Pediatrics and Human Development, College of Human Medicine, Michigan State University, East Lansing, Michigan; Director, Pediatrics Program, Director, Adolescent Medicine Fellowship Program, Kalamazoo Center for Medical Studies, Michigan State University, Kalamazoo, Michigan

Siri Kjos, M.D., Women's Hospital, University of Southern California School of Medicine, Los Angeles, California

Diana Koster, M.D., Medical Director, Rio Grande Planned Parenthood, Albuquerque, New Mexico

Deb Ludka, R.N., O.G.N.P., Program Development Director, Planned Parenthood of Wisconsin, Milwaukee, Wisconsin

Dorris Morrissette, M.D., Private Practice, Fort Worth, Texas

John Peterson, M.D., Medical Director, Planned Parenthood of East Central Indiana, Inc., Muncie, Indiana

Michael Rosenberg, M.D., M.P.H., President, Health Decisions, Inc., Chapel Hill, North Carolina; Adjunct Professor of Obstetrics/Gynecology, School of Epidemiology, School of Public Health, Clinical Associate Professor of Obstetrics and Gynecology, School of Medicine, University of North Carolina, Chapel Hill, North Carolina; Associate, Department of Population Dynamics, Johns Hopkins University School of Hygiene and Public Health, Baltimore, Maryland

Sirish Shah, M.D., Medical Director, Planned Parenthood of Northwest Ohio, Inc., Toledo, Ohio

Steven Sondheimer, M.D., Director, Family Planning Service, Co-Director, Premenstrual Syndrome Program, Associate Professor, Department of Obstetrics and Gynecology, Hospital of the University of Pennsylvania, Philadelphia, Pennsylvania

Gary Stewart, M.D., M.P.H., Associate Clinical Professor, Department of Obstetrics/Gynecology, School of Medicine, University of California at Davis, Sacramento, California; Instructor, Maternal and Child Health Program, School of Public Health, University of California at Berkeley, Berkeley, California; Medical Director, Planned Parenthood of the Sacramento Valley, Sacramento, California

Peter Vargas, M.D., Medical Director, Planned Parenthood of the Rocky Mountains, Aurora, Colorado

Special thanks to:

Eileen Hoffman, M.D., Director of Education, Women's Health Program, Mt. Sinai Hospital, New York, New York

Staff Reviewers at Planned Parenthood Federation of America, Inc.:

Jill Cobrin, Esq., Vice President for Insurance

Judith Greenstein, Director, Health Care Product Development

From the People's Medical Society:

Charles B. Inlander, President

Karla Morales, Vice President of Editorial Services

Janet Worsley Norwood and Andrea Monticino Riffle, Editorial Project Managers

Michael A. Donio, Director of Projects

Major editorial contributors to the book were: Kathleen Blease, Kelly F. Diefenderfer, Kaye Fitzgerald, Justine M. Johnson, Nancy J. Moffett, Deanna J. Moyer, and Maureen P. Sangiorgio. Special thanks go to Cynthia K. Moran, editor for People's Medical Society.

People's Medical Society staff deserving special recognition include Karen Kemmerer, Jennifer Hay, Gayle Ebert, Julie Bryfogle, and Lori Kulp.

Thanks also to Ann Snyder for helping to launch the project.

Special thanks also go to Jerry O'Brien for the book's design and Donna Nielsen for her illustrations.

Special kudos to Bill Betts, copyeditor; Sally Lutz, indexer; and Nancy Bailey, proofer, for making a manuscript into a book.

Thanks to Gail Ross for making this project possible.

We are indebted to Ann Patty, editorial director at Crown Publishers, for her commitment and support in this project, and to Crown senior editor, Karen Rinaldi, for her cogent comments and wise suggestions.

Many individuals provided materials that have been used or incorporated into this book. Thanks to: Terri Lowe, National Abortion Rights Action League; Alice Kirkman, American College of Obstetricians and Gynecologists; Mari Kempner, Choice in Dying, Inc.; Jean Rubel, Th.D., Anorexia Nervosa and Related Eating Disorders, Inc.; Dan Kendrick, Arthritis Foundation; Elsevier Science, Inc; the American Cancer Society; American College of Nurse-Midwives; National Women's Health Network; American College of Plastic and Reconstructive Surgeons; and American Society for Reproductive Medicine.

INTRODUCTION

Why has Planned Parenthood created this book? We have been dedicated to the health of women for 80 years—dedicated to giving women the straight facts they need to stay healthy. While health-care information today is often confusing, Planned Parenthood strives to provide easy-to-understand health information for all women—regardless of age or lifestyle.

Women's health is in the spotlight. Since the early 1990s, when it was publicly recognized that medical research had not paid enough attention to the health and medical needs of women, much has changed. For example, major research projects looking at such diverse topics as heart disease, cancer, menopause, and aging are being finished at last throughout the nation. Federal dollars finally are being directed to women's health research, now that it is recognized that similar diseases and conditions often affect women and men differently.

Women use the health-care system far sooner in life and more often than men do. Beginning in her teens with her first gynecological examination, a woman uses the health system on a regular basis throughout her lifetime. Women are also the primary decision makers when purchasing health care for their families.

Planned Parenthood has served in the vanguard in women's health since 1916, when our founder Margaret Sanger opened America's first birth control clinic and published *What Every Girl Should Know.* The police closed the clinic within weeks, and Anthony Comstock banned the booklet for years, but Planned Parenthood has been there for women, providing uncensored information about their health ever since. It is our firm commitment, established by Margaret Sanger more than 80 years ago, that women have a fundamental right to health information and the ability to take charge of their health-care management.

As a result of the devotion, courage, and commitment of Planned Parenthood staff and volunteers nationwide, Planned Parenthood is now the largest provider of health care to women in the United States. Millions of women, men, and teenagers visit Planned Parenthood health centers every year for preventive health-care services, treatment, counseling, and information. We distribute more information about women's health concerns than any other health-care organization in America.

The *Planned Parenthood Women's Health Encyclopedia* is a unique text designed specifically for women. You will find more than 120 entires on women's health, from birth control to yoga, in the *Women's Health Encyclopedia.* Let it help guide you in your quest to manage your own health. Let it serve as your primary resource for practical preventive health-care information. Consult it whenever you have a health question or concern.

We urge you to use this book as an adviser. Use it as a starting point when you begin planning a pregnancy or when you are challenged with a life-altering loss. Use it to decipher the cryptic notes on a prescription or a medical chart. Refer to it when you need to sort through a maze of information about insurance or malpractice. For further information, guidance, referral, and service, consult the resources listed at the end of most entries and the suggested readings at the back of the book. On-line sites and addresses have been included where available.

It is also important to note that the information found in the pages that follow comes from a wide list of sources. The medical information comes from published medical literature. Different viewpoints on controversial health issues are also included so that the reader has a wide range of options from which to make a health or medical decision. In other words, this is your book, not ours. It is designed for you to use as the need arises.

We have also attempted to make the book easy to use. While there is a table of contents and all entries are in alphabetical order by general topic, there are some additional features that make access to all of the information even easier. First, many entries conclude with a cross-reference guide to other topics that may expand your knowledge of a particular subject. This feature directs you quickly to a related topic. Second, the book has an extensive index that suggests a wide range of related topics you might otherwise have overlooked in your search. In addition, boldface type is used to highlight important terms within each topic.

We believe you will find, line for line, more information about women's health care in the *Planned Parenthood Women's Health Encyclopedia* than in any other publication of its kind. We are pleased that you have chosen it for your bookshelf, and we hope you will use it often and use it in good health.

The History of the Planned Parenthood Federation of America

Planned Parenthood Federation of America, Inc., is the world's oldest and largest voluntary reproductive health-care organization. Tracing its origins to the first birth control clinic in America, founded in 1916 by Margaret Sanger, Planned Parenthood is dedicated to the principle that every individual has the fundamental right to choose when or whether to have children.

On October 16, 1916, in the Brownsville community of Brooklyn, New York, Margaret Sanger, her sister Ethel Byrne, and an associate, Fania Mindell, opened the first family planning clinic in America. They provided contraceptive advice to desperately poor, immigrant women.

A month later, all three women were charged with violating New York's antiobscenity statutes. Their arrest focused attention on federal and local Comstock laws that defined contraceptives and abortifacients as "obscene." To protest the laws, Sanger refused to pay the fine and chose instead to spend 30 days in prison.

Aided by Sanger's leadership, the birth control movement grew rapidly in size and impact during the years before and after World War I. In 1936, after two decades of reproductive-rights activism, the U.S. Circuit Court of Appeals found that birth control could no longer be classified as obscene. In the years that followed, Sanger's controversial ideas ceased to be shocking and gradually became a part of American public life.

In 1942 the organization that Sanger founded took the name Planned Parenthood Federation of America (PPFA). Since then, PPFA has provided family planning counseling and reproductive health care in hundreds of communities nationwide.

In 1965 the right of all married couples to use contraception was finally upheld when the U.S. Supreme Court ruled, in *Griswold v. Connecticut,* that laws prohibiting the use of birth control by married couples violated the right of marital privacy. The Supreme Court's decision bears the name of Planned Parenthood of Connecticut's executive director of the time, Estelle Griswold, who was sued by the state for dispensing contraceptives and contraceptive information.

The right of *unmarried* people to use contraceptives was won only 25 years ago, when the U.S. Supreme Court, in *Eisenstadt v. Baird* (1972), struck down a Massachusetts statute that barred the distribution of contraceptives to unmarried people.

On January 22, 1973, the U.S. Supreme Court handed down its landmark decision, *Roe v. Wade,* which struck down restrictive abortion laws throughout the nation and declared that U.S. women had a constitutional right to choose abortion.

An antichoice constituency of about 20 percent of the American public has begun to wield considerable political influence in U.S.

legislative and judicial systems. The terrorist arm of the antichoice movement uses increasingly violent methods to prevent women from exercising their constitutional rights. The majority of Americans, however, continue to believe that individuals should be able to make their own reproductive health decisions without government interference.

Despite alarming threats, Planned Parenthood's 21,000 volunteers and staff members nationwide continue to provide medical, educational, and counseling services to meet the family planning needs of more than 5 million Americans each year. Supported by the gifts of 400,000 donors, Planned Parenthood also serves as a vigorous advocate for reproductive freedom for every individual.

Planned Parenthood Federation of America comprises 152 affiliates with 938 health centers in 49 states and the District of Columbia; a national office in New York City; a legislative and public information office in Washington, D.C.; and three U.S. regional offices (Atlanta, San Francisco, and Chicago). PPFA's international family planning efforts maintain three regional offices (Nairobi, Kenya, for Africa; Bangkok, Thailand, for Asia and the Pacific; and Miami, for Latin America and the Caribbean).

For more than three-quarters of a century, Planned Parenthood has pursued its history-making tradition, advocating reproductive rights for women and men around the world. Providing health services to American women and their families is the foundation of that heritage and has earned Planned Parenthood its reputation as America's most trusted name in women's health. To make an appointment at the Planned Parenthood health center nearest you, call 800-230-PLAN.

ABORTION

Women have turned to abortion to terminate unwanted pregnancy throughout the ages. According to the Alan Guttmacher Institute, approximately 1.6 million women choose abortion each year in the United States. Most are under 25 years old and unmarried. Women who are separated from their husbands and poor women are more likely to choose abortions than other women. A woman may choose an abortion because:

- She is not ready to become a parent.
- She cannot afford a baby.
- She has all the children she wants.
- She or the fetus has a health problem.
- She was the victim of rape or incest.
- She doesn't want to be a single mother.
- Her husband, partner, or parents want her to have an abortion.
- She doesn't want anyone to know she has had sex or is pregnant.
- She is too young and immature to have a child.

SURGICAL ABORTION

Abortion is the ending of a pregnancy. When a woman decides to end her pregnancy, the procedure is called **induced abortion. Spontaneous abortion,** or **miscarriage,** occurs when the embryo or fetus dies in the womb and is expelled by the body. A **stillbirth** occurs when the fetus is dead at birth.

The three most common methods for surgical abortion are menstrual regulation, suction curettage, and dilation and evacuation. Each of the methods interrupts pregnancy by removing the embryo or fetus from the uterus. Most abortions are performed under a local anesthetic, although some health-care facilities offer general anesthesia. They may be done by a practitioner in an office, in a clinic or health center, or in a hospital. An assistant is usually present before, during, and after the procedure to reassure the woman by answering questions, holding hands, and talking.

During surgical abortion, many women experience some cramping and a tugging feeling during the suction procedure. The majority of women experience little pain and light bleeding after an abortion. Heavy bleeding, pain, and fever are not normal effects; if a woman experiences these symptoms, she should contact her practitioner immediately.

Menstrual regulation, or **menstrual aspiration,** is performed within two weeks of a missed period. In this procedure, the uterus is emptied using the gentle suction of a syringe. There is a risk of incomplete abortion because the preembryo or embryo is so small it can be missed. The procedure is also not widely available. Most experts believe that a later abortion, at about eight weeks, involves less discomfort and less chance of complications than menstrual regulation.

Suction curettage is performed six to 14 weeks following a missed period. This procedure, also known as **vacuum curettage** or **vacuum aspiration,** takes about five minutes. With this method:

- The vagina is washed with an antiseptic solution.

■ Usually, a local anesthetic is injected into or near the cervix.

■ The opening of the cervix is gradually stretched using a series of increasingly thick rods called dilators, which are inserted into the opening. The thickest dilator is about the width of a pen.

■ After the opening is stretched, a blunt tube is inserted into the uterus. This tube is connected to a suction machine.

■ The suction machine is turned on, emptying the uterus by gentle suction.

■ The suction tube is removed, and a narrow metal loop called a curette is used to gently scrape the walls of the uterus to ensure that it has been completely emptied.

Before 1960, **dilation and curettage (D&C),** a procedure in which the cervix was dilated and the fetus and tissues were removed with a curette, was commonly performed for early abortion. However, suction curettage has now largely replaced it.

In the second trimester of pregnancy, a **dilation and evacuation (D&E),** is performed in two steps. First:

■ The vagina is washed with an antiseptic solution.

■ Absorbent dilators are put into the cervix and remain there for several hours, often overnight. The dilators absorb fluids from the cervical area and gradually stretch the cervix as they thicken. Women who are to go home with the dilators in place are given instructions for self-care until they return for the abortion. They may be given antibiotics to prevent infection.

In the second step of a D&E, which takes 10 to 15 minutes:

■ Intravenous medications to ease pain and prevent infection may be given.

■ A local anesthetic is injected into or near the cervix.

■ The fetus and placental tissues are removed from the uterus with instruments and suction curettage.

Following an abortion, the woman rests in a medically supervised room, where she is observed for any complications. This recovery time usually lasts about an hour. The clinic may require that the woman be accompanied when she leaves the clinic because she may be weak or disoriented from the medication or anesthetic. While normal activity can be resumed the day after an abortion, douches, tub baths, tampons, and sexual intercourse should be avoided for two weeks. A follow-up consultation is often scheduled after an abortion, and contraception may be discussed and prescribed.

So-called **self-help** procedures for very early abortions done at home are not advised. Serious risks include **incomplete abortion,** in which the embryo or fetus and other tissues are not completely removed and may cause infection; heavy bleeding; infection; and perforating, or making a hole in, the wall of the uterus. Complications can lead to serious injury or death.

MEDICAL ABORTION

Any drug, herb, or chemical agent that can cause abortion is known as an **abortifacient.** These substances work by causing uterine contractions, or labor, which forces the embryo or fetus and placental tissues out of the body. Plants of various types have been used since ancient times to induce abortion, although herbal abortifacients are often toxic and may have unpredictable results.

An advantage of abortifacients is that they place control with women and eliminate the feelings of invasiveness that many women undergoing surgical abortions endure. Because surgery is not involved in medical abortions, the risks of surgery are removed, and the risk of infection is lowered. In addition, medical abortions are more private, providing women with an alternative to reproductive health centers and the harassment of antichoice activists that may surround them.

Prostaglandins, synthetic versions of natural hormones, are used to induce labor after the 24th week of pregnancy if the woman's health would be jeopardized by carrying the fetus to term, or if the fetus is severely deformed. They may also effectively terminate pregnancies of four to six weeks. The prostaglandins are in the form of a vaginal suppository. Fewer than 3 percent of abortions in the United States are induced using prostaglandins.

Mifepristone, formerly known as **RU-486,** is an abortifacient developed in France that may soon be available in the United States. It is effective in inducing abortions when given as late as the sixth week of pregnancy and offers an alternative to menstrual aspiration.

Mifepristone is an antiprogesterone drug that works by blocking the receptors of progesterone, which is a key hormone in the establishment and maintenance of human pregnancy. The physical side effects of mifepristone include uterine cramps, bleeding, nausea, and fatigue—which are similar to those of a spontaneous miscarriage.

Researchers are also investigating another option for medically inducing abortions: a combination of two drugs currently available in the United States. The drugs are **methotrexate,** which is used to treat cancer, arthritis, and ectopic pregnancies, and **misoprostol,** an ulcer drug. Methotrexate breaks down the uterine lining, while misoprostol causes uterine contractions that expel the embryo. Studies are still being conducted on the use of these drugs for abortion.

ABORTIONS AFTER 24 WEEKS

Only one out of every 10,000 women—between 100 and 200 each year—has an abortion after 24 weeks of pregnancy. These are usually done

AVAILABILITY OF MIFEPRISTONE

Mifepristone was approved for use in France in September 1988, for use in the United Kingdom in 1991, and for use in Sweden in 1992 under the brand name RU-486 (Roussel-Uclaf formulation 486). Under the Bush administration, mifepristone was placed on a list of drugs banned by the Food and Drug Administration (FDA) from importation into the United States.

In January 1992 the Clinton administration asked the FDA to reevaluate this import ban. As a result, the pharmaceutical firm that developed the drug, Roussel-Uclaf, donated the patent for the drug mifepristone to the Population Council, a New York–based non-profit research institution. At the time of publication, the FDA is expected to approve the use of mifepristone in the near future. However, it may not be available from all practitioners even after approval.

For further information about mifepristone, contact the Planned Parenthood Federation of America: in New York, 212-261-4665; in Washington, D.C., 202-785-3351.

because of genetic abnormalities detected late in the pregnancy or because of serious maternal health problems.

The **induction method** uses an injection of salt solution into the uterus to cause contractions, or labor, that results in a stillbirth. Labor can also be induced with a prostaglandin. The method is done in a hospital with the woman staying overnight or longer. The chance of complications is higher than that of early abortion or D&E but may outweigh the risk of carrying the pregnancy to term.

In rare cases, major surgery is performed because the induction method cannot be used or because it was ineffective. In a **hysterotomy,** an incision is made in the abdomen, the fetus and placenta are removed, and the incision is closed. Hysterotomy requires general anesthesia and five to seven days in the hospital. It does not prevent the woman from having children in the future.

COUNSELING

Reproductive health centers and hospitals that provide abortions should have trained counselors to discuss the three options—parenting, adoption, and abortion—available to women facing unwanted pregnancies. The counselor should also ensure that the woman is not being pressured into her choice by a parent, partner, or friend.

Health centers and hospitals require the woman to sign an "informed consent" form before she has an abortion. The form ensures that she has been informed about all of the options; that she understands the abortion procedure, its risks and benefits, and how to care for herself afterward; and that she has chosen abortion of her own free will.

EFFECTS OF EARLY ABORTION

According to the Alan Guttmacher Institute (AGI), a special affiliate of Planned Parenthood that is involved with reproductive health research, policy analysis, and public education, early abortion is safer than a shot of penicillin and about 11 times safer than carrying a pregnancy to term. Fewer than five out of 1,000 women suffer serious complications from early abortions. However, the risk of rare and serious complications—which may lead to death—increases the longer the pregnancy is allowed to progress. Complications that may arise include:

■ Allergic reactions to anesthetics or other medication

■ Incomplete abortion

■ Blood clots in the uterus

■ Uterine infections

■ Heavy bleeding that requires medical treatment

■ A cut or torn cervix

■ Perforation of the wall of the uterus

Though choosing an abortion may be a difficult decision for many women, research studies indicate that the most common emotional response to abortion is relief. Overall, emotional responses to induced abortion are generally positive, according to the AGI. Although mild, transient depression immediately following the procedure occurs in fewer than 20 percent of all women who have had abortions, AGI reports that up to 98 percent of the women who have abortions have no regrets and under similar circumstances would make the same choice again.

Of women who have had an abortion, 10 percent experience some lingering depression, but severe psychiatric disturbances occur in fewer than .02 percent of women following abortion. Young women who choose abortion generally do better in the future, economically and educationally, and they have fewer subsequent pregnancies than young women who do not.

THE COST OF ABORTION

Fees for abortion vary depending on how far along the pregnancy is when the procedure takes place. Charges usually cover one examination and laboratory tests, the anesthetic, the procedure, the follow-up exam, and a birth control method. Costs at clinics range from $250 to $400 for abortion in the first trimester. Costs at hospitals will be higher depending on how long the woman stays and what anesthetics are used. There may be additional charges if extra tests or medications are required.

Private insurance companies have varying policies on the coverage of abortion. In most states, Medicaid funding of abortion is restricted to abortion in which the life of the woman would be endangered if the pregnancy were carried to term, or when pregnancy is the result of rape or incest.

MANDATORY PARENTAL INVOLVEMENT AND WAITING PERIODS

Most states do not require women to tell their partners or husbands before having an abortion. However, 38 states do require women under the age of 18 to notify or get the permission of at least one parent before an abortion. If a minor in one of those states chooses not to tell a parent, she must appear before a judge, who decides whether she has the maturity to make the deci-

THE ABORTION CONTROVERSY

For decades, abortion has been a source of heated debate in the United States. Those who favor the right of women to choose abortion are called **pro-choice**. Pro-choice advocates are driven by the belief that women have the right to decide when and whether to have a child, based on their own moral and religious beliefs. Those who oppose abortion describe themselves as **pro-life** and argue that life begins at the moment of fertilization and that abortion, therefore, is murder. Advocates of both points of view often cite strong moral and religious beliefs to reinforce their positions.

In its 1973 decision in *Roe v. Wade*, the United States Supreme Court ruled that a woman's right to choose abortion is constitutionally protected. Having failed to overrule *Roe v. Wade*, antichoice groups have been working to further restrict access to abortion. At the same time, pro-choice advocates are working to repeal legislation, such as the 24-hour waiting period requirement that curtails access to abortion.

sion on her own. If the judge decides she does not, the judge must determine whether an abortion is in the young woman's best interests.

Most teenagers voluntarily involve their parents in the abortion decision. Many of those who feel they cannot involve their parents obtain confidential abortion services out of state. The delays associated with judicial bypass and the time spent seeking abortion in another state can sharply increase both physical and mental health risks for the teen.

A number of states have implemented or are considering legislation that would require a waiting period, usually of 24 hours after counseling, before a woman may have an abortion. The waiting period is intended to ensure that the woman is not making an uninformed decision. Studies show that the waiting period can cause problems by necessitating a second trip to the clinic and can add to cost and the stress of having an abortion.

SEE adoption; contraception, emergency.

For more information on abortion, contact:

Alan Guttmacher Institute
120 Wall St.
New York, NY 10005
212-248-1111
information@agi-usa.org

National Abortion and Reproductive Rights Action League
1156 15th St., N.W., Suite 700
Washington, DC 20005
202-973-3000
naral@naral.org

National Abortion Federation
1436 U St., N.W.
Washington, DC 20009
Abortion Hotline
800-772-9100
202-667-5881
http://www.prochoice.org/naf

Planned Parenthood Federation of America, Inc.
810 Seventh Avenue
New York, NY 10019
For the Planned Parenthood nearest you, call
800-230-PLAN
http://www.ppfa.org/ppfa

ACUPUNCTURE

A cupuncture is an ancient Chinese healing art in which very thin needles are inserted under the skin in order to treat illness and restore good health. A practitioner of this art is an acupuncturist. Dating from 1600 to 1500 B.C., acupuncture attracted renewed attention and interest in the West after the opening of China in the early 1970s. The number of Western practitioners using acupuncture is growing. Acupuncture can be used to treat a variety of disorders, including menstrual problems, infer-

tility in women and men, fibroids, migraine headaches, and stress. People trying to quit smoking have also benefited from acupuncture.

Acupuncture is used to harmonize a person's life energy, or Qi (pronounced *chee*). In Chinese medicine, good health relies on the balance between female and male, light and dark, or yin and yang forces, to ensure a flow of Qi throughout the body.

The Qi flows along paths known as meridians, sets of invisible pathways that cover the body in set patterns. When illness occurs, the acupuncturist examines the meridians by evaluating the body's various pulses and then carefully selecting acupuncture sites. Extremely thin needles made from gold, silver, or copper are placed into sites just below the skin by the acupuncturist. A gentle twisting or pricking of the needle helps to ensure that it is properly placed and will correct the flow of Qi along the meridians.

Acupuncturists believe that currents, or impulses, begin to flow along the meridians where the needles are placed. This current travels through the nervous system and goes to the organ that is out of balance. Once the obstruction or hindrance is removed, the life forces are free to circulate once again, and balance is restored.

Reports from China indicate that major surgery has been performed while using acupuncture as the only anesthetic. Acupuncture can be done in conjunction with herbal medicine, disease-specific and preventive nutritional measures, relaxation skills, exercise, t'ai chi (an ancient Chinese art that combines meditation and exercises), and specific advice on health behaviors.

To date, acupuncture is licensed in more than half of the 50 states. In states where there is no licensing board, only licensed medical and osteopathic physicians may practice acupuncture, or the acupuncturist must operate under physician supervision or referral. For information about licensing in a particular state, contact the National Commission for Certification of Acupuncturists, listed below.

SEE Chinese medicine.

For more information on acupuncture, contact:

American Association of Acupuncture and Oriental Medicine
433 Front St.
Catasauqua, PA 18032
610-433-2448
aaaom1@aol.com

National Commission for Certification of Acupuncturists
P.O. Box 97075
Washington, DC 20096-7075
202-232-1404

Traditional Acupuncture Institute
American City Building
10227 Wincopin Circle, Suite 100
Columbia, MD 21044
301-596-6006

ADDICTION

Addiction is the compulsive need for and use of a habit-forming substance. It is characterized by tolerance, meaning the individual becomes less responsive to the substance the longer it is used, and consequently needs more of it to produce the desired effect. Some substances that are habit-forming are alcohol, illegal drugs and some prescription drugs, nicotine, and caffeine. Self-medication in the form of drugs or alcohol to relieve conditions such as stress or depression is often the basis of an addiction.

Withdrawal symptoms, which occur when the amount of a habit-forming substance is decreased drastically, appear in those who are addicted because the body becomes dependent on the continuous presence of the drug in the body's system. When the drug is eliminated or reduced, the body experiences mental and physical symptoms. Common symptoms include aches and pains, anxiety, diarrhea, insomnia, and nausea.

ALCOHOL AND ADDICTION

Many people enjoy responsibly consuming alcoholic beverages from time to time. But the overconsumption of alcohol can lead to numerous problems, including a disease called alcoholism.

Alcoholism affects a growing number of American women. Women who use alcohol often do so as a form of self-medication—to relieve stress, fight depression, or deaden the pain of physical or sexual abuse. In addition, as

more women work outside the home, they also have more opportunities to drink, more money of their own to spend on alcohol, and more daily stress. Some experts also point out that previous statistics of women and alcoholism were not accurate, since alcoholism research had been principally conducted on men until the last 15 years.

DEFINITION OF ALCOHOLISM

Alcoholism is a disease that is characterized by a person's periodic or continuous inability to control drinking, a preoccupation with alcohol, the use of alcohol despite its consequences, and distortions in thinking, most notably denial, according to the National Council on Alcoholism and Drug Dependence (NCADD). The symptoms of alcoholism, a long-lasting illness, develop in stages and create problems in work, family and social life, health, and economic functioning.

Programs that identify alcoholics often overlook women who need treatment. Women often drink in the privacy of their own homes because of the stigma attached to an alcoholic woman. In addition, some programs favor men, who are more likely to be identified through employee assistance programs or by the police due to public drunkenness or fighting under the influence. Alcoholic women also tend to pass unnoticed through health-care facilities.

The myth that alcoholics are simply weak-willed people is harmful because it can contribute to denial of the problem. Acknowledging the problem is the first step in treating the disease. Knowing that alcoholism is a disease makes it easier for the alcoholic to seek treatment and for the family to admit the problem and seek help.

DANGERS OF ALCOHOL

Because the average woman's volume of total body water is lower than that of men, the same drink given to men and women will have a greater and faster effect on women. Tolerance to alcohol also varies according to the menstrual cycle, with the highest tolerance during menstruation.

In addition, heavy drinking can cause serious, irreversible birth defects. Babies born of alcoholic mothers are at risk for developing **fetal alcohol syndrome,** a pattern of physical and mental defects that includes severe growth deficiency, heart defects, malformed facial features,

ACCORDING TO THE NATIONAL COUNCIL ON ALCOHOLISM AND DRUG DEPENDENCE:

■ Sixty percent of adult women 18 and over drink. Of the women who drink, 55 percent have fewer than 60 drinks per month, while 5 percent are considered heavy drinkers, having more than 60 per month. Roughly one-third of people who abuse alcohol or who are alcohol-dependent are women.

■ Women make up 34 percent of Alcoholics Anonymous membership.

■ Regular drinking is common among high school girls, and a sizable number engage in heavy drinking.

■ Women frequently engage in the high-risk practice of abusing other drugs in combination with alcohol.

■ Among alcoholic women, the incidence of suicide attempts exceeds that of the general population of women as well as that of alcoholic men.

■ An increased risk of breast cancer may be associated with alcohol consumption.

■ Women are likely to develop liver disease due to alcohol more quickly and with less alcohol consumption than men.

■ Women who drink heavily or are alcoholic are more likely to become victims of alcohol-related aggression such as date rape.

■ Women are now heavily targeted for the marketing of alcoholic beverages. Women spent an estimated $30 billion on alcoholic beverages in 1994 compared with $20 billion in 1984.

■ Drinking behavior differs with age, life roles, and marital status of women. A woman's drinking habits usually resemble those of her partner, siblings, or close friends.

■ Women who have never married or who are divorced or separated are more likely to drink heavily and experience alcohol-related problems than women who are married or widowed.

■ Of all women, unmarried women living with a partner are the most likely to engage in heavy drinking and to develop drinking problems.

a smaller head, abnormalities of fine motor coordination, and mental retardation. Miscarriages can occur when a pregnant woman drinks four to seven drinks a week. Since it is not known exactly how much alcohol intake endangers a fetus, it is generally recommended that a pregnant woman restrict herself to no more than two ounces of table wine a day. However, some authorities warn that even this amount can be detrimental in some individuals, and, to be absolutely safe, no alcohol should be consumed during pregnancy, an opinion endorsed by the U.S. Surgeon General's Office in 1981. Any alcohol consumed by the mother can also be passed to the baby during breast-feeding.

The use of alcohol also lowers inhibitions, which may encourage some women to engage in sex without a condom or other contraceptive, exposing the woman to the risks of pregnancy and sexually transmitted infections, including AIDS/HIV.

Traffic accidents are another serious consequence of alcohol abuse. According to the NCADD, almost half of all traffic fatalities are alcohol-related. People between the ages of 21 and 24 cause the highest number of fatal crashes due to driving under the influence.

Drinking and driving do not mix, and liquor affects everybody differently. The best rule is to never drive after drinking.

Do You—or Does Someone You Know— Have a Drinking Problem?

The following questions developed by the National Institute on Alcohol Abuse and Alcoholism may be used to help determine if you or someone you know has a drinking problem or may be an alcoholic:

■ Do you think and talk about drinking often?

■ Do you drink more now than you used to?

■ Do you sometimes gulp drinks?

■ Do you often take a drink to help you relax?

■ Do you drink when you are alone?

■ Do you sometimes forget what happened when you were drinking?

■ Do you keep a bottle hidden somewhere at home or at work for a quick "pick-me-up"?

■ Do you need a drink to have fun?

■ Do you ever start drinking without really thinking about it?

■ Do you ever drink in the morning to relieve a hangover?

■ Do you ever feel that you need a drink?

■ Do you become irritable when drinking?

■ Do you drink with the intention of getting drunk?

■ Has your drinking harmed your family or friends in any way?

■ Does drinking change your personality, creating an entirely new you?

■ Are you more impulsive when you are drinking?

If you answered yes to any of these questions, you may have a drinking problem. Consider seeking professional help.

CAUSES OF ALCOHOLISM

Alcoholism is thought to have a variety of causes, and research is being done to help better understand this complex disease. Alcohol is an addictive depressant drug that can become habit forming. Abuse may begin as innocent attempts at self-medication to relieve stress, with increasing amounts leading the user to dependency. The addiction results from a feeling of painful physical withdrawal when alcohol is no longer in the system. The manifestations of withdrawal, which include convulsions, tremors, nausea, chills, and fever, can be fatal.

There may also be a family or genetic predisposition to alcoholism. Studies show that a person whose parents or other relatives were alcoholics are more likely to become alcoholic than people with abstinent parents or relatives. The cause is not known—it may be genetic, environmental, or both. The problem might be genetic if a person is unable to properly metabolize alcohol because of heredity. Such drinkers could build a tolerance and eventually form an addiction to alcohol.

Some studies have shown that antisocial behavior and other negative personality traits may be linked to alcoholism in men. In women, alcoholism is usually related to depression.

SIGNS OF PROBLEM DRINKING

If a woman misuses alcohol—for example, uses it to forget a problem, to get through the day, to escape, or simply to become intoxicated—she may have an alcohol problem. While only 10 percent of people who drink become alcoholics according to NCADD definition, people should be warned that consuming more than four drinks (a drink being defined as 12 ounces of beer, four ounces of wine, or 1½ ounces of liquor) in a row, three days a week, every week, can be considered prealcoholic. A habit of three drinks per day for most women (six for most men) can do considerable damage to bodily organs. An estimated 4 million people in the United States are prealcoholic today (an estimated 6 million are alcoholics).

People should keep in mind that not everyone who enjoys drinking is an alcoholic and that not everyone who drinks every day is an alcoholic. Alcohol can be safe when consumed in moderation. On the other hand, there are alcoholics who do not drink every day.

GETTING HELP

By the time a problem drinker searches for help, he or she has probably become addicted to the substance and may require it in order to function. For this reason, he or she may need physical and emotional assistance to stop drinking.

An alcoholic can turn to many people for help. Medical practitioners, members of the clergy, or community health or social workers can help an alcoholic seek treatment. Most hospitals have inpatient or outpatient clinics to aid alcoholics. There are also public and private hospitals exclusively designed for the treatment of alcoholism.

Most alcohol recovery programs are based on male models of confrontation and do not reflect the needs of women. Programs often ignore the important precipitating factors behind alcoholism, such as incest survival or abuse, and never get to the heart of the problem. There is also no mechanism in place for dealing with the woman's children or family responsibilities. In fact, treatment for alcoholism may endanger a woman's legal status as a mother.

Alcoholics Anonymous (AA) is a group that emphasizes mutual support, a commitment to abstinence, and anonymity in a 12-step program toward recovery from alcoholism. AA has helped millions of people suffering from alcoholism to overcome their disease.

Families of alcoholics can seek help from Al-Anon, a group for alcoholics' spouses, and Alateen, a group for teenage children of alcoholics. These groups can help families of alcoholics understand and deal with their problems, even if the alcoholic family member has not yet sought help.

The local phone book lists organizations for alcoholics. These groups accept anonymous calls any time of the day or night.

DRUGS AND ADDICTION

Drugs, when used for nonmedical purposes or for reasons other than their intended purposes, can lead to dependency. At all social levels and backgrounds, there are women who use drugs and who are dependent upon them to alter moods or the perception of reality, to gratify physical desires, and to enhance abilities. The dependency often escalates and endangers a woman's health and well-being. Withdrawal symptoms, which may include vomiting, chills, tremors, convulsions, insomnia, and even psychotic behavior, occur if the drug dosage is drastically reduced or stopped.

DRUG USE AND WOMEN

Mood-altering prescription drugs have long been aimed at—and used by—women. In the nineteenth century, patent medicines containing dangerously large amounts of opiates were sold to women for relief of "female troubles." Today, physicians prescribe two-thirds of all legal psychoactive (mood-altering) drugs to women. More than 1 million American women report dependence on them.

DRUG ADDICTION

Addiction, the compulsive need for a substance, results after continued exposure to certain drugs. Some drugs are more addictive than others—narcotics and cocaine, for example, have highly addictive properties.

In general, users take drugs at regular, short intervals and exercise little or no self-control over their drug usage. Drugs may offer the users a euphoric sense or "high"; relieve feelings of inadequacy, depression, and pain; improve performance or abilities (such as with anabolic steroids); or give the user a way to escape from reality, stressful problems, or an unpleasant environment.

No matter which reason prompts them to take drugs, users continue using drugs to experience a certain state of euphoria and well-being and eventually need them to maintain and cope with everyday life. This type of drug dependence can lead to many health complications, including disease (hepatitis and lung and heart disease, for example), mental problems, and even AIDS if intravenous drug equipment is shared or if sexual favors are bartered for drugs.

TYPES OF DRUG DEPENDENCE

Drug abuse is normally characterized by certain drug-dependent states in which the user finds him- or herself functionally dependent, psychologically dependent, and physically dependent.

Functional dependence describes the body's need for a certain drug to perform a certain function. For example, a person may become functionally dependent on laxatives or nasal sprays. **Psychological dependence** (or habituation) is a type of compulsive behavior that fulfills an emotional need and craving for drugs to maintain a sense of well-being. **Physical dependence** (or true addiction) is a state in

RECOGNIZING DRUG ADDICTION

Drug users may eventually develop addictions and become physically and psychologically dependent on a drug.

The signs and symptoms of drug use vary from person to person, but general signs of addiction can be recognized:

■ Changes in personality or behavior, such as violent mood swings that include euphoria, apathy, depression, secretiveness, and lying

■ Discovery of drugs or drug paraphernalia: hypodermic needles, tubes, plastic bags, or other suspicious articles found on or around the user

■ Decline in job performance or academic performance

■ Changes in physical habits or appearance, including weight loss, loss of appetite, and sleeping habits

■ Withdrawal from parents, family, and friends

■ Frequent intoxication of user. The user is consistently intoxicated or high and exhibits abnormal or hazardous behavior.

Drug addiction may also be suspected if a reduced dosage or complete cessation of the drug produces pronounced withdrawal symptoms.

which the body physically needs the drug, and withdrawal symptoms appear if the dosage is decreased or stopped. Increased tolerance of the drug also occurs, meaning that increasingly higher doses of the drug are needed to achieve the same drug effect.

TYPES OF DRUGS

Drugs are classified into these general categories:

■ Depressants. Drugs that slow down and relax signals passing through the central nervous system and that may cause physical dependency: alcohol, barbiturates, sedatives, tranquilizers

■ Narcotics, or narcotic analgesics. Painkillers that are addicting and produce an intense high: opium, codeine, heroin, morphine

■ Stimulants. Addicting drugs that speed up signals to the central nervous system and produce alert, energetic behavior: cocaine, amphetamines, caffeine, nicotine

■ Hallucinogens. "Psychedelic" drugs that produce hallucinations or changes in sensory perceptions: LSD, ecstasy, mescaline, PCP, psilocybin, and cannabis (marijuana, hashish)

The treatment of drug dependence and abuse consists of various treatment programs, most of them employing gradual detoxification and continued psychotherapy treatment.

NICOTINE AND ADDICTION

In 1988 the Surgeon General's Office issued the warning that nicotine is as addictive as heroin and cocaine. The warning summarized the research of more than 50 scientists and 2,000 scientific articles indicating that smoking must be viewed as a life-threatening addiction and not merely as a dangerous habit.

While most smokers know that smoking causes an array of health problems, they continue to smoke because of the addictive properties of nicotine. Following are some of the effects of nicotine on the brain and the mind:

■ It increases the availability of an important brain chemical involved in feelings of reward and well-being.

■ Smoking makes task performance easier, improves memory, reduces anxiety, increases pain tolerance, and reduces hunger.

■ By taking short puffs or by inhaling deeply, the smoker can be either emotionally aroused or calmed.

■ Because nicotine stimulates the release of the brain's opiates, the endorphins, smokers find activities pleasurable that might otherwise be boring.

■ Smoking tends to reduce the desire for sweet-tasting, high-calorie foods.

An estimated 22 million American women were smokers in 1993. Of these, 73 percent wanted to quit smoking. However, attempts to quit smoking and to remain abstinent are hindered by nicotine addiction and by the subsequent effects of nicotine withdrawal, according to a study performed by the Centers for Disease Control and Prevention. Withdrawal symptoms may include insomnia, anxiety, nausea, tremors, and chills.

Currently, several organizations are petitioning the Food and Drug Administration to regulate products containing levels of nicotine that cause or satisfy addiction. The decision is pending court rulings. Regulating nicotine is an important step in minimizing the serious health conditions that smoking causes.

CAFFEINE

Caffeine is a bitter substance found in certain leaves and beans (such as cocoa and coffee beans) and made into products like coffee, tea, cola drinks, and chocolate. Its effect on the central nervous system not only keeps people alert but also, after only one cup of coffee, provides an improvement in mood that may last for as long as two hours. Medically, caffeine is used as a stimulant and diuretic (a drug that increases urination). It is also an ingredient of some pain relievers because it tends to constrict expanded blood vessels that cause the nerve irritation that brings on vascular headaches.

By triggering the release of adrenaline and increasing its presence in the bloodstream, caffeine speeds up the heart and stimulates the brain. However, it produces an extreme "high," which is then followed by a "crash," or feeling of letdown. While some women appear to suffer no mental or physical ill effects from absorbing large amounts of caffeine, others experience caffeine intoxication after drinking several cups of coffee or some other caffeine product. Symptoms include rapid heartbeat, headache, sleep disturbance, heartburn, irritability, anxiety, and frequent urination. The most logical treatment of these symptoms is to cut down caffeine consumption to the point where the side effects subside or to abstain from caffeine altogether.

Withdrawal symptoms occur in those who are addicted to caffeine when they sharply decrease or stop caffeine consumption. These symptoms include drowsiness, an inability to concentrate, a disinclination to work, excessive yawning, headache, and in more extreme cases, depression. A woman may want to cut back slowly while quitting caffeine in order to avoid these side effects.

Because high caffeine intake can increase blood pressure by about 14 percent and is also suspected of raising blood cholesterol levels, women with hypertension or coronary problems should control their caffeine intake. Caffeine in large amounts also places the user at risks higher than the normal for pancreatic and bladder cancer. Because caffeine constricts the blood vessels, there is an association between heavy intake and nighttime leg cramps. There may also be an increase in the severity of migraine headaches.

Because some studies have indicated a higher risk of miscarriage and prematurity in women who consumed large quantities of caffeine, many practitioners advise women to cut down their coffee consumption to one cup a day (or the equivalent in other forms).

SEE alcohol; smoking.

For more information on alcoholism, contact:

Al-Anon and Alateen Family Groups Headquarters
1600 Corporate Landing Pkwy.
Virginia Beach, VA 23454
800-356-9996 (information)
800-344-2666 (meeting information)
800-443-4525 (Canada)

Alcoholics Anonymous
475 Riverside Dr.
New York, NY 10115
212-870-3400
http://www.alcoholics-anonymous.org

Coalition on Alcohol and Drug Dependent Women and Their Children
National Council on Alcoholism and Drug Dependence
12 W. 21st St., 7th Floor
New York, NY 10010
800-423-4673
212-206-6770
http://www.ncadd.org

For more information on drug addiction and recovery programs, contact:

Drug Abuse Information and Treatment Referral Line
11426 Rockville Pike, Suite 200
Rockville, MD 20852
800-662-4357
800-662-9832 (Spanish)
800-228-0427 (deaf access)

National Clearinghouse for Alcohol and Drug Information
Substance Abuse Prevention
P.O. Box 2345
Rockville, MD 20847-2345
800-729-6686
301-468-2600
http://www.health.org

For more information on smoking, or help with quitting, contact:

American Lung Association
1740 Broadway
New York, NY 10019
800-LUNG-USA
212-315-8700
http://www.lungusa.org

International Network of Women Against Tobacco
American Public Health Association
1015 15th St., N.W., Suite 300
Washington, DC 20005-2605
202-789-5622

Smokenders
4455 E. Camelback Rd., Suite D150
Phoenix, AZ 85018
602-840-7414
smokenders@aol.com

ADOPTION

There are approximately 50,000 adoptions of children within the United States, and at least 8,000 adoptions of foreign children, each year. In addition, an estimated 10,000 children with special needs are adopted each year.

Adoption is the placement of a child with someone other than a biological parent to provide for its upbringing. The American Society for Reproductive Medicine estimates that 2 to 4 percent of the United States population are adopted. Many individuals, single and married, choose to adopt if they are unable to have children of their own. Relinquishing children for adoption is also an option for pregnant women that serves as an alternative to parenting or abortion. But some women find that the pain of being separated from their children is deeper and more long lasting than they expected.

Adoptions may be arranged through agencies (licensed and unlicensed) or may be done independently, through an attorney. In **agency adoption,** the agency provides counseling, handles legal matters, makes arrangements for a child's birth, and selects a home for the child. In **independent adoption,** the legal arrangements are done privately, by an attorney, and adoptive parents often agree to pay medical bills and possibly living expenses during the pregnancy. A woman considering relinquishing her child for an independent adoption should seek her own lawyer, even though one may be offered by the adoptive couple. Some states prohibit independent adoption because there is a risk that both parties may be exploited.

While an independent adoption may take less time, an agency adoption is less likely to fail due to legal problems and may offer counseling and follow-up services. Adoptions by relatives must be approved by a judge in a family or surrogate court.

TYPES OF ADOPTION

Adoption may be "closed" or "open." In a **closed adoption,** which was the standard in the past, the names of the biological parents and the adoptive parents were not revealed to one another. Agencies believed that keeping the information unavailable to all the parties involved created a necessary separation between the adoptive and biological parents. Advocates believe that the separation preserves the privacy of the birth parents and enhances the stability of the adoptive family and the permanency of the adoption.

In an **open adoption,** which has been gaining acceptance, there is an exchange of limited information between the biological parents and the adoptive parents. In some arrangements, the birth parents may choose the adoptive parents, and the parties may choose to keep in contact with each other. Those who support open adoption believe adoptees have a right to know their origins and should have access to family medical and genetic histories for health reasons. Both closed and open adoptions are legal and binding provided they are put into effect in accordance with state laws, which vary from state to state.

In **interracial adoptions,** adoptive parents are of a different race than the child. Counseling and discussion are very helpful in dealing with the cultural problems that may arise from such diversity. The child's point of view must be considered at all times. Many agencies do not recommend interracial adoptions, and there may be restrictions in various locales.

A **domestic adoption** means that the adoptive child is a citizen of the country in which the adoption takes place. An **international adoption** involves a child who is a citizen of a different country than that of the adoptive parents. Naturalization and immigration laws must be followed.

Special needs adoption refers to the adoption of a child who has an emotional or physical

CHOOSING ADOPTION: QUESTIONS TO CONSIDER

A pregnant woman considering adoption should speak with a counselor about her options, her motivations, and her resources while making her decision. The National Council for Adoption suggests the following issues be explored:

■ The circumstances surrounding the pregnancy

■ The availability of money and other resources, presently and in the future

■ The needs of a child and the needs of the woman

■ What the future will be like for the woman if she chooses adoption, parenting, or abortion

■ The importance of family support and the consequences of the woman's decision on others

■ The necessity for good prenatal care

In addition, pregnant women considering adoption should discuss the following issues with an adoption counselor, an adoption agency representative, and, if possible, a lawyer experienced in adoption:

■ Resources, such as medical care and housing, available during the pregnancy and birth of the child

■ The birth mother's role in selecting the adoptive home

■ The choice of open or closed adoption. While most states can maintain anonymity for birth parents, a few require that the records remain open, or open them to adoptees once they reach 18 years of age. Some provide nonidentifiable information, such as medical records, to adoptees. In general, states open records if both the birth parents and the adopted child agree.

■ The birth mother's options in revoking consent to the adoption, should she change her mind

■ An explanation of the home study of prospective adoptive parents, and an explanation of what steps are taken to ensure a happy home for the child

■ The role of the biological father in the adoption process. In most states, the biological father must sign the relinquishment papers also, or a court must terminate his right to the child.

■ Postpregnancy services, including emotional counseling and support groups for birth mothers. Relinquishing a child for adoption can have a great emotional impact, causing feelings such as regret, jealousy, and self-doubt that should be addressed. A woman should consider how she will feel regarding the adoption.

✓ CHOOSING AN ADOPTION AGENCY

Before choosing an adoption agency, be sure to:

■ Call the department or office in your state that licenses adoption agencies. Find out if the agency you are considering has a current license and when the agency was last visited by a representative of the department. Ask if any unresolved complaints about the agency exist, including those of a financial nature.

■ Call various organizations that work in the human services field to see if the agency is a member in good standing with them.

■ Check with different support groups for adoptive parents about the reputation of the agency.

■ Ask the agency for a copy of its fee schedule for various services, including any costs related to an adoption that may not be included (medical bills for the birth mother and baby; travel fees). Also get a copy of the agency's written policy on refunds should the adoption fall through.

■ Request the names of some past and current clients of agencies in your area and ask them about their experiences.

---

disability. While many parents find special needs adoption rewarding, raising a special needs child can be emotionally and financially draining. There must be discussion and a realistic understanding of the child's problems and the family's resources. Support groups are available to help adoptive families deal with the problems they encounter.

THE ADOPTION PROCESS

Each adoption agency—domestic and international—has different requirements concerning issues such as age, race, religion, marital status, and sexual orientation, and each may have different waiting periods. In addition, state laws on adoption are under constant revision. An individual interested in adoption should contact a qualified attorney for information on specific laws and visit adoption agencies for an overview of their policies and attitudes.

According to the National Council for Adoption, most adoption agencies adhere to the following requirements:

■ Marital status. Adoption is easier for married couples than for single people. A minimum of three years of marriage is common. Previously divorced individuals are considered if their current marriage is stable.

■ Age. The minimum age is generally 18. Most agencies estimate there should be no more than 40 years difference between the age of the child and that of the younger of the adoptive parents.

■ Fertility status. Generally, infertile couples receive priority for adoption.

■ Previous children. Since most agencies will not place more than two children with one family, a family with one child, by birth or by adoption, can be selected to adopt a second child.

■ Finances. Adoptive parents must be able to pay the required fees, though sliding-scale fees are available based on need. Adoptions can be expensive, costing more than $10,000. The family should be able to manage its budget and support the child.

■ Background check. Applicants are checked to be sure they have no criminal record.

Upon accepting an application, an agency may ask for references from prospective parents and will require a **home study,** in which a home worker examines the environment in which the child will live. During this period, a child will be identified and the individual or couple will make the decision about whether to adopt. There will then be a supervisory period, during which the child lives with the adoptive parents, who accept responsibility for the child. After a period determined by state law, the child is legally adopted by an adoption decree.

The costs of adoption vary. The fees may be collected in a lump sum or in periodic payments. Independent adoptions are often more expensive than agency adoptions. Expenses may also include medical bills for the birth mother and the baby as well as travel expenses.

SEE abortion; infertility, procedures for.

For more information about adopting or making adoption plans, contact:

Adopt a Special Kid (ASK)
2201 Broadway, Suite 702
Oakland, CA 94612
510-451-1748

Adoptive Families of America
3333 Hwy. 100 N.
Minneapolis, MN 55422
612-535-4829

Children Awaiting Parents
700 Exchange St.
Rochester, NY 14608
716-232-5110

Independent Adoption Center
391 Taylor Blvd., Suite 100
Pleasant Hill, CA 94523
510-827-2229
http://www.adoptionhelp.org/nfediac

National Council for Adoption
1930 17th St., N.W.
Washington, DC 20009
202-328-1200
info@ncfa-usa.org

AGING

Though society today extols the value of youth, the privileges and experiences that come with age are cherished by the older population. Women are living longer lives today than they ever have before, with an average life expectancy from birth of 79 years. If a woman reaches age 65, she can expect to live 20 more years—almost one-fourth of a lifetime. Though aging brings its share of difficulties and adjustments, with the years come added opportunities, and great potential for personal growth, friendship, and love.

HEALTH AND AGING

The first thing most people think of when they consider aging is the deterioration of health. However, older women are, overall, relatively healthy. The United States Census Bureau reports that eight out of 10 people over the age of 65 report that their health is "good" or "excellent." In addition, the death rates for older women have dropped significantly over the past 40 years.

Health maintenance is an important part of feeling good throughout the later years of life. Over the years, people are encouraged to stay out of the sun, practice good dental hygiene, cut back on high-fat foods and alcohol, get enough vitamins and minerals, and quit smoking. For many, these preventive measures pay off: such recommendations can help prevent osteoporosis, heart disease, skin cancer and wrinkles, gum disease, and tooth loss in later life. Regular exercise also helps to build bone mass and helps to maintain flexibility and strength as the body ages.

Even for those who didn't keep up with such recommendations while they were younger, it is never too late. Exercise, for example, greatly benefits older women by strengthening muscles and improving flexibility, countering the effects of osteoporosis. Changes in diet and quitting habits like smoking can also make a considerable difference and may add even more years to life. Other health problems that come with age, such as vision and hearing loss, are often treatable conditions, and there are many resources available to prevent disability and to help those who are disabled improve the quality of their lives.

An important key to health during the later years is the cooperation of a qualified practitioner. Good medical care, plus access to information on preventive measures and self-care, is an indispensable part of living a healthy life. Older women should make an effort to find a qualified practitioner. A board-certified specialist in geriatric medicine may be the best choice for someone over age 65 because training programs on women's health are not yet standardized or easy to find. Qualifications aside, a practitioner should have good communication skills and make an effort to answer questions, discuss problems, and provide information for the woman. A woman can ask her friends and family for recommendations for a practitioner, or she can contact the American Board of Medical Specialties at 800-776-CERT for information on board-certified physicians in her area.

BEAUTY AND AGE

Age brings with it changes to the body. After menopause, the skin loses some of its elasticity, giving way to wrinkles. The breasts may become less full, and hair may lose its color. The changes in personal appearance are difficult for some to adjust to, especially in a society that associates beauty with images of youth.

For those who are uncomfortable with the signs of aging, cosmetics and hair products are available for temporarily smoothing out wrinkles and covering gray hair. For dry skin, moisturizers are available to help restore elasticity and perhaps reduce the appearance of wrinkles. Cosmetic surgery may be an option for some women.

However, many women and men believe that the signs of aging do not detract from beauty and may even add to it. Some see the

ALZHEIMER'S DISEASE

Alzheimer's disease is a progressive degeneration of brain cells. Believed to affect more than 4 million Americans, and more women than men, Alzheimer's results in a loss of memory, confusion, anxiety, depression, and eventually death. The disease, which is thought to be caused by an inherited gene, has no cure, although some medical treatments may slow degeneration.

An early symptom of Alzheimer's is loss of short-term memory—not just simple forgetfulness. It is also characterized by difficulty thinking and possibly by personality changes. Eventually, the Alzheimer's patient will be completely dependent on others for care. One of the challenges facing many American women is that of caring for elderly parents with the disease.

Diagnosis for Alzheimer's must be done carefully, because many other neurological disorders (which are treatable) may be confused with Alzheimer's. A practitioner should perform a complete physical and neurological exam, blood tests, a thyroid test, and a spinal tap or lumbar puncture (to check for infections of the nervous system). In addition, an electroencephalogram (which measures brain activity) and a CAT scan (computerized axial tomography scan, a three-dimensional x-ray of the brain) should also be done.

The drug tacrine (THA) is the main treatment for Alzheimer's today, although other experimental drugs are currently being tested. THA works by increasing the levels of the chemical acetylcholine, which carries messages among nerve cells in the brain. Side effects include liver damage.

For more information on Alzheimer's, contact:

Alzheimer's Association
919 N. Michigan Ave., Suite 1000
Chicago, IL 60611-1676
800-272-3900
http://www.alz.org/

American Health Assistance Foundation
15825 Shady Grove Rd., Suite 140
Rockville, MD 20850
800-437-2423
301-948-3244
http://www.ahaf.org

changes as the mark of maturity and wisdom, holding more value than youthful beauty.

SEXUALITY AND AGE

There is no decrease in sexual ability for either men or women that comes with the natural process of aging, although it may take longer for both men and women to become aroused. For a woman over age 65, it may take as long as five minutes to become lubricated. Men take longer to achieve an erection, but the erection lasts longer before orgasm, which can complement the slower arousal time for women. While menopause means the end of worries about birth control, the possibility of sexually transmitted infections is still present, even for older women, so a condom should be used with any partner outside of a mutually monogamous relationship.

If the effects of age make sex difficult, a change in position may make it easier. For example, the "spoon" position, in which the partners lie front-to-back, on their sides, relieves the pressure that one body on top of another may cause. Holding, cuddling, or caressing a partner is an intimate, pleasurable, meaningful act as well. Masturbation, done alone or with a partner, and manual stimulation can also be sexually satisfying.

DEALING WITH GRIEF AND DEATH

While the life expectancy of both men and women has increased, women are still outliving men by an average of seven years. In fact, women make up the majority of the over-65 population and outnumber men in the over-80 population by two to one.

The downside to women's increased lon-

gevity is that they often have to cope with the deaths of their partners, friends, and family members. Deaths of family and friends may mean not just handling grief but also financial problems and possibly a change in residence.

Those over 65 are encouraged to seek counseling for grief and other difficulties. Statistics show that few older women seek care for their problems, perhaps because many members of their generation grew up in an era where people did not speak openly about their problems. Some seniors also feel such counseling is expensive, although this concern is increasingly less valid. Before 1990 Medicare only covered payments of psychiatrists. However, Medicare payments now extend to psychiatric and clinical psychologists and licensed and accredited social workers, enabling older people to seek the help they may need.

Older women who have lost a partner do not have to remain socially isolated. One solution is to maintain close, emotionally supportive ties to others. By staying involved with religious, civic, and social groups, many women find the practical help, companionship, and emotional support that help make living enjoyable.

POVERTY

Some of the greatest challenges that older women face are economic ones. The national poverty rate for women 65 and over is almost twice that of men. Older women living alone are even more likely to be poor than those living with a partner or others. In fact, according to the Business and Professional Women's Foundation, marital status is the most significant indicator of whether a woman will have a comfortable retirement or a life ending in poverty. Consider the following statistics:

■ A widowed woman is four times more likely to live in poverty after retirement than a married woman.

■ Single or divorced women are five times more likely to live in poverty after retirement than married women.

■ Eighty percent of widows now living in poverty were not poor before the death of their husbands.

■ Elderly women living alone had annual median incomes of $9,513 in 1990.

Although Social Security benefits are intended to provide a reasonable level of financial support for the retirement years, women often do not receive the same level of payment as men. The primary reason for lower benefits is the generally lower earnings women receive, a difference explained by the wage gap, occupational segregation, and the years out of the labor force that women often spend tending to family responsibilities—years when their Social Security accounts are not being credited.

The best way to avoid financial difficulties in later years is to plan ahead for retirement. A woman should not rely on the possibility of remarriage as a form of economic rescue, but instead should try to take control of the situation. A number of organizations can provide information on Social Security and finances, and many work with women to help change difficult financial situations.

INDEPENDENCE

Many women do not experience independence until the later years of life. At this time, children are grown and out of the house, and retirement allows more free time. These situations provide opportunities unavailable in the past.

One of the greatest freedoms older women have is from stereotypes. No longer do they have to fit the image of the wife or homemaker or comply with the standards of beauty and conventionality. Many feel that older women have earned the right to speak their minds. What may be considered unorthodox from a younger woman is considered character in an older woman.

On the other hand, with people living longer, a woman may find herself in the role of caretaker, caring for an older or younger family member. Many women—75 percent of all caregivers are women—accept this challenging position in addition to a full-time job. While caregiving has many rewards, it commonly leads to fatigue and stress. Many support groups and organizations provide help for caregivers facing "burn-out."

WELL-BEING

In addition to physical health, emotional well-being is important to the older woman, and remaining involved in all aspects of life is an important part of maintaining that emotional health. Though some people have the impression that aging means slowing down and cutting back on activity, this does not have to be the case. Retirement provides plenty of time to pursue opportunities that may not have been feasible in the past. An older woman may want to pursue an education, volunteer for a local organization, or start her own business. If finances allow, travel may be possible.

New friendships and relationships are also a valuable part of growing older. During the later years, many women form strong friendships with other women, and some may find a new partner. Again, by taking control of their lives, women give themselves the best opportunities for happiness and health in later life.

CHALLENGING AGEISM

While biological changes occur over a lifetime, the natural aging process does necessarily reflect society's concept of "getting old." Ageism is prejudice or discrimination because of age. It is based on the belief that a person's worth and abilities are determined solely by chronological age. It is an attitude that threatens the continuing creative and mental growth of both younger and older women.

Research shows that intellectual capacity remains stable throughout life and that the ability to learn new things does not disappear with age. Women are thought to suffer ageism more than men because the attitude that the primary purpose of a woman's life is to have and raise children persists, and therefore women are considered obsolete once their childbearing potential ends. Many contemporary women may feel themselves free from such beliefs; yet they, too,

LATE-ONSET SUBSTANCE ABUSE

Older women may turn to alcohol and drugs to ease psychological and physical pain—just as young people do—often resulting in late-onset substance abuse.

For information on helping those over 65 who may have a substance abuse problem, contact:

Hopedale Hall
P.O. Box 267
Hopedale, IL 61747
800-354-7089
800-344-0824 (Illinois)

LOOKING AHEAD TO RETIREMENT

The Pre-Retirement Education Planning Program (PREP) is an activity of the National Center for Women and Retirement Research designed to encourage women to look ahead to their financial future and to provide them with the skills they need to plan effectively. For more information, contact:

National Center for Women and Retirement Research
Long Island University
Southampton Campus
Southampton, NY 11968
800-426-7386
ncwrr@sand.liunet.edu

often suffer the legacy of discrimination when they enter or reenter the workforce in their middle years.

The baby boomers, now aged 32 to 50, are currently the largest age group in the population. Their concerns about aging will profoundly influence attitudes and policies about aging in the coming decades. In spite of the difficulties many older women currently face, the outlook may be improving for future generations, as women continue to be better educated, better paid, and healthier physically and mentally.

Today a number of older women are combating ageism as members of such activist groups as the American Association of Retired Persons (AARP), Older Women's League (OWL), and the Gray Panthers.

SEE board certification; death and dying; disabilities; insurance; long-term care; physical fitness; practitioners, how to choose.

For more information on aging and women, contact:

Gray Panthers
2025 Pennsylvania Ave., N.W.
Suite 821
Washington, DC 20006
202-466-3132
dixieh1064@aol.com

National Academy on Aging
1275 K St., N.W., Suite 350
Washington, DC 20005
202-408-3375
http://www.geron.org

For information on Social Security and finances, contact:

Clearinghouse on Pensions and Divorce
    Pension Rights Center
918 16th St., N.W., Suite 704
Washington, DC 20006
202-296-3776

National Senior Citizens Law Center
1815 H St., N.W., Suite 700
Washington, DC 20006
202-887-5280
hno538@handsnet.org

Older Women's League
666 11th St., N.W., Suite 700
Washington, DC 20001
202-783-6686

Social Security Administration
Office of Public Inquiries
6401 Security Blvd.
Baltimore, MD 21235
410-965-8882

Womoney
Sharon Rich, Ed.D.
76 Townsend Rd.
Belmont, MA 02178
617-489-3601

AIDS/HIV

Acquired immunodeficiency syndrome (AIDS) is the final stage of HIV disease, a condition that results from the destruction of the body's immune system by the human immunodeficiency virus (HIV). This virus can weaken the body's ability to fight off infection and diseases. Women, especially young women, are the fastest-growing group of people with AIDS.

ARE YOU AT RISK?

According to the Centers for Disease Control and Prevention, there is evidence that HIV has been in the United States since at least 1978. If you answer yes to any of the following questions, and they apply to you since 1978, consult your practitioner about HIV testing and counseling.

■ Have you shared needles or syringes to inject drugs or steroids?

■ Did you receive blood transfusions or blood-clotting factor between 1978 and 1985?

■ Have you had any other sexually transmitted infections (STIs)?

■ Have you had unprotected sex with someone whose HIV status was unknown to you?

■ Have you had unprotected sex with someone who may have used IV drugs or who had sexual contact with partners who may have used IV drugs?

When a virus enters the body, the immune system's job is to produce antibodies that seek and destroy the invader. However, HIV, like other viruses, has the ability to protect itself from antibodies by camouflaging itself as part of the genetic makeup of its host cell.

The host cells that HIV infects, called **T-cell lymphocytes,** work as part of the immune system to prevent disease. The HIV virus multiplies as the T-cell multiplies, and eventually destroys the T-cell, leaving the body completely vulnerable to opportunistic infections and diseases. An **opportunistic infection** is an infection that is normally destroyed by a healthy immune system but instead "takes advantage of" an unhealthy system. Opportunistic infections destroy the immune system and are fatal.

There is no cure for AIDS, but medical developments have helped delay the onset of AIDS symptoms or lessened their effects, thereby prolonging the life expectancies of some people with AIDS.

HOW HIV IS TRANSMITTED

HIV thrives in certain bodily fluids and secretions, especially in semen, blood, and breast milk. The virus enters the body through cuts and sores as well as the moist lining of the vagina, penis, rectum, and even the mouth. A woman may give the virus to her fetus during pregnancy or birth. Breast-feeding may also pass the virus to an infant. Although there are traces of HIV in sweat, saliva, and tears, there is not enough of the virus in these fluids to cause infection.

The most common ways HIV is spread are by:

■ Having vaginal or anal intercourse

■ Sharing needles or syringes. This includes needles used in piercing or tattooing as well as those used in intravenous drug use.

■ Receiving a transfusion of blood. Methods of screening blood supplies have made this avenue of transmission much less prevalent.

■ Having donor insemination using the sperm of a man with the virus. Again, screening has made this rare.

■ Being accidentally punctured or cut with a needle or surgical instrument contaminated with the virus. This is called a needle stick.

■ Receiving organs donated by someone with the virus

HIV *cannot* be contracted by:

■ Visiting, socializing, working with, or going to school with someone who has it

■ Being sneezed or coughed on by a person who has it

■ Sweating with or crying with someone who has it

■ Being bitten by a mosquito or another insect

■ Touching or sharing things that a person with HIV has touched. This includes doorknobs, toilets, telephones, swimming pools, eating utensils, and drinking glasses.

■ Giving blood

AIDS STATISTICS

When AIDS was first diagnosed in the United States in 1981, nearly all those infected were gay men or intravenous drug users. Today, the profile of an individual at risk of contracting HIV and developing AIDS is far more diverse. In fact, infection through heterosexual contact with an HIV-infected man is the fastest-growing mode of transmission. According to the Centers for Disease Control and Prevention (CDC), in 1994 women represented 18 percent of the new AIDS cases reported among adults. Of the women who contracted AIDS in 1994, 41 percent reported that their source was sharing needles while using intravenous drugs, and 38 percent reported that they contracted HIV from a male partner.

The CDC also reports that AIDS is killing more women than ever. In 1982, soon after the disease was discovered in the United States, AIDS was the 10th leading cause of death among all American women between the ages of 25 and 44. Currently, AIDS has risen to the rank of fourth leading cause of death. Among African-American women aged 25 to 44, AIDS has become the number one killer.

AIDS disproportionately affects minority women. The rate of black women contracting the disease is 16 times higher than that of white women. For Latinas, the rate is seven times greater. In 1994, 75 percent of the women who contracted AIDS were African American or Latina, although they make up only 21 percent of the population.

TESTING FOR HIV

The tests developed to detect HIV are actually designed to detect the antibodies that are produced to fight the virus. These antibodies are ultimately ineffective in fighting the virus, but their presence indicates HIV infection. The body takes up to six months to produce the antibodies; therefore, any HIV antibody test that is negative should be confirmed with another test after six months. If a woman's test result shows the presence of the antibody, she is referred to

✓ REASONS FOR AIDS TESTING

HIV testing may be chosen for any number of reasons, including:

■ Both you and your partner have chosen to be exclusively monogamous and want to stop practicing safer sex.

■ You want to become pregnant.

■ You suspect that you have been exposed to the virus.

■ You may be tested as a requirement for health insurance or life insurance.

■ You want early treatment for HIV disease if you are infected.

■ You are applying for the armed services, Job Corps, Peace Corps, or another agency that requires testing.

as HIV-positive. Testing is available on a confidential basis (meaning a private record is kept of the test) or on an anonymous basis (meaning that the woman does not need to give her name). Antibody tests are available through most practitioners, hospitals, health clinics, and local, state, and federal health departments. Confidential counseling should be provided by these sources at the time results are disclosed.

SAFER SEX

The only foolproof protections against HIV infection are not sharing needles and not having sexual intercourse. Sex between long-term, mutually faithful, uninfected partners is also "safe."

Outside of this type of relationship, practicing "safer sex" by using a latex condom or vaginal pouch during sexual intercourse, from start to finish, can greatly reduce your risk. Condoms labeled "lambskin" or "natural membrane" may be too porous to provide a barrier against the virus. Anal or vaginal intercourse without a condom has caused millions of reported cases of HIV infection.

Very low risk behaviors include masturbation, mutual masturbation, touching, kissing and deep kissing, and oral sex on a man with a condom, or oral sex on a woman with a barrier such as plastic wrap or a cut-open condom covering the genitals. There are no reported cases of HIV transmission from these behaviors.

Oral sex, vaginal intercourse with a condom or vaginal pouch, and anal intercourse with a condom or vaginal pouch have low risk. Reported cases due to these behaviors are rare.

SYMPTOMS OF HIV

Having HIV is not the same as having AIDS. Having HIV means being infected by the virus that may eventually become a full-blown case of AIDS. (No one is sure if everyone with HIV will develop AIDS.) There are several stages of HIV disease:

1. People with HIV usually develop detectable antibodies within six months of infection. Some of them have symptoms during this time that usually are not severe. Slight fever, headaches, fatigue, muscle aches, and swollen glands may last for a few weeks.

2. There is usually a long period without symptoms after antibodies develop. This "latent period" may last many years—the average is 10. Although there are no symptoms, the immune system and various body tissues become damaged during this time.

3. People with HIV often have swelling of the lymph glands in the throat, armpits, and

TALKING ABOUT AIDS

With the incidence of AIDS on the rise, now more than ever, it is important to consider a prospective partner's HIV status before beginning a sexual relationship. Don't be embarrassed to talk about safer sex before the heat of passion; if you are close enough with your partner to have sex, you should be close enough to discuss these facts honestly. Partners should care about each other and be interested in each other's pleasure, comfort, and health.

■ Be open. Let your partner know your health concerns and sexual health history. Encourage your partner to be open, too.

■ Be direct. Talk about your sexual needs and expectations.

■ Be persistent. Don't let your partner remain silent on these issues.

It is also important to educate children and young adults about AIDS and HIV, but it may not be easy to start a conversation and provide all the facts. The Centers for Disease Control and Prevention (CDC) provides a variety of educational material that will help. Along with posters and brochures, they also offer a booklet entitled "Putting the Facts to Use: Talking with Young People About HIV Infection and AIDS." It covers deciding what to say to younger children (late elementary and middle school age) and to teenagers (junior and senior high school age). Call the CDC National AIDS Hotline at 800-342-AIDS or write to: CDC National AIDS Clearinghouse, P.O. Box 6003, Dept. G, Rockville, MD 20849.

The Planned Parenthood Federation of America offers a parent's guide entitled "Kids and AIDS," available by sending $3 to PPFA, 810 Seventh Avenue, New York, NY 10019.

---

groin. This may be the only symptom of HIV infection for a number of years. This is called persistent generalized lymphadenopathy.

4. When HIV seriously damages an immune system, a condition some practitioners call **AIDS-related complex (ARC)** and others call **pre-AIDS,** may occur. The symptoms of this stage include:

■ A fungal infection causing a white coating of the vagina, mouth, or throat (this is commonly called thrush)

■ Viral infections that affect the skin and mucous membranes of the anus or genital area

■ Severe and frequent viral infections like herpes or pelvic inflammatory disease

5. AIDS is the final stage of HIV disease.

It may take 12 or more years after HIV infection for AIDS symptoms to develop.

SYMPTOMS OF AIDS

AIDS begins when a person with HIV develops one of the defining opportunistic infections or conditions. These include a variety of viral, bacterial, fungal, and parasitic opportunistic infections as well as certain cancers. Other conditions included in the definition of AIDS are:

■ HIV-wasting syndrome, an involuntary loss of 10 percent or more of normal weight, with chronic diarrhea, or weakness and fever caused by conditions other than HIV disease

- HIV infection of the brain, also called AIDS- or HIV-dementia or HIV-encephalopathy
- Pneumonias
- Tuberculosis
- Cervical cancer in women

TREATMENT OF AIDS/HIV

To date, there is no completely effective treatment or vaccine for AIDS. AIDS drugs include zidovudine (AZT), dideoxyinosine (DDI), zalcitabine (DDC), and lamivudine (3TC), which are often used in combination. These drugs are intended to slow the progress of HIV disease. Many of these treatments are toxic, and they may cost thousands of dollars a year. As we go to press, drugs called protease inhibitors have been found to show great promise in decreasing the viral load when combined with AZT and 3TC.

Alternative treatments, such as acupuncture, herbal and homeopathic remedies, and yoga, have also been used against AIDS, though they are mainly effective in relieving pain. Some people with HIV disease or AIDS turn to experimental drugs for treatment.

HIV, AIDS, AND PREGNANCY

Fifteen to 30 percent of children born to HIV-positive women are infected with the virus. The virus is transmitted through pregnancy, labor, or breast-feeding. Thousands of infants are infected with the virus each year. In the United States, HIV is currently the seventh leading cause of death in children. Nearly 90 percent of all AIDS cases reported among children and virtually all new HIV infections among children in the United States are now attributed to perinatal transmission.

Recent evidence shows that the risk of prenatal transmission can be reduced with the use of the drug zidovudine (also called AZT) in women who are in the early stage of HIV disease. By beginning a regimen of AZT sometime between 14 and 34 weeks of gestation and continuing through the pregnancy, labor, and in the infant during its first six weeks of life, practitioners have found that the risk of HIV transmission from a woman to her baby can be reduced from 25.5 to 8.3 percent.

RECOMMENDATIONS FOR PREGNANT WOMEN

The United States Public Health Service recommends HIV counseling and voluntary testing for all pregnant women in the United States. Any woman who is pregnant and has been at risk of contracting HIV should consult her practitioner for HIV antibody testing and the advantages and disadvantages of AZT. The earlier in the pregnancy treatment begins, the more effective it is.

SEE death and dying; long-term care; pregnancy—prenatal concerns; safer sex; sexually transmitted infections.

For more information about HIV infection or AIDS, contact:

AIDS Clinical Trials Hotline
800-TRIALS-A
800-243-7012 (deaf access)

Centers for Disease Control and Prevention National AIDS Hotline
800-342-AIDS
800-344-7432 (Spanish)
800-243-7889 (deaf access)
http://sunsite.unc.edu/asha/

Project Inform National Hotline
AIDS Treatment Information
800-822-7422

Lesbian and Gay Rights AIDS Project
American Civil Liberties Union
132 W. 43rd St.
New York, NY 10036
212-944-9800 ext. 545
lgrp@aol.com

National AIDS Clearinghouse
Centers for Disease Control and Prevention
P.O. Box 6003
Rockville, MD 20849
800-458-5231
800-243-7012 (deaf access)
http://www.cdcnac.org

National Institute of Allergy and Infectious Diseases
National Institutes of Health
31 Center Dr., MSC 2520
Bldg. 31, Room 7A50
Bethesda, MD 20892-2520
301-496-5717
niaidoc@niaid.nih.gov

ALCOHOL

Alcohol is a depressant drug, absorbed by the blood, that has both physical and mental effects. Alcohol affects everyone differently, though it does tend to affect women more quickly and powerfully than it affects men. This is because women have less water in their systems than men, and therefore any alcohol in the system is stronger and less diluted. Women also have less of the enzymes that break down alcohol than men. In addition, the hormonal changes that occur during menstruation and affect metabolism play a role in how alcohol is absorbed and tolerated by the female body.

DRINKING HABITS

People drink for various reasons. The **social drinker** tends to drink slowly, limit alcohol intake, and show responsible drinking habits. The **problem drinker** tends to drink to get intoxicated and thereby escape problems. A problem drinker may also experience personality changes when he or she drinks and may show irresponsible drinking habits such as driving or going to work while intoxicated. **Alcoholics** spend time planning their drinking, drink secretly, and are often unaware of the amount they have drunk. They may often drink alone, deny drinking, suffer withdrawal symptoms when not drinking, and cause problems because of their drinking.

Often a woman's drinking habits reflect those of her partner, friends, or siblings. A woman's drinking habits also hinge on psychological factors in her life, such as depression, isolation, abuse, or stress. Studies have shown that a woman who has never married or who is divorced or separated is at a higher risk for heavy drinking than a woman who is married or widowed. Those women who are unmarried but living with a partner are at the highest risk of heavy drinking habits.

BENEFITS OF ALCOHOL

Although people tend to think of alcohol consumption as negative, it may have benefits under certain circumstances. A recent study showed that one to three drinks per week may be beneficial to women aged 50 to 70 who have a risk for heart disease. Women who have a risk for heart disease and drink moderately have a lower rate of mortality than those who have a risk for heart disease and drink either heavily or not at all. In the same study, women who were under the age of 50 and drank had a higher risk of death.

RISKS OF ALCOHOL

Alcohol consumption should never be mixed with any other drug or medication. This is the number one cause of drug-related deaths in the United States. While drinking can cause and complicate a number of health conditions, it can also react negatively with medications, such as amitriptyline (an antidepressant) and methotrexate. The possible effects of alcohol should be discussed with the practitioner whenever a drug is prescribed.

Studies have shown that drinking more than three drinks a week, by a person of any age, results in a higher mortality rate. In women, the alcoholic death rate is 50 to 100 percent higher than for male alcoholics. There have also been links between heavy drinking and the rise in breast cancer. Long-term, heavy alcohol intake can result in an increase in the risk for heart disease, circulatory problems, peptic ulcers, cancer, brain damage, and cirrhosis of the liver. Cirrhosis of the liver was listed as the 11th leading cause of death in the United States in 1992 when eight out of every 100,000 people died of liver disease and cirrhosis.

Repeated, extensive drinking to the point of intoxication can cause harmful and irreversible damage both physically and emotionally. Being intoxicated can lead to injuries, automobile accidents, fights, unintended pregnancy, sexually transmitted infections, and date rape. It also increases the risk of suicidal behaviors that may result in death.

Alcohol consumption poses health and social risks. Even moderate amounts of alcohol can reduce coordination and awareness. It is very important not to drive, operate machinery, or play certain sports after consuming even moderate amounts of alcohol. Consuming large amounts of alcohol can diminish concentration, intensify negative behaviors, slur speech, cause staggering and double vision, promote mood swings, and result in unconsciousness. The indirect effects of heavy drinking are also associated with such adverse consequences as dysfunctional family life, unemployment, poverty, and being at risk for sexual and physical abuse.

BLOOD ALCOHOL LEVELS

Blood alcohol level, BAL, refers to the amount of alcohol in a person's bloodstream as recorded in milligrams of alcohol per 100 milliliters of blood. If a person is said to have a blood alcohol level of .2, then 2 percent of his or her blood is alcohol. The human liver can only break down the alcohol of one drink (12 ounces of beer, four ounces of wine, or 1½ ounces of liquor) per hour, the equivalent of a .02 blood alcohol level. The faster one drinks, the higher his or her blood alcohol level will be. A person's blood alcohol level also depends on the amount of blood or size of the person. A BAL of .08 is considered legally drunk in many states; a BAL of .5 usually results in death.

HOW LONG TO WAIT BEFORE DRIVING

Drinking and driving can have serious consequences, and liquor affects everyone differently. As a rule, it is a good idea not to drive at all if you have been drinking. The following table is a general guideline for how long to wait after drinking alcohol before attempting to drive. A drink is defined as 12 ounces of beer, four ounces of wine, or 1½ ounces of liquor. For example, if you weigh 130 pounds and have consumed three drinks, you should wait five hours before driving.

Hours to Wait Before Driving

Weight	1 Drink	2 Drinks	3 Drinks	4 Drinks	5 Drinks	6 Drinks
100–119	0	3	6	10	13	16
120–139	0	2	5	8	10	12
140–159	0	2	4	6	8	10
160–179	0	1	3	5	7	9
180–199	0	0	2	4	6	7
200–219	0	0	1	3	5	6
Over 200	0	0	1	3	4	6

A BAL self-monitor can be purchased from various organizations. They are miniature tests, which you blow into for a reading. These tests are within .02 accuracy of the amount of alcohol in one's blood. However, they are not recommended for use in determining whether driving is safe or not.

Source: U.S. Department of Health and Human Services.

BLOOD ALCOHOL LEVELS (BY PERCENT) AND PHYSICAL REACTIONS

.02   A mellow feeling with slight warmth

.05   Noticeably relaxed; less alert and self-focused; impaired coordination

.08   Legally intoxicated and unfit for driving; definite impairment in coordination and judgment

.10   Noisy; possibly behaving in an embarrassing manner; mood swings; reaction time reduced

.15   Impaired balance or movement; clearly intoxicated

.30   Many people become unconscious.

.40   Most people become unconscious. Breathing slows and may stop.

.50   Breathing stops. Death occurs.

SPECIAL CONCERNS FOR PREGNANT WOMEN

Experts advise that all alcohol consumption be eliminated during pregnancy. Even the lowest levels of alcohol consumption during a pregnancy have been known to affect the fetus. However, in rare cases, a woman may be advised by her practitioner to have an occasional glass of wine, but any such alcohol use should be carefully monitored.

Drinking alcoholic beverages during a pregnancy often causes fetal alcohol syndrome, which affects one in every 750 newborns. **Fetal alcohol syndrome,** or FAS, is a group of abnormalities that occurs in children whose mothers consumed alcohol during the pregnancy. FAS children have abnormalities affecting growth, the central nervous system, and facial features.

Linked with FAS are **fetal alcohol effects.** These also occur when alcohol is consumed during a pregnancy. Children with fetal alcohol effects have learning and behavioral problems as well as hearing and birth defects. The period of highest risk occurs around the time of conception.

SEE addiction.

For more information on alcohol, contact:

National Clearinghouse for Alcohol and Drug Information
P.O. Box 2345
Rockville, MD 20847-2345
800-729-6686
301-468-2600
http://www.health.org

National Council on Alcoholism and Drug Dependence
12 W. 21st St., 7th floor
New York, NY 10010
800-622-2255
212-206-6770
http://www.ncadd.org

ANDROGENS

Most women don't realize it, but their ovaries and adrenal glands produce more than "female" hormones; they also produce a class of "male" hormones, called **androgens.**

These hormones, the principal of which is testosterone, are the powerful stimulators of sexual desire. Androgens can be triggered by emotions or thoughts about love or sex and by foreplay. During sexual arousal, nerve impulses cause blood supply to sexual organs to increase, the clitoris to become erect, and the vagina to become lubricated. In addition, during pregnancy, two androgens known as androstenedione and dehydroisoandrosterone are converted into estrogen by the placenta.

Women whose ovaries have been removed, or who are past menopause, experience a drop in blood androgen levels just as they do in estrogen levels. Androgens have shown to be effective in the treatment of some menopausal symptoms, including hot flashes, headaches, decreased sex drive, and hormone-related depression.

However, androgens are only prescribed by practitioners for menopause symptoms when estrogen/progestin hormone replacement therapy is unsuccessful, or for specific problems such as hair loss or diminished sex drive. In general, hormone replacement therapy containing estrogen and progestin is as effective as androgen therapy in relieving the symptoms of menopause, with fewer side effects.

Common side effects of androgens include the growth of facial hair, an enlargement of the clitoris, and deepening of the voice. These side effects can be minimized by regulating dosage. Side effects are fewer if the hormone is given by intramuscular injection, every four to six weeks, rather than orally.

Several estrogen-testosterone and testosterone-only drugs are approved for use for menopausal symptoms by the Food and Drug Administration. They have not been shown to increase a woman's risk for heart disease.

SEE endocrine system; estrogen; hormone replacement therapy.

ANEMIA

Anemia is a deficiency of red blood cells that results from a variety of conditions. It is diagnosed when a blood test shows the number of red blood cells to be less than 37 percent of the total blood volume or when the blood's hemoglobin (a protein found in red blood cells) value is less than 12 grams per 100 milliliters of blood. Anemia is more common in women than it is in men because women's iron levels are depleted by menstruation and pregnancy. It is most likely to occur in women of African-American descent, young and elderly women, and poor women. Anemia often occurs because of poor nutrition or malnutrition.

SYMPTOMS

The symptoms of anemia include:
- Tiredness
- Headache
- Dizziness or fainting spells
- Hair loss
- Brittle, pale fingernails
- A pale complexion
- Sore tongue or mouth sores
- A loss of appetite and a craving for non-foods, such as ice, dirt, and clay

A complete blood count is necessary to confirm the presence of the disorder. There are

SICKLE-CELL ANEMIA

Sickle-cell anemia is a genetic disorder that affects mainly men and women of African descent. About .3 percent of all African Americans have the condition, while another 12 percent have one gene for the disease. Sickle-cell anemia is the result of a recessive gene disease, meaning that both parents must have the gene to pass it on to their child. If both parents have the gene, there is a 25 percent chance the child will have the disease.

In sickle-cell anemia, there are red blood cells in the blood that are sickle-, or crescent-, shaped. These cells are unable to pass though small blood vessels and thus accumulate as clots, which may cause **infarcts**—areas where the tissue dies because of lack of oxygen. Sickle-shaped cells also break down easily and often cause severe anemia.

Symptoms of sickle-cell anemia include painful joints and abdominal pain. The symptoms appear during a child's first year and progressively worsen. Those with sickle-cell anemia rarely live beyond age 50, and many die earlier.

It is recommended that women with sickle-cell anemia avoid pregnancy. The condition usually becomes more severe during pregnancy, and there is a high risk (one-third to one-half) of miscarriage. Pregnant women with the disease also often develop dangerous blood clots in the lungs.

Sickle-cell anemia and the gene for the disease can be detected with blood tests. If a woman becomes pregnant, the fetus can be tested for the disease through amniocentesis or chorionic villus sampling.

many women who do not realize they have anemia, and there are others who believe they are anemic when they are not.

TYPES OF ANEMIA

Iron-deficiency anemia is the most common form of anemia. Iron is used in the body to create hemoglobin, the protein in red blood cells that enables the delivery of oxygen to other cells. If not enough iron is being received by the body, the amount of red blood cells decreases.

For most women, the iron lost in menstrual flow is restored during the rest of the month. However, heavy menstrual flows, which may result from fibroids or the use of an intrauterine device (IUD), sometimes cause anemia. Internal bleeding, perhaps caused by a stomach ulcer, can result in anemia. Women often become anemic during pregnancy because nutritional demands are not being met.

Pernicious anemia, or Addison's anemia, is generally caused by deficiencies of certain B vitamins, folic acid and B_{12}, which are needed to help form red blood cells. This form of anemia is rare, since these vitamins are found in sufficient amounts in animal products. However, women who are strict vegetarians should consider a vitamin supplement. Oral contraceptives may also create a deficiency of folic acid in some women.

Some people suffer from pernicious anemia because their bodies do not absorb vitamin B_{12} easily. This may result from certain diseases, such as celiac disease, or from previous stomach or intestinal surgery that can interfere with the passage of the vitamin into the bloodstream.

Hemolytic anemia occurs when the body destroys its own red blood cells. This may happen because of Rh disease, incompatible blood transfusions, or exposure to some chemicals and medications. **Aplastic anemia** results from a disease within the bone marrow, where red blood cells are created. It may also occur after radiation, chemotherapy, or exposure to some other chemicals and medications.

Conditions such as tuberculosis, hepatitis, and rheumatoid arthritis may also play a role in the development of anemia. Large amounts of aspirin, ibuprofen, or nonsteroidal anti-inflammatory drugs (NSAIDs) may also contribute. A woman using large amounts of these medications may want to discuss the possibility of anemia with her practitioner.

SELF-CARE FOR ANEMIA

To prevent anemia, or to treat anemia that is caused by a poor diet:

■ Eat foods rich in iron, folic acid, and vitamin B_{12}.

—For iron, try eggs, red meat, liver, raisins, prunes, chicken, dried fruits, and cheese.

—For folic acid, try leafy green vegetables, such as spinach and turnip greens, sunflower seeds, soybeans, avocados, beets, and wheat germ.

—For vitamin B_{12}, try liver, organ meats, beef, pork, eggs, and nonfat dry milk.

■ Avoid alcohol, caffeinated tea, and coffee, which can interfere with the absorption of vitamins by the body.

■ Avoid antacids and phosphates. Phosphates are found in candy bars, beer, soda, and ice cream. These also block iron absorption.

TREATMENT

Anemia should not be treated without the supervision of a practitioner. Anemia caused by an underlying factor (such as a stomach ulcer or Rh disease) may be relieved by treating that condition. If a medication is causing absorption problems, prescriptions may be changed to avoid anemia. IUDs are not recommended for women with severe anemia.

If anemia is a result of poor nutrition, a diet containing iron and iron supplements (such as ferrous sulfate, ferrous fumerate, and ferrous gluconate) should be followed. The iron and vitamins in food sources are absorbed into the body much more easily than those in prepared supplements. For women with a malabsorption problem, injections of vitamin B_{12} may be necessary.

Pregnant women are sometimes advised to take iron supplements. However, many experts now believe that a balanced diet should be enough to prevent iron deficiency from occurring, since blood volume doubles during pregnancy. Folic acid supplements, because they help prevent neural tube defects (defects in which the brain and spinal cord do not develop properly), are recommended for pregnant women.

SEE nutrition.

For more information on anemia, contact:

Cooley's Anemia Foundation
129-09 26th Ave., Room 203
Flushing, NY 11354
800-522-7222
ncaf@aol.com

Sickle Cell Disease Association of America, Inc.
200 Corporate Pointe, Suite 495
Culver City, CA 90230-7633
800-421-8453

ANTIBIOTICS

Antibiotics are medications derived from cultures of bacteria that are used to kill other bacteria that cause infections. Used mainly for treating infections, antibiotics include penicillin, ampicillin, neomycin, metronidazole, and tetracycline.

Some antibiotics are designed to fight a specific type of infection in a specific location, while others, known as broad-spectrum antibiotics, destroy all types of bacteria throughout the body. If a course of one type of antibiotic is ineffective, a practitioner may prescribe other types until one is found that fights the infection.

Antibiotics should be taken only with the supervision of a practitioner. When antibiotics are prescribed, all of the pills should be taken according to the practitioner's instructions, even if improvement occurs after only a few days. Unless the full course of drugs is taken, the infection may recur.

While they are usually effective in treating infections, antibiotics may cause side effects. In addition, bacteria often rapidly become resistant to antibiotics, requiring higher dosage for the same effect. The amount of penicillin required to treat an infection today is 50 times greater than it was 30 years ago.

ANTIBIOTICS AND WOMEN

In women, antibiotics are often administered after childbirth involving a cesarean section, episiotomy, or other invasive procedure, in order to prevent infection, especially if the women have known heart murmurs. They are also commonly used to treat bacterial vaginal infections, pelvic inflammatory disease, and

SIDE EFFECTS OF ANTIBIOTICS

Side effects of antibiotics vary from medication to medication. However, possible side effects include:
- Anxiety
- Nausea
- Diarrhea
- Allergic reactions, such as rash, swelling, wheezing, or sensitivity to the sun
- Confusion
- Dizziness
- Insomnia
- Vaginal or oral yeast infections
- General unwell feelings
- Weight gain or loss
- Yellow eyes and skin
- Anemia
- Hyperactivity

sexually transmitted infections. An antibiotic is often used to prevent infection during the insertion of an IUD. Antibiotics may also cause bleeding between menstrual periods, known as breakthrough bleeding.

ORAL CONTRACEPTIVES

There is controversy about whether or not prolonged use of some antibiotics can decrease the effectiveness of oral contraception. In fact, some pharmacies attach warnings to the antibiotic medications. But, while there are many anecdotal claims for such an effect, there is no pharmacological evidence to support those claims—with one exception. The antibiotic rifampin (Rifadin, Rimactane), which is used in the treatment of tuberculosis, has been proven to reduce the effectiveness of oral contraceptives.

Women who are taking the Pill should discuss with their practitioners the potential interaction of any medication that is prescribed for them. If necessary, medications can often be adjusted to avoid combinations that are known to negatively interact.

YEAST INFECTIONS

Some types of antibiotics affect the growth of yeast in the body. The yeast organisms, along with a number of other healthy bacteria, are commonly present in the digestive tract. When broad-spectrum antibiotics—antibiotics that kill a variety of different bacteria—are administered, they destroy the healthy bacteria but leave the yeast organisms, which are immune to antibiotics, unaffected. As a result, the yeast organisms multiply, causing yeast infections. (In addition, some experts feel that chronic yeast infections gradually weaken the immune system, which would result in more infections and therefore more antibiotic use.) To prevent antibiotic-related yeast infections, antibiotics may be administered in conjunction with an antifungal medication.

See medications.

ARTHRITIS

According to the Arthritis Foundation, two-thirds of the 40 million Americans who have arthritis are women. Arthritis is a condition that causes pain, swelling, and stiffness in one or more joints. Most forms of arthritis cause inflammation of the joints. Some cause inflammation of other parts of the body.

Two of the most common forms of arthritis (there are more than 100 different forms) are osteoarthritis and rheumatoid arthritis; both are chronic conditions that cause pain in the joints and inhibit movement. Another type of arthritis, called **gout,** occurs when uric acid crystals form in one or two joints (usually the big toe), causing inflammation. **Infectious arthritis,** caused by an infection elsewhere in the body that affects the joints, is unlike other forms of arthritis; it is not chronic and can be treated with antibiotics.

Women are about as likely to get osteoarthritis as men are, but they are three times more likely to get rheumatoid arthritis.

Osteoarthritis, or **degenerative arthritis,** develops in a joint over many years. Sometimes called wear-and-tear arthritis, or degenerative joint disease, it involves the breakdown of cartilage and other tissues in a joint. In the process, the cartilage cushioning the bone softens and cracks, intruding upon the fluid capsule that lubricates the joint. New bone growth narrows the capsule further and causes it to fill with bits of cartilage and bone. Later, cysts develop and bony growths, called bone spurs, distort the capsule, restricting or immobilizing the joint. Symptoms of osteoarthritis include a mild aching in the joint, especially during movement. The joint tends to hurt after periods of inactivity or overuse.

Rheumatoid arthritis (RA) may develop at any age, but most often strikes between ages 20 and 45 (other experts say ages 35 to 50) and has no known cause. A chronic disease that causes inflamed joints, it can affect other parts of the body, too, including connective tissues and the tissues that surround organs such as the heart and lungs. It affects the most flexible joints—usually the arms, hands, legs, and feet—by inflaming the synovial membranes that line the joint capsules. The delicate membranes thicken and become fibrous, causing symptoms that include pain, stiffness, weakness, swelling, tenderness, and disability.

Rheumatoid arthritis begins with stiffness

DIET AND ARTHRITIS

The food-arthritis link is highly controversial, and most practitioners believe there are not enough hard facts (such as good, controlled clinical studies) to say for sure that food sensitivities can cause arthritis, especially when it comes to rheumatoid arthritis.

However, though the link between arthritis and nutrition has not been proved—indeed, only one type of arthritis, gout, has been definitely connected with diet—some research findings do suggest that food plays a role in other types of arthritis as well, or at least in some sorts of joint inflammation that may resemble arthritis.

In a small number of sensitive people, certain foods may provoke an allergic inflammatory reaction in joint tissue, just as it might cause hives or asthma in other sensitive people. The kinds of fat a person eats seem to influence the body's inflammatory response. Researchers believe that some fats promote the manufacture of inflammation-producing biochemicals, while other fats, such as fish oil, interfere with the manufacture of inflammation-producing biochemicals.

Although research is scant on what foods are most likely to cause symptoms of arthritis, in several studies milk and cheese were found to cause symptoms. Corn, shrimp, nitrates, beef, and wheat have also been implicated in some cases. Some researchers believe, too, that a certain family of vegetables, called nightshades, can cause symptoms of joint inflammation for some people. These include potatoes, eggplants, tomatoes, bell peppers, and chili peppers. Norman F. Childers, Ph.D., creator of the no-nightshade diet, claims that 70 percent of arthritis sufferers can find relief by avoiding nightshades.

Foods high in purines—protein compounds found in anchovies, organ meats, mushrooms, and other foods—elevate levels of uric acid in the system and should be avoided by gout sufferers.

Arthritis sufferers are also advised to:
■ Maintain a healthy—ideal—body weight.
■ Get the recommended dietary allowance of every nutrient.
■ Keep fat intake low (25 percent or less of daily calories from fat).
■ Drink eight glasses of water a day.
■ Reduce intake of fried foods and foods with vegetable oils, such as safflower, sunflower, corn, sesame, and soy. They contain omega-6 fatty acids, which produce inflammatory chemicals in the body.
■ Increase intake of fatty fish, such as mackerel, sardines, and salmon. The fish oils contain omega-3 fatty acids and are thought to produce anti-inflammatory chemicals.

of the feet and hands, and fine finger movements, such as buttoning, may become difficult. Joint deformity, caused by the erosion of joint cartilage and bone, can occur within a year or two of the onset of the condition. Oral contraceptive users have a lower incidence of rheumatoid arthritis, and recent research indicates that estrogen may be of use as a treatment.

DIAGNOSIS AND TREATMENT

Because of the number of different types of arthritis, a certain diagnosis can be difficult to pinpoint. Diagnostic tests for arthritis include blood tests, x-rays, radioisotopic scanning (a specialized form of imaging), electromyography (examination of electrical impulses emitted by muscles and nerves), arthroscopy (examination of the inside of the joint by insertion of a thin viewing tube), analysis of the joint fluid, and biopsy.

Treatments include drugs, physical therapy, occupational therapy, psychological counseling, surgery, and some alternative approaches. There is no treatment that cures rheumatoid arthritis or osteoarthritis. Medical care, instead, focuses on relieving pain and reducing inflammation, slowing the progress of the disease, preventing permanent joint damage, improving the function of a joint through surgery if necessary, and keeping the woman and her joints functional throughout her lifetime.

Nonsteroidal anti-inflammatory drugs (NSAIDs), such as aspirin, ibuprofen, and an array of prescription drugs, work immediately to help relieve joint pain. Drugs used almost exclusively for the treatment of RA also include steroid drugs, such as prednisone and cortisone. However, steroid drugs are seldom used for osteoarthritis because they are not helpful for this condition and have potentially serious side effects, especially in large doses over a long period of time (a regimen no longer recommended). These side effects include lowered resistance to infection, weight gain, muscle wasting, and mood changes. Remittive agents, such as gold salts, penicillamine, and methotrexate, which work over the course of a few weeks, may help alter, change, or slow the course of the disease. Arthroscopic surgery can also be done to cut away inflamed tissue within the joint. As a last resort, all or part of a joint can be surgically replaced to relieve pain and improve function.

There are also nonmedical treatments for arthritis. Exercise, physical therapy, and the application of heat, cold, and mineralized water can help relieve symptoms by loosening joints. Alternative therapies, such as acupuncture and massage, have also proved effective in treating some people's arthritis pain.

SEE fibromyalgia.

For more information on arthritis, contact:

Arthritis Consulting Services
4620 N. State Rd. 7, Suite 206
Fort Lauderdale, FL 33319
800-327-3027

Arthritis Foundation Information Line
30 W. Peachtree St.
Atlanta, GA 30309
800-283-7800
404-872-7100
http://www.arthritis.org

BIOPSY

Biopsies, the removal of small bits of body tissue for diagnosis, are widely used to determine whether a growth is cancerous. A pathologist, a specialist in diagnosing problems of tissues, examines a prepared slide of the collected sample under a microscope to study the cells for disease. The material removed from the body may also be stained or processed for special studies to obtain more information on the diagnosis and prognosis and as a guide to treatment.

Usually, practitioners target a suspicious area for biopsy using a scope, such as a laparoscope (inserted through an incision in the abdomen) or a colposcope (used to view the vagina). In addition, an x-ray or ultrasound may be done to locate an area for biopsy. When no targeting procedure is done, the biopsy is known as a **blind, or random, biopsy**. In this case, the practitioner samples an area without the advantage of a complete or magnified view of the tissue. Because of the lack of precision in the way the sample is collected, this procedure is not commonly recommended. Needle aspiration and needle biopsy, two forms of breast biopsy, may be done with or without the aid of an x-ray or other viewing technique.

PROCEDURES

The following procedures are among the common types of biopsies that women undergo:

Aspiration endometrial biopsy. In this short procedure, a plastic tube is inserted into the uterus to suction tissue from the endometrium (the lining of the uterus) for microscopic exam-

ination. This procedure may be performed in a practitioner's office and takes a few minutes. It is only useful when a small sample of tissue is needed. An aspiration endometrial biopsy may be performed to diagnose endometrial cancer as well as fertility problems, hormonal irregularities, and other disorders.

Cervical biopsy. Cervical biopsy involves the removal of samples of tissue from the cervix, using a magnifying instrument called a colposcope that allows the practitioner to view the lesions that need to be sampled. Since the cervix has few nerve endings, the procedure causes little pain and is generally done without an anesthetic. When cells are scraped off the cervical canal for biopsy, the procedure is known as **endocervical curettage.** In a **punch biopsy,** bits of tissue about the size of half a grain of rice are removed from the cervix, using an instrument that resembles a paper punch.

After a cervical biopsy, there may be some light spotting and cramping. Most practitioners recommend avoiding intercourse, douching, and tampons for a short time after the procedure in order to allow the cervix to heal.

Conization. Conization, or cone biopsy, is a procedure in which a cone-shaped piece of tissue is surgically removed from the center of the cervix. The procedure requires a local or general anesthetic and may be done in a hospital, outpatient clinic, or even in a practitioner's office. It may be performed for the diagnosis and sometimes the treatment of cervical cancer.

A new procedure, called **loop electrosurgical excision procedures (LEEP),** can also be used for conization, employing a low voltage radio wave to remove the tissue for examination in one piece. This procedure may also be done in a practitioner's office.

Heavy bleeding that lasts a week or longer may follow conization. This type of biopsy can interfere with a woman's fertility and ability to carry a pregnancy to term. A woman can undergo more than one conization, but most practitioners don't like to do more than two.

Vulvar biopsy. Vulvar biopsy is the removal of tissue from the vulva (the fleshy lip of the vagina) for the diagnosis of cancer of the vulva. The procedure usually involves a local anesthetic and a punch biopsy, in which a surgical instrument similar to a small paper punch is used to extract a plug of the suspicious tissue. The site of the biopsy is usually too small to require any stitches.

SEE breast biopsy; colposcopy; dilation and curettage (D&C); hysteroscopy; laparoscopy; medical testing (appendix B); specific cancers.

BIRTH DEFECTS

Birth defects are abnormalities in babies that are present from birth. There are two main sources of birth defects. **Genetic disorders** result from abnormalities of the baby's genes or chromosomes. **Developmental disorders,** which are not inherited by the fetus, involve external factors, such as medication used by the woman during pregnancy, the woman's exposure to toxins (including alcohol and other drugs), damage during delivery (in the case of cerebral palsy), malnutrition, and various infections, such as rubella and syphilis. Most causes of birth defects, however, are unknown.

GENETIC DISORDERS

Each cell of the body contains genetic material that dictates its structure and characteristics. The material is arranged in units called chromosomes; every cell (with the exception of reproductive cells) contains 46 chromosomes arranged in 23 pairs, with one pair (called the sex, or X and Y, chromosomes) dictating the gender of the child. Half of the chromosomes are inherited by the child from the mother and half from the father.

Some 3 percent of newborns are affected by genetic defects. There are three types of genetic defects: chromosomal defects, single-gene defects, and multifactorial, or polygenic, disorders.

Chromosomal defects are usually familial; that is, they are inherited by the child from its parents. In some cases, certain defects may be the result of a spontaneous mutation during sperm and ovum formation. Chromosomal defects result from either an excess or a lack of chromosomal DNA, the genetic material that dictates how the body is to be formed. Such defects include Down syndrome.

(continued on page 48)

RISK FOR BIRTH DEFECTS BY MOTHER'S AGE

Woman's Age	Risk for Down Syndrome	Total Risk for Chromosomal Abnormalities*
20	1:1,667	1:526
21	1:1,667	1:526
22	1:1,429	1:500
23	1:1,429	1:500
24	1:1,250	1:476
25	1:1,250	1:476
26	1:1,176	1:476
27	1:1,111	1:455
28	1:1,053	1:435
29	1:1,000	1:417
30	1:952	1:385
31	1:909	1:385
32	1:769	1:322
33	1:602	1:286
34	1:485	1:238
35	1:378	1:192
36	1:289	1:156
37	1:224	1:127
38	1:173	1:102
39	1:136	1:83
40	1:106	1:66
41	1:82	1:53
42	1:63	1:42
43	1:49	1:33
44	1:38	1:26
45	1:30	1:21
46	1:23	1:16
47	1:18	1:13
48	1:14	1:10
49	1:11	1:8

* These occurrences of abnormalities range from very mild or near normal to severe.
Source: ACOG Technical Bulletin 108, September 1987.

14 COMMON BIRTH DEFECTS

Most pregnancies are free of birth defects. Preparation for pregnancy with good nutrition, vitamin supplements, and avoidance of alcohol and other drugs can reduce the risk of any problems. Prepregnancy counseling and early prenatal care, available through your practitioner, can further reduce the risk of birth defects. Further, many advancements in prenatal testing, such as ultrasound and amniocentesis, allow the detection of defects early in the pregnancy, before birth. Such procedures allow parents to have a choice in continuing the pregnancy and/or to prepare for a child with a defect. (For more information on prenatal concerns, preconception concerns, and prenatal testing, see these topics, listed under "Pregnancy.")

Cerebral palsy (CP). Cerebral palsy is characterized by physical and mental disabilities that are caused by brain damage. Speech and intellectual development may also be impaired. CP is often expressed by abnormal muscle control, loss of sensation, and some degree of hearing impairment. Physical and speech therapy is available for those with the condition, which may slowly progress over time.

Cleft lips and palate. This occurs with incomplete fusion in lip or palate (roof of mouth). Problems in an infant's ability to suck are common, as are speech disorders. These conditions can be corrected with reconstructive surgery. Heredity factors are identifiable in 25 percent of cases. Nongenetic factors may be identified and include maternal diabetes, alcohol abuse, anticancer drugs, and seizure medications.

Cystic fibrosis (CF). Cystic fibrosis is the most common fatal genetic disease among Caucasians. It is caused by a recessive, single-gene disorder, which causes a malfunction in the workings of the lungs and the pancreas. In those with the condition, thick mucus builds up in the lungs, making breathing difficult and encouraging the growth of bacteria, which then leads to pneumonia and other bronchial diseases. Some cases are not diagnosed until age four. While ultimately fatal, people with CF can live longer lives well into adulthood with the help of treatments that introduce healthy genes and enzymes into the system. Prenatal testing reveals the disease in many cases.

Down syndrome. Down syndrome occurs when the #21 chromosome pair does not divide normally at conception. Children with the disorder have short stature; slanting eyelids; broad, flat noses; small ears; short, stubby fingers; and moderate to severe mental retardation. Congenital heart defects are also common. Down syndrome can be prenatally detected by screening programs and testing, most notably amniocentesis. In the United States, 5,000 children with Down syndrome are born each year; the older a woman is during pregnancy, the greater the chance of having a child with the condition. Despite limitations, those with Down syndrome have potential to become productive members of society. There are many support groups available to help cope with Down syndrome.

Duchenne-type muscular dystrophy. This fatal condition is carried by women, though only men can develop it. It appears in boys between ages three and nine. The disease causes the deterioration of muscles over time. Muscles degenerate, and a child must usually use a wheelchair by the teen years. It affects all muscles, including the heart and those used in breathing. Although orthopedic devices are available for those with the disease, there is no cure.

Fetal alcohol syndrome (FAS) and drug-addicted infants. Severe birth defects can be brought on by a woman's abuse of alcohol and illicit drugs during pregnancy. Alcohol passes through the placenta to the developing fetus. Infants with FAS are undersized at birth and have small heads, mild to moderate retardation, short attention spans, and behavioral problems. They may have joint abnormalities and congenital heart disease. Infants born to drug-addicted women are often born addicted themselves, may suffer withdrawal symptoms, and may have subsequent developmental problems.

Hemophilia. In hemophilia, blood does not clot normally, and even minor scrapes can lead to uncontrolled and possibly fatal bleeding. The disease is carried by women, although it affects men almost exclusively. Those with hemophilia must avoid activities, such as contact sports, that increase the risk of bleeding. Treatment can be done with transfusions that contain a blood-clotting factor. Screening is available for women who may carry the disease.

Huntington's disease. This rare disease is an inherited dominant, single-gene disorder not apparent at birth. Early symptoms—clumsiness or tics—appear between the ages of 35 and 45. Symptoms worsen to include twisted facial expressions, uncontrollable writhing of the body, and severe emotional problems that resemble manic depression or schizophrenia. Ultimately, the disease is fatal. Genetic testing can be used to detect carriers of the disease.

Neural tube defects (NTDs). Spina bifida and anencephaly, both neural tube defects, are among the most common birth defects in the United States. Anencephaly (missing brain) is always fatal. Spina bifida, which results in a gap in the bone that surrounds the spinal cord, can be slight or severe. Mild cases may result in nothing more than a dimple in the skin or a purple membrane over the spine. Severe cases include paralysis, lack of bladder and bowel control, and hydrocephalus (water on the brain). NTDs are caused by a combination of hereditary and environmental factors. Over 95 percent of the cases of NTDs can be detected by alpha-fetoprotein screening early in pregnancy.

Phenylketonuria (PKU). This rare enzyme deficiency prevents proper breakdown of the amino acid phenylalanine. PKU, an inherited disease, can lead to severe mental retardation and physical problems. However, a special diet low in this amino acid can avert problems. It is routinely screened for at birth.

(continued on page 48)

14 COMMON BIRTH DEFECTS—*CONTINUED*

Rubella. Severe birth defects can result if a woman is exposed to rubella (German measles) in early pregnancy. Defects associated with rubella include blindness, deafness, microcephaly (small-sized head), mental retardation, cerebral palsy, and congenital heart defects. The woman is immune to rubella if she has already had the disease or if she is vaccinated prior to becoming pregnant. A blood test should be done before pregnancy to determine whether a woman is immune or if she needs a vaccination.

Sickle-cell anemia. This inherited disease occurs when the body produces crescent-shaped, rather than round, red blood cells. These abnormal cells are more likely to stick together and clog blood vessels, leaving a person with a shortage of red blood cells and thus a shortage of oxygen. Symptoms, such as painful joints and abdominal pain, may not appear until six months of age. Sickle-cell disease is usually found in people of African descent; one out of 12 African Americans have the disease. Clots of sickle cells caught in the arteries can result in injury to the brain, lungs, and kidneys. It may be fatal. Blood tests are available to diagnose carriers of the trait.

Talipes (clubfoot). Talipes is the second most common birth defect in the United States. With talipes, one or both feet are twisted inward and downward, or upward and outward. It is thought to occur when the fetus holds a fixed position in the uterus for a long period of time, possibly when fetal movement is limited by insufficient amniotic fluid.

Tay-Sachs disease. Tay-Sachs is a recessive genetic disorder that creates in the body an inability to produce an enzyme that normally breaks down fatty deposits in the brain and nerve cells. It is most common in Jews, especially of Eastern European origin. Symptoms, which include behavior changes, paralysis, and blindness, may not appear until six months of age. There is no treatment available; death usually occurs before age three or four.

Single-gene defects are familial, caused by one or a pair of abnormal genes. The mutant genes may be either **dominant,** meaning they will cause a defect when only one of a pair is present, or **recessive,** meaning that two abnormal genes must be present. There are over 1,200 dominant-gene disorders, including Huntington's disease and primary hyperlipemia, a predisposition to premature arteriosclerosis. About 950 types of recessive-gene disorders exist, among them Tay-Sachs disease, sickle-cell anemia, and phenylketonuria. Recessive genes that are linked to the X chromosome are the cause of approximately 150 disorders. These include hemophilia and Duchenne muscular dystrophy.

Multifactorial disorders result from the interaction between genetic factors and environmental factors, without a clear inheritance pattern. Many congenital defects are of this type of disorder, such as cleft lip and cleft palate, talipes (club foot), and spina bifida. While there is an inherited factor or tendency, the expression of the defect does not always occur. Although subsequent children are at increased risk for recurring multifactorial disorders, they do not usually occur.

CHECKING FOR ABNORMALITIES

New techniques are emerging daily allowing the diagnosis of many genetic and structural disorders. Amniocentesis, chorionic villus sampling (CVS), and the alpha-fetoprotein (AFP) test are prenatal tests that a practitioner may perform to check for fetal abnormalities. **Amniocentesis** involves extracting a sample of fluid from the amniotic sac (sac that surrounds the fetus) with a long, thin needle. It is performed in the second trimester and is used to detect chromosomal defects, including Down syndrome, and structural problems, such as neural tube defects. **Chorionic villus sampling,** performed in the first trimester, is the removal of placental tissue for analysis either through the cervix with a thin tube or through the abdomen with a needle. It can detect Down syndrome, hemophilia, and Tay-

LOWERING THE RISKS OF BIRTH DEFECTS

To promote a healthy pregnancy, the following regimen is recommended:

■ Get good prenatal care. Find a qualified practitioner with good communication skills and schedule regular appointments throughout your pregnancy.

■ Eat a well-balanced diet. The diet should include foods high in nutrients but low in fat. Good food choices include whole grains (for vitamin B and fiber), non-fat dairy products (for calcium and riboflavin), and poultry, lean meats, and tuna packed in water (for iron and zinc).

■ Take folic acid supplements. The United States Office of Public Health recommends that all women of reproductive age get 400 micrograms of folic acid daily. Several recent studies have shown that this important B vitamin (also known as folate) can reduce the risk of birth defects of the spine and brain by about 60 percent. Women should supplement their diets with 400 micrograms of folic acid by taking a multivitamin every day. Food sources include lentils, garbanzo beans, spinach, black beans, and black-eyed peas.

■ Reduce or eliminate alcohol intake. Alcohol can cause fetal alcohol syndrome, a combination of birth defects including low birth weight and mental retardation. The period of highest risk occurs around the time of conception.

■ Don't smoke. Smoking affects the fetus from the time of conception. It can cause birth defects and inhibit the fetus's growth, yet it is one of the most preventable causes of such problems. Women who smoke are far more likely to give birth to low-birth-weight babies, and the risk of sudden infant death syndrome is 10 times greater for their children than for the children of nonsmokers.

■ Drink eight glasses of chemical-free water a day.

■ Avoid chemicals in food. Be aware that processed foods often have hidden ingredients that may not be healthful.

Sachs disease. **Alpha-fetoprotein** is a substance produced by the fetus that is found in the woman's bloodstream and in the amniotic fluid. It can be measured through a blood test to check for structural abnormalities, including neural tube defects. Alpha-fetoprotein screening may be done in conjunction with a test for hormones in the woman's blood. This test, referred to as **alpha-plus,** or **triple screening,** is used to determine the risk for Down syndrome. **Ultrasound,** a procedure used to create an image of the fetus with sound waves, may reveal structural defects, but it cannot detect genetic or chromosomal disorders in the fetus. (For more information on these procedures, see "Pregnancy—Prenatal Testing.")

EXTERNAL FACTORS

Birth defects may be caused by a variety of external factors. During a preconception examination, a medical exam done before pregnancy to screen for possible disorders, a woman should discuss with her practitioner any medications—both prescription and over-the-counter—she is taking. The practitioner will recommend changes that should be made prior to or during the pregnancy.

Other agents, or teratogens, known to be dangerous to the fetus, are:

■ Methyl mercury, found in contaminated fish, which can cause cerebral palsy

■ Radiation exposure. While high levels of radiation may put a fetus at risk, diagnostic x-rays (10 rads or less) have no proven ill effects.

■ Infections, including rubella, measles, mumps, herpes simplex, syphilis, gonorrhea, viral hepatitis, cytomegalovirus, and influenza. These can cause fetal infections as well as mental retardation, malformations, and defects in the organs.

■ Androgens. These male hormones, sometimes prescribed for women, can cause pseudo-hermaphroditism (development of male genitalia) in girls and advanced development of the penis and testes in boys.

■ Alcohol, which causes growth retardation, mental retardation, and various major and minor malformations

SEE alcohol; disabilities; medications; nutrition; pregnancy—preconception concerns; pregnancy—prenatal concerns; pregnancy—prenatal testing; smoking.

For more information on birth defects, contact:

American Association on Mental Retardation
444 N. Capital St., N.W., Suite 846
Washington, DC 20001-1512
800-424-3688
202-387-1968
aamr@access.digex.net

Cleft Palate Foundation
1218 Grandview Ave.
Pittsburgh, PA 15211
412-481-1376
cleftline@aol.com

Children's Wish Foundation
P.O. Box 28785
Atlanta, GA 30358
800-323-9474
404-393-9474 (Georgia)

Cystic Fibrosis Foundation
6931 Arlington Rd.
Bethesda, MD 20814
800-344-4823
301-951-4422

Huntington's Disease Society of America
140 W. 22nd St., 6th Floor
New York, NY 10011-2420
800-345-4372
212-242-1968
curehd@hdfa.ttisms.com

March of Dimes Birth Defects Foundation
1275 Mamaroneck Ave.
White Plains, NY 10605
914-428-7100

National Down Syndrome Congress
1605 Chantilly Dr., Suite 250
Atlanta, GA 30324
800-232-6372
ndsc@charitiesusa.com

National Down Syndrome Society
666 Broadway
New York, NY 10012
212-460-9330
http://www.pcsltd.com/ndss/index.html

Spina Bifida Association of America
4590 MacArthur Blvd., N.W., Suite 250
Washington, DC 20007-4226
800-621-3141
http://www.infohiway.com/spinabifida

United Cerebral Palsy Association
1660 L St., N.W., Suite 700
Washington, DC 20036
800-USA-5UCP
202-776-0406
http://www.ucpa.org

BLOOD PRESSURE

Blood pressure is the force the blood exerts against the walls of the arteries as it flows through the body. When the left ventricle (the lower left chamber) of the heart contracts (a beat), oxygenated blood is literally shot into the arteries. As the blood travels through the body, it presses against the walls of the blood vessels it passes through. The vessels stretch and contract to maintain blood flow. If the vessels are narrowed, increasing the resistance to blood flow, blood pressure rises.

Approximately 61 million people have high blood pressure, or **hypertension.** If the condition is untreated, it may lead to heart attack, stroke, and kidney or eye damage. In women, high blood pressure may occur during pregnancy. Hypertension occurs almost twice as frequently in African Americans as in European Americans, and African Americans suffer more illness and death from their elevated blood pressure. High blood pressure occurs more often in white men under 50 than in white women of the same age, but after 50 the situation is just the reverse. Among blacks there is no difference in occurrence between men and women. About a quarter of all whites over 65 have high blood pressure; the rate is 50 percent for blacks.

MEASURING OF BLOOD PRESSURE

Systolic pressure is the measurement of blood pressure when the heart contracts and the blood's force against the vessel walls is at its greatest strength. **Diastolic pressure** is the measurement of the force of the blood after that contraction, when the heart is more or less relaxed.

Blood pressure is measured using a **sphygmomanometer,** or blood pressure cuff, that is wrapped around the upper arm and inflated with air. The pressure of the air pushes a column of liquid mercury up a numbered scale marked in millimeters. When the cuff is fully inflated, the practitioner places a stethoscope against the inside of the elbow. As the cuff's air pressure begins to decrease and the mercury drops, the practitioner hears a beat through the stethoscope, and the reading on the mercury at that moment indicates the approximate systolic pressure. As the pressure in the cuff continues to decrease, the sound of the beat disappears, and the scale is read again for diastolic pressure. Thus, blood pressure readings come in two numbers, usually expressed as a fraction. For example, in the reading 120/80 (read "120 over 80"), the first number is the systolic pressure, and the second number is the diastolic pressure.

BLOOD PRESSURE GUIDELINES

Blood pressure varies depending on age, gender, and other factors, and the guidelines for normal blood pressure readings vary as well. However, most medical experts consider blood pressure, in people under 40 years old, that remains at 140/90 over a period of time (usually at least two readings over three days, or after several hours of rest) to be hypertension.

In people over 40, 160/95 is considered hypertension.

Hypotension, or **low blood pressure,** is blood pressure that measures below 100/70. This condition usually does not require treatment unless other symptoms exist.

HYPERTENSION

Hypertension is considered a disease. Medical experts are unsure of its cause but believe that a combination of factors (or just one in some cases) may trigger the disease. They include:

■ Heredity

■ A history of kidney disease

■ Sleep apnea (sudden stoppage of breathing during the night)

■ Chronic dehydration

■ Obesity

■ A history of heart disease. Arteriosclerosis, or hardening of the arteries, occurs when fatty deposits build up within the arteries and may cause high blood pressure.

■ Stress

■ Excessive alcohol use

There are usually no obvious symptoms of hypertension, and for this reason many people call it the silent killer. Most people only discover they have hypertension when they have their blood pressure checked or when life-threatening conditions, such as heart attacks or angina pains, occur.

CONSEQUENCES OF HYPERTENSION

If high blood pressure is left untreated, the following conditions may result:

■ Heart attack. People with high blood pressure are twice as likely to suffer heart attacks as those without it.

■ Stroke. People with hypertension are eight times as likely to suffer strokes as those with normal blood pressure.

■ Kidney damage. High blood pressure causes kidney damage, which may eventually prevent the body from eliminating waste products from the blood efficiently.

■ Eye damage. Hypertension can cause retinal hemorrhaging and even blindness.

TREATMENT OF HYPERTENSION

While medical experts are uncertain about the specific biological reactions that cause hypertension, they do know what factors contribute to development and progression of the disease. By taking measures to control or eliminate these factors, people with hypertension can often reduce their blood pressure.

Medication is also a means of lowering blood pressure, usually recommended for people who have a diastolic pressure greater than 105. There are four major categories of medication for high blood pressure.

Diuretics are medications that cause the body to excrete excess salt and water from the body, reducing the blood volume. As a result, the heart does not have to work as hard. Diuretics can have side effects, including higher cholesterol, triglyceride, and blood sugar levels. Commonly prescribed diuretics include Diuril, Dyazide, Lasix, and Hygroton. Diuretics used to be the first choice in hypertension medication; however, the availability of newer drugs has changed that.

Beta blockers act directly on the heart, blood vessels, and nervous system. In general, the drugs interfere with the way the adrenaline chemicals affect the heart and arteries, preventing the constriction of the small arteries that control blood pressure. Side effects may include depression and fatigue. Commonly prescribed beta blockers include Inderal, Corgard, Lopressor, Catapres, Aldomet, and Minipress.

Vasodilators cause the peripheral blood vessels to open for less restricted, less resistant blood flow. These drugs also have side effects, including rapid heartbeat, water retention, dizziness, nausea, vomiting, and diarrhea, which especially affect highly allergic people. Apresoline and Loniten are the most commonly prescribed vasodilators.

Calcium channel blockers are drugs that prevent calcium, which triggers constriction of the arteries, from entering the cells. Taking of these drugs must be carefully monitored, as they can lead to heart failure in rare cases. The most commonly prescribed calcium channel blockers include Procardia XL, Cardizem, and Calan SR.

HYPERTENSION AND ORAL CONTRACEPTIVES

Oral contraceptives raise blood pressure in a few women who take them. The progestins in the Pill cause the body to produce more of a substance called angiotensin, which in turn elevates the blood pressure. The rise is usually slight but may increase over time. Increases in blood pressure that are due to the Pill occur more often in women with a family history of high blood pressure or those with a history of hypertension during pregnancy.

High blood pressure produced as a result of the Pill usually returns to normal once the woman stops taking it. Women with a history of high blood pressure should be monitored by a practitioner while taking the Pill. All women who take the Pill should have their blood pressure checked after the first three months on the Pill and at least once a year after that.

HYPERTENSION AND PREGNANCY

A mild increase in blood pressure is common during pregnancy. However, about 7 percent of all expectant mothers develop **preeclampsia,** pregnancy-induced hypertension. High blood pressure, excessive swelling, and protein in the urine characterize this condition. If preeclampsia is not treated, it can lead to **maternal eclampsia,** an extremely serious condition that can result in convulsions, failure of various organ systems, coma, and even maternal death.

Preeclampsia usually occurs during a first pregnancy, although it can happen in later ones, and the problem typically does not begin until the second trimester, when the maternal blood volume is reaching its peak. Those at greatest risk for preeclampsia are expectant women over 35, women with a family history of the condition, and women who have diabetes or are overweight.

The cause of pregnancy-induced hypertension is unknown, although researchers believe that hormones produced during pregnancy may have a direct effect on blood vessels. There is no known cause of the condition, and there is

SELF-CARE FOR HYPERTENSION

Most medical experts recommend that people with hypertension do the following:
■ Drink eight glasses of water a day.
■ Begin a moderate exercise program with your practitioner's supervision.
■ Quit smoking.
■ Lose extra weight.
■ Eat a diet low in fat and salt and high in fiber, supervised by your practitioner.
■ Avoid caffeine and alcohol.
■ Avoid stress and practice relaxation techniques.

no way to prevent it. However, eliminating major risk factors such as obesity and attending regular appointments with a practitioner may reduce a woman's chances of developing hypertension during pregnancy. Women who have high blood pressure before becoming pregnant should discuss special measures to prevent preeclampsia with their practitioners.

SEE heart disease; pregnancy—prenatal concerns.

For more information on blood pressure, contact:

American Heart Association
7272 Greenville Ave.
Dallas, TX 75231-4596
800-AHA-USA1
214-373-6300
http://www.amhrt.org

Coronary Club, Inc.
9500 Euclid Ave.
Cleveland, OH 44195
800-478-4255
216-444-3690

High Blood Pressure Information Center
National Heart, Lung, and Blood Institute
P.O. Box 30105
Bethesda, MD 20824-0105
301-251-1222
http:\\www.nhlbi.nih.gov/nhlbi/nhlbi.html

National Hypertension Association
324 E. 30th St.
New York, NY 10016
212-889-3557

BOARD CERTIFICATION

woman choosing a physician should consider the concept of board certification when making her decision. Board certification is a standard that designates physicians who have had additional training in a specific field of study. Most doctors who consider themselves specialists in a particular body system, age group, or disorder hold board certification; however, a licensed physician may practice any specialty and call himself a specialist in a particular field, whether or not he or she is actually board-certified in that specialty.

To obtain board certification, a doctor must hold a valid medical license, complete the required number of years of specialty training in a particular field (called a residency), and pass a rigorous examination administered by a specialty board—a national board of professionals in that specialty field. Some physicians continue their education by completing an additional two- or three-year program and become subspecialists within a specialty. For example, maternal and fetal medicine is a subspecialty of obstetrics and gynecology.

A doctor who passes the board examination is given the status of *Diplomate*. Most board-certified doctors become members of their medical specialty societies, and any doctor who meets the full requirements for membership is called a *Fellow* of the society and may use the designation. For instance, the title "FACOG" after a doctor's name denotes that that person is a Fellow of the American College of Obstetricians and Gynecologists.

The training and education requirements are similar for osteopathic physicians (D.O.'s) and allopathic physicians (M.D.'s), though they are certified by different boards. Allopaths are certified by one or more of the 24-member boards of the American Board of Medical Specialties (ABMS); board-certified osteopathic physicians are designated by the department of certification of the American Osteopathic Association (AOA). The training programs for ABMS-recognized specialties are only offered at accredited medical schools with approved programs. There are also self-designated medical specialty boards, which are not recognized by the ABMS or the AOA and may not have the same standards and training requirements as the national boards.

Board certification is only one of the many criteria that may be useful in choosing a physician. It indicates that a physician has completed a course of study in accordance with the established educational standards. Board certification has been called a minimum standard of excellence. It is not a test of competence, only of knowledge. Board certification is, however, a good sign that the physician is up-to-date on the standards of practice, procedures, theories, and success-failure rates utilized within the specialty.

There are many reasons a doctor may not be board-certified. A noncertified doctor may have been trained at a small hospital that did not meet training program requirements; she may have failed her board exams (she gets three tries); she may feel that board certification is irrelevant to her practice; or she may have obtained her training in a foreign country and be ineligible for the exam. Women dealing with a specialist who is not board-certified should ask why he or she is not.

A listing of board-certified physicians can be

found in the *Official ABMS Directory of Board Certified Medical Specialists,* published by Marquis Who's Who, available in most local libraries. Most county medical societies and some doctors also have a copy of this directory. The directory lists all of the ABMS board-certified specialists in the country that chose to be included; the listings cover state, specialty, education, training, and membership in professional organizations of their specialty. This book can be used to learn two other important facts about doctors:

■ Where they did their residency training. Was it at a major university hospital? A community hospital?

■ How long they have been practicing as doctors, based on when they completed their residency training. Are they fresh out of school? Older than age 70?

A copy of the *American Medical Directory:* *Physicians in the United States* may also be available at a local library. This lists every doctor who is a member of the American Medical Association: year of license, primary/secondary specialty, type of practice, board certification, and premedical and medical school education.

The American Board of Medical Specialties' number, 800-776-CERT, can also be called to find out if a particular doctor is ABMS board-certified.

For more information on osteopathic certification, contact:

American Osteopathic Association
Department of Certification
142 E. Ontario St.
Chicago, IL 60611
800-621-1773
312-280-5845

SEE childbirth—choosing a practitioner; practitioners, how to choose.

BREAST BIOPSY

When a suspicious breast lump is found or a mammogram (an x-ray of the breast) shows a mass or calcification, a sample of tissue may be needed to determine whether or not the abnormality is cancerous or benign (harmless). The removal of this tissue for diagnosis is called a biopsy. Biopsies may also be recommended for other symptoms, such as nipple discharge, puckering or dimpling of the skin of the breast, and hard, swollen lymph glands in the armpit.

NEEDLE BIOPSIES

A nonsurgical breast biopsy can be performed using fine-needle aspiration or the needle-core method. These procedures are simple and take about 15 minutes. These methods are usually used when the lump is close to the surface of the skin and can be felt by hand. These procedures may also be performed with the aid of x-ray or ultrasound images to help guide the needle to the suspicious site.

Fine-needle aspiration, done when the lump is thought to be fluid-filled, can be done in a practitioner's office without an anesthetic. A long, thin, hollow needle is inserted through the breast tissue into the lump. If the lump contains fluid, it is drained through the needle and can be analyzed. Clear fluid usually means the lump is a cyst and is noncancerous. If the fluid is bloody or thick, or if the cyst does not drain completely and collapse, there is more of a chance the lump is cancerous.

If the lump is solid, a **needle-core biopsy** may be done. This procedure requires a local anesthetic to numb the breast. A larger needle, which is often equipped with a cutting tip, is inserted through a small incision, and a small piece of the lump's tissue is removed. The tissue is then analyzed for cancer cells.

Needle-core biopsy causes some concern because with only a small segment of the lump removed, it can miss cancerous cells in other areas of the lump. While a positive result is always definitive, a negative biopsy has some margin of error.

OPEN BIOPSIES

Open, surgical biopsies offer more accurate results, since a larger section or the entire lump is removed for analysis. There are two methods of open biopsies in which a cut is made in the breast—incisional and excisional. An incisional biopsy removes part of the lump. The excisional method removes the entire lump. Open biopsies are often performed when there is a greater likelihood that the lump is malignant. Often, the analysis of the biopsy is done as the surgery is continuing; if the results show cancer, the lumps are removed during the same procedure.

RISKS ASSOCIATED WITH BIOPSIES

Needle biopsies have little risk attached to them. They are simple procedures performed with no anesthetic or with a local anesthetic. **Open biopsies** are surgical procedures, possibly requiring a general anesthetic, and carry the normal risks of surgery.

The two most common complications that occur with open biopsies are infection and hematoma, a pocket of blood that forms beneath the skin. **Hematoma** is caused by bleeding inside the surgical area and will happen within a day or two of the procedure. A blood blister forms, turns blue, and creates a lump under the skin. The body will usually absorb this blood, as it does with bruising, unless the hematoma is burst accidentally.

Redness, swelling, and fever are indications of **infection**, which may occur within a few days after surgery. A practitioner should be contacted immediately if any of the symptoms appear. Antibiotics are usually prescribed to counter the infection.

Complications occur in about 10 percent of breast biopsies but are not life-threatening and do not have long-term effects. Both incisional and excisional biopsies will result in some scarring. Most surgeons use stitches that dissolve, minimizing scarring, and are careful to place the incision where it will be least visible.

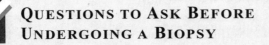

QUESTIONS TO ASK BEFORE UNDERGOING A BIOPSY

- Why do I need a biopsy?
- What kind of biopsy will be done?
- Who will do the biopsy?
- What might the biopsy show, and when will I know the results?
- Will this be an inpatient or outpatient procedure?
- What happens if the biopsy shows cancer?
- What kind of care will I need after the procedure?
- What is the cost of the procedure?

During the procedure, a cut is made in the breast, about 1½ inches long, through which the entire lump, or a section of the lump, is removed. Unless the lump is very deep in the breast or very large, these methods can be done using a local anesthetic on an outpatient basis.

When a lump is not present but calcifications (microscopic lesions) have been found on a mammogram, a **needle-guided biopsy,** also called a **wire-localization biopsy,** is performed. Before the procedure begins, a long needle is inserted into the breast to the site of the abnormality by a radiologist as it is observed on x-ray. A wire may then be placed through the needle to mark the tissue site, and another mammogram is taken to confirm accurate placement. Then the needle is removed, anesthetic is provided, and the surgeon makes an incision and removes tissue from the site at the tip of the wire. This tissue is x-rayed while the site is open to be sure the calcifications or lesions have been removed.

An **ultrasound-guided biopsy** is similar to a needle-guided biopsy but uses ultrasound (a diagnostic test that uses sound waves to create an image of the breast) instead of a needle to locate the abnormality. The skin over the lesion is marked; surgery is performed, and a second ultrasound confirms that the suspicious area has been removed.

ANALYSIS

The tissue or fluid taken from the breast using either needle or surgical methods is examined under a microscope by a specialist known as a pathologist. Biopsy samples are highly accurate. Of the methods mentioned, open biopsy methods are more accurate than the needle techniques because the sample is larger and therefore easier to interpret. There may be false-negative results (meaning cancer is not diagnosed when it is present) because abnormal cells are missed during collection.

Samples taken during biopsy may be processed by one or both of two methods. In a **frozen section analysis,** the sample is quick-frozen, sliced, stained, and examined under a microscope immediately after the biopsy. In a **permanent section analysis,** the sample is cut into small pieces, dehydrated, then fixed in paraffin wax and sliced into thin pieces. Each slice is put on a slide; the wax is melted away and the tissue is stained. When the slides are ready in 24 to 36 hours, the pathologist examines them and makes a diagnosis. Although a frozen section is 95 to 98 percent accurate, the results may not be as accurate as a permanent section analysis.

SEE biopsy; breast—fibrocystic conditions; breast lumps, benign; breast surgery; cancer, breast; mammography.

BREAST-FEEDING

Breast-feeding, or nursing, is the oldest form of feeding a human baby. Nearly half of newborns in the United States are breast-fed at birth. By six months, only about 11 percent are being breast-fed, and only about 2 percent are being breast-fed at one year.

BREAST MILK AND NUTRITION

According to the American Academy of Pediatrics, a baby's nutritional needs during the rapid-growth period of infancy are greater than at any other time in life. Most babies will triple their birth weight during their first year.

Breast milk contains many of the valuable nutrients a baby needs to grow and gain weight, all in a properly balanced form for the baby. The main ingredients in human milk are sugar (lactose), easy-to-digest protein (whey and casein), and fat (digestible fatty acids). Human milk also helps boost a baby's immune system and is least likely to cause allergic reactions.

Experts recommend that a woman increase her fluid intake to 12 glasses of water a day and that she pay special attention to her calcium intake, in order for her and her baby to receive the greatest benefits from breast-feeding.

BREAST MILK AND PROTECTION AGAINST DISEASE

For the first three or four days after delivery, a woman secretes colostrum, an antibody-rich yellow fluid that precedes milk production. It is colostrum that passes a woman's antibodies, substances that protect against infection, on to the breast-fed baby. Breast milk is protein rich and contains minerals, vitamins, and enzymes that are important for a baby's growth and health.

Evidence shows that breast-fed infants have fewer incidents of diarrhea and fewer allergies than children who are fed with formula. Breast milk has also been found to protect infants from painful ear infections (otitis media) and upper respiratory tract infections.

PRACTICAL BENEFITS

Besides nutritional content, there are practical reasons to breast-feed a baby. Breast-feeding is very inexpensive—most women are encouraged to increase their daily caloric intake by 500 calories while breast-feeding, which costs

59

only about one-third the price of commercial formula. (However, a woman may need to buy a breast pump and bottles while breast-feeding, and she will also have to invest her time.)

Moreover, breast milk is available at any time, at any place. While some women prefer privacy during feedings, other women feel comfortable nursing in public.

PSYCHOLOGICAL BENEFITS

There are also psychological and emotional benefits to breast-feeding. Nursing provides direct skin-to-skin contact, which most mothers find soothing for both themselves and their babies. Pediatricians believe that the same hormones that trigger milk production may also promote feelings that enhance nurturing feelings in the woman. And many women report that breast-feeding helps them feel closer to their child and more able to protect and take care of their baby. There are also deep-seated erotic feelings that may make nursing very pleasurable.

HEALTH BENEFITS TO THE MOTHER

Some preliminary studies have suggested that breast-feeding may be protective against breast cancer. According to a study of more than 16,000 women at the University of Wisconsin–Madison, premenopausal women who breast-feed for several months may lower their risk by about 30 percent. Some 25 percent of all breast cancers occur in premenopausal women. Women who have breast cancer should consult their practitioners before breast-feeding.

KEEPING THE FAMILY INVOLVED

To promote bonding between other family members and the child, women can involve them in other aspects of the baby's care. Here are some tips:

■ Talk it out. Before the baby arrives, open the lines of communication and discuss the feeding issue to help prevent misunderstandings and jealous feelings.

■ Let your partner console the baby. Ask your partner to help comfort a crying baby.

■ Learn to let go. Under supervision, have sisters and brothers hold and carry the baby.

■ Split the tasks. Ask everyone to take turns changing diapers.

■ Share in the feeding. Babies can be bottle-fed with breast milk expressed with a breast pump. This not only allows the rest of the family to bond with the baby; it can also take the pressure off an exhausted or stressed mother.

La Leche League International, a support group for nursing women, reports that mothers who breast-feed usually lose weight after pregnancy more easily than mothers who do not breast-feed. When a woman is pregnant, she gains several pounds specifically for breast-feeding. A recent study showed that the group of mothers who breast-fed lost more weight without dieting by the time their babies were six months old than did a similar group of women who bottle-fed their babies and who had been consuming fewer calories. Another study found that women's usual tendency to store fat on their thighs was reduced when they were breast-feeding.

Research has also indicated that breast-feeding women can safely exercise and diet. According to a 1994 study in the *New England Journal of Medicine,* when mothers performed aerobic exercise four or five times per week beginning six to eight weeks after their babies were born, they experienced no adverse effect on lactation in terms of volume or composition of breast milk. In addition, a study in a 1994 South African medical journal suggested that breast-feeding may provide maternal protection against osteoporosis later in life.

CONTRACEPTION

Complete and continuous breast-feeding is a natural contraceptive, although it must be frequent and prolonged. Breast-feeding suppresses ovulation and menstruation for some time. However, it is possible to ovulate and become pregnant while breast-feeding, even if there has not been a menstrual period. Women should use a barrier contraceptive while breast-feeding. Starting six weeks after delivery, Norplant or Depo-Provera may be used as contraception.

DISADVANTAGES OF BREAST-FEEDING

According to the American Academy of Pediatrics, when breast-feeding is going well, it has no known disadvantages for the baby. The only possible negative is the impact nursing has on the rest of the family, especially the mother. Because only women can breast-feed, the mother will have most of the responsibility at feeding times and may have to be awake and available whenever the baby is hungry. (However, breast milk can be expressed from the breast with a small pump, allowing others to take over some of the feedings.) Moreover, because babies digest human milk more quickly and thoroughly than formula, more frequent feedings are required than for bottle-fed babies.

Because of this responsibility, many women who breast-feed become exhausted and experience stress. In addition, breast-feeding can lead to sore breasts, clothing soiled by leaking milk, and possibly breast inflammation (known as mastitis) caused by infection.

Breast-feeding can also make the rest of the family feel left out. They can't experience the joy of holding the baby and watching the baby eat, and some partners may feel jealous of the close relationship between mother and child.

Women should keep in mind that breast-feeding is an option. There are many very nutritious commercial formulas available for use by women who do not wish to breast-feed for whatever reason.

HOW TO BREAST-FEED

In order for babies to nurse properly, they must take the entire areola (the darkened area around the nipple) and the nipple into the mouth. Sometimes, according to the American Academy of Pediatrics, it takes a few days for a baby to catch on. This is normal, and is common especially in newborns who have been given bottles or pacifiers.

For feedings, the baby can be cradled in the arm below the breast. The infant can also be held gently underneath the arm, with the wrist and hand supporting the baby's head in front of the breast, a position sometimes called the football hold. A woman can also lie on her side with her baby lying in front of her breast. This position may be more comfortable for a woman who has had a cesarean.

When the infant is sucking correctly, the motion will stimulate nerve fibers in the nipple. This triggers the "let-down process," a complex reflex that induces milk secretion.

For the first week after delivery, pediatricians recommend that a woman nurse her infant whenever the baby is hungry. After the first week, most newborns will want to nurse every two to three hours, day and night. Nursing this often can prevent engorgement, in which both breasts become very full. Babies will let their mothers know when they are hungry by crying or nuzzling at the breast.

Both breasts should be emptied every two to four hours. Each feeding should start with about 10 minutes on one breast, then burping, then 10 minutes on the other breast. As the infant grows older and starts sleeping longer during the night, the feeding pattern can be adjusted.

Experts advise against breast-feeding:

■ When the mother has active tuberculosis or chicken pox. However, common infections—such as a cold—cannot be passed to the infant through breast milk. A practitioner should be asked about which conditions preclude breast-feeding.

■ When the mother has HIV. Women at risk for HIV infection should be tested before nursing.

■ When the mother is taking anticancer drugs or radioactive medications

If a woman is taking either prescription or over-the-counter drugs, she should let her baby's pediatrician know before nursing. The doctor can best advise if any of the drugs could pass through the breast milk and harm her baby.

In addition, barbiturates, large quantities of alcohol (more than six ounces a day), and certain antibiotics and tranquilizers should be avoided.

BREAST-FEEDING FOR WOMEN WHO WORK OUTSIDE THE HOME

A woman who wishes to breast-feed her child does not need to give up the option of breast-feeding because she works outside the home. A mother can help regulate her infant's feeding schedule to some extent, and supplemental bottles of human milk or formula can be stored in the refrigerator or freezer for times when she is unable to feed the child herself. It is important to sterilize all containers and all unused refrigerated breast milk should be discarded after 48 hours; formula should be discarded within 24 hours. If breast milk needs to be kept longer, it may be stored frozen, but for no longer than two weeks.

Many workingwomen express their milk to be used to feed their baby while they are at work; breast milk can also be expressed to keep the woman's milk supply flowing if she is unable to breast-feed for a few days. Milk can be expressed either by hand or by pump. To express by hand, fingers are placed above and below the areola, and the breast is pressed toward the chest wall with a rhythmic motion until the milk flows or squirts out. The milk should be caught in a wide mouth, sterile container, then poured into a bottle.

There are two types of breast pumps: hand and electric. Hand pumps use negative pressure to collect the breast milk. Electric pumps are used to induce lactation when a mother will not be able to feed her infant directly for a few days. Prices range from $75 to $1,000. Pumps may be rented from a medical supply store or hospital. A lactation consultant, a professional who specializes in breast-feeding, provides information and services to breast-feeding mothers, especially those who work outside the home.

FIRST FEEDING—FIRST CONTROVERSY?

Breast-feeding can begin immediately after delivery, although many hospitals won't let mothers nurse their newborn until eight hours or longer have passed after delivery, usually because of hospital protocol. This is a controversial issue. Some experts believe breast-feeding should begin as soon as possible after a normal, healthy delivery. To help guard against any misunderstandings, discuss the issue with your obstetrician and the staff at the hospital or birthing center where you plan to deliver. Here are questions that you can ask them:

■ Do you encourage breast-feeding?
■ Do you allow the woman to breast-feed immediately following birth, while she's still in the delivery room (assuming both the mother and the baby are healthy)?

If the hospital has policies or schedules that postpone or prohibit breast-feeding, discuss the problem with your obstetrician or a hospital administrator to see if a change can be made. If the issue is important to you, you may want to make other arrangements for care if your wishes cannot be accommodated.

SEE breast inflammation (mastitis); reproductive system and sex organs of the woman.

For more information on breast-feeding, contact:

American Academy of Pediatrics
141 Northwest Point Blvd.
P.O. Box 927
Elk Grove, IL 60009-0927
847-981-7945
http:\\www.aap.org

La Leche League International
1400 N. Meacham Rd.
P.O. Box 4079
Schaumburg, IL 60168
800-LA-LECHE
847-519-7730
http://www.prairienet.org/llli/

BREAST—
FIBROCYSTIC
CONDITIONS

Fibrocystic conditions, characterized by the growth of usually harmless, fluid-filled cysts in the breasts, occur in as many as 30 percent of women between the ages of 35 and 55, and in 60 to 90 percent of all women. The growths in the breast (also known as fibrocystic changes, cystic disease, chronic cystic mastitis, and mammary dysplasia) consist of a combination of long, threadlike fibers and cysts, irregular sacs that contain fluid or semisolid material. The cysts, considered normal because they are so common, usually appear in both breasts and feel like clusters of grapes or peas, although they may become as large as golf balls.

SYMPTOMS

Fibrocystic lumps are tender with irregular densities. They are thought to occur in response to unusually high or low levels of the hormone estrogen in the body and are affected by cyclical changes in the levels of estrogen. In the few

PRECANCEROUS CONDITIONS

While a fibrocystic condition alone does not increase a woman's risk of breast cancer, certain lesions that sometimes accompany breast cysts may. In 2 to 4 percent of biopsies done on women with fibrocystic conditions, **atypical lobular** or **ductal hyperplasia** is found. These precancerous conditions, characterized by excessive growth of abnormal cells, carry an increased risk of breast cancer.

Women with no family history of early breast cancer have a one in five chance of developing breast cancer over the course of their lifetime if they have atypical hyperplasia. Those with early breast cancer in their family may have odds as high as 50 percent.

Only a biopsy will determine if hyperplasia is present. Hyperplastic masses are usually not surgically excised, since they can spread throughout the entire breast via the milk ducts, making removal impossible. Women with hyperplasia may need to be checked by their practitioner every six months and have a mammogram yearly.

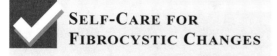

SELF-CARE FOR FIBROCYSTIC CHANGES

The cyclical swelling of fibrocystic breasts and the development of more lumps and cysts may be preventable. To help prevent or relieve symptoms:

■ Try vitamin E. It has been shown to be effective in reducing discomfort and the size and number of breast lumps. Daily oral doses of 600 international units (IU) of vitamin E have shown good results in studies. However, vitamin E can be toxic and should be taken with a practitioner's supervision.

■ Breast-feed your children after they are born. This has been shown to relieve symptoms and prevent cysts from occurring.

days before the menstrual cycle, they may swell and become painful in some women. This discomfort usually disappears a few days after the period begins. Some women experience discomfort throughout the menstrual cycle. Often, the lumps disappear or shrink after menopause.

DIAGNOSIS

Eighty percent of breast abnormalities are found to be noncancerous, or benign. In addition, women who have fibrocystic conditions are not at increased risk for breast cancer, as was once thought. While cysts are soft and sometimes tender, cancerous lumps are usually painless and hard and do not change during the menstrual cycle.

To be sure a lump is benign, a sample of the tissue is collected through a procedure known as a **biopsy,** then analyzed. An **ultrasound,** a test that uses sound waves to create an image of the breast, or a **mammogram,** an x-ray of the breast, might also be helpful in selected cases, though a biopsy is most accurate. Fibrocystic lumps cannot be detected using thermography, a test that locates abnormal areas by temperature.

Monthly self-examination is important for women with fibrocystic breasts. Any lumps or thickening that do not fit the usual pattern should be seen by a practitioner.

TREATMENT OF FIBROCYSTIC LUMPS

If lumps are benign and cause minimal discomfort, they may not require treatment and may disappear on their own after menopause. A cyst may be drained with a hollow needle through a procedure known as **needle aspiration.** If the cyst fills again, it may be surgically removed. In extreme cases, all breast tissue may be removed and replaced with breast implants.

A painful fibrocystic condition may also be treated with drugs. A drug known as **danazol** is sometimes effective in reducing swelling and relieving breast pain. **Oral contraceptives,** which provide a constant, low dose of estrogen, may also relieve symptoms. Some alternative therapies, such as acupuncture and herbal and homeopathic medicines, may also be effective in treating symptoms.

SEE breast biopsy; breast lumps, benign; breast self-examination; mammography.

BREAST INFLAMMATION (MASTITIS)

Breast inflammation, or mastitis, is the result of an infection in the breast. While bacteria (most often *Staphylococcus aureus*) may enter through a cut or bite on the nipple to cause inflammation, infections most often occur in women who are breast-feeding. Most infections begin with a blocked milk duct. Symptoms of infection include:

- Fever
- Swelling of the skin or nipple
- Redness
- Tenderness
- A tired, achy feeling

Infection is usually treated with antibiotics that are safe for women who are breast-feeding and with the application of heat in the form of a hot bath, shower, or heating pad. With these treatments, the condition usually eases in 48 hours. If the infection is not treated, it may develop into an abscess, which may have to be surgically drained. Rarely, infections cause scarring or nipple distortion.

Nursing women with breast infection should continue nursing to drain the breast of milk. The infection will not harm the baby (because the bacteria are usually from its mouth), and keeping the breast empty discourages further growth of the organisms. If nursing cannot be continued, the breast milk should be evacuated manually or with a breast pump.

Herbal remedies applied to the nipple may ease discomfort. They include poultices from elderberry blossom and olive oil; grated raw potato; and fresh ginger root. Garlic (a natural antibiotic) may be placed under the tongue for relief.

SEE breast-feeding.

BREAST LUMPS, BENIGN

Many women experience noncancerous breast lumps at some time during their menstrual years. These lumps usually form within the lobes of the milk-secreting glands of the breast, embedded in the fatty tissue. Some 80 percent of all lumps biopsied are found to be benign. Harmless lumps can be tender, movable, and affected by the menstrual period. Cancerous lumps may be painless, hard, and unaffected by the menstrual cycle.

Breast self-examinations should be performed on a monthly basis (the best time is two or three days after the menstrual period has ended), and any changes should be noted. If any lumps are found in the breast, a practitioner should be notified as soon as possible for evaluation. Breast exams are known to save lives by identifying early signs of breast cancer. A mammography, an x-ray of the breast, or an ultrasound, in which an image of the breast is created with sound waves, may also be done to detect the presence and nature of breast lumps.

Cysts (small fluid-filled sacs) in the breast tissue—known as a **fibrocystic condition**—are the most common type of benign lump found. However, several other kinds of harmless breast lumps exist. They are fibroadenomas, lipomas, intraductal papillomas, breast calcification, and traumatic fat necrosis.

Fibroadenomas. Fibroadenomas are usually found in women who are in their teens or 20s, rarely in those 30 and older. They are round and solid, movable and painless, and are not affected by changes in the menstrual cycle. Stationary lumps must be biopsied to distinguish them from cancerous growths.

Some health experts recommend removal of all fibroadenomas. Others recommend surgery only if the growths become large enough to change breast shape or if a woman is 30 or older. The cause of the fibroadenomas is unknown, and there is no way to prevent their formation. Fibroadenomas do not increase a woman's risk of breast cancer.

Lipomas. Lipomas are benign tumors made of fat tissue. They appear alone, rather than in groups, and are painless. Once confirmed by a biopsy, lipomas do not need to be treated or removed. However, if there is any doubt about the diagnosis, lipomas should be surgically removed. Lipomas do not increase a woman's risk of breast cancer.

Intraductal papillomas. These small, wartlike lumps grow in the lining of the milk ducts, usually near the nipple. Intraductal papillomas can produce dark, sometimes bloody discharge from the nipple. The discharge may block the duct, leading to infection and inflammation. Papillomas are usually removed because they are difficult to distinguish from cancer.

Breast calcification. Small calcium deposits may develop in the breasts, visible only through mammography. There are two types of calcifications: macro- and microcalcifications. A **macrocalcification** is considered benign and represents degenerative changes in the breasts. A biopsy is usually not required. The National Cancer Institute reports they are found in 50 percent of women over age 50 and in 10 percent of younger women. A **microcalcification** is a tiny speck of calcium found in the breast. A group of microcalcifications in one area may indicate cancer and should be removed.

Traumatic fat necrosis. These painless, round lumps are composed of the dead fat cells that collect after an injury to the breast or after breast biopsy or surgery. The skin around the lump may be red. This condition appears occasionally in older women or those with large breasts and is not linked to cancer. Removal is not usually necessary.

SEE breast biopsy; breast—fibrocystic conditions; breast self-examination; mammography.

BREAST SELF-EXAMINATION

The most effective way to combat breast cancer is to perform regular self-examinations. A woman becomes her own best defense against breast cancer if she becomes familiar with her breasts and their unique character. Since breasts are made of fatty and glandular tissue, it is not unusual for them to feel lumpy under normal conditions. That is why it

PERFORMING BREAST SELF-EXAMS

The breasts should be examined at the same time each month. The National Cancer Institute recommends that the self-examination be done two or three days after the end of the menstrual period. At this time, the breasts are less likely to be tender or swollen. Postmenopausal women should pick a particular day—the first day of the month, for example—to perform the exam.

To perform a breast self-examination (BSE), lie down and place a pillow under your right shoulder. Place your right arm over your head. With the three middle fingers of your left hand, begin to feel for lumps or thickening, pressing hard enough to know exactly how your right breast feels.

To examine your left breast, place the pillow under your left shoulder, put your left arm over your head, and use the three middle fingers of your right hand to feel for lumps or thickening in the left breast.

There are three different patterns you can follow to perform the BSE. Whichever pattern you use, use the same one each month:

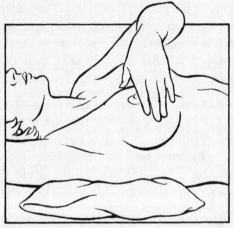

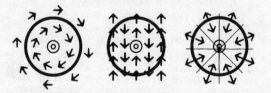

■ You can press your fingers in a circular motion, beginning at the nipple and moving out in concentric circles.

■ You can make straight lines across your breast.

■ You can make a starburst pattern, radiating from the nipple, then out.

is important to know which lumps are persistent and which are not. Once a woman begins to know what is normal for her, she can also notice changes and bring them to the attention of her practitioner.

The breast self-examination (BSE) is a self-help tool that makes finding suspicious lumps more likely. Some 80 percent of breast cancers are first detected by the woman through BSE. However, by the time they can be felt, growths measure at least one centimeter. A mammogram, an x-ray of the breast, can detect abnormalities even earlier, before they can be felt through self exam.

Caught in the early noninvasive stages, still confined to the ducts or lobes, breast cancer has a good prognosis. In most cases, the cancer is highly curable by surgical removal when found in the early stages.

In addition to the BSE, women aged 20 to 40 should have a professional examination at least every three years, or during an annual

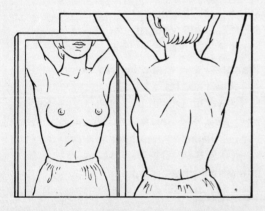 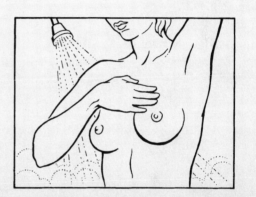

After checking the breast for lumps, examine the nipple for any changes and squeeze gently. Report any discharge to your practitioner.

While standing in front of a mirror, you should also check your breasts for any puckering or unusual swelling. First look at them with your arms at your sides, then stretch your arms above your head and look for any changes. Finally, stand with your hands on your hips and flex your chest muscles. Report any changes to your practitioner.

Perform BSE every month so you can get to know your breasts and what regular changes they go through in conjunction with your menstrual cycle. Many women prefer doing the BSE in the shower or bathtub, since fingers slide readily over wet and soapy skin, making it easier to detect changes.

Since early detection improves the success of cancer treatment, especially if the cancer is caught in the early stages, it is important to seek medical attention immediately if a lump is found. Do not wait until the end of the next menstrual cycle to see if a lump or thickening is due only to menstrual-related changes.

Source: American Cancer Society. Illustrations reprinted from "How to Do Breast Self-Examination," 1992.

gynecological exam. Women over 40 should have a professional exam every year.

Mammograms, low-dose x-rays of the breast, reveal abnormal changes that are too small to be felt through a manual examination. However, they cannot show everything.

According to the American Cancer Society, about 10 to 15 percent of the cancers that can be felt do not show up on a mammogram. It is important, therefore, that a woman continue a schedule of mammograms, professional examinations, and self-examinations.

SEE breast—fibrocystic conditions; breast lumps, benign; cancer, breast; mammography.

For more information on breast self-examination, contact:

American Cancer Society
1599 Clifton Rd., N.E.
Atlanta, GA 30329
800-ACS-2345
404-320-3333
http://www.cancer.org

National Cancer Institute
Cancer Information Service
9000 Rockville Pike, Suite 414
Bethesda, MD 20892
800- 4-CANCER
800-638-6070 (Alaska)
800-524-1234 (Hawaii)
http://wwwicic.nci.nih.gov

Planned Parenthood Federation of America, Inc.
810 Seventh Avenue
New York, NY 10019
For the Planned Parenthood nearest you, call:
  800-230-PLAN
http://www.ppfa.org/ppfa

BREAST SURGERY

Breast surgery involves the removal or alteration of the breast tissue for treatment of disease, usually cancer, or for reconstructive or cosmetic reasons.

The type of surgery performed to treat breast cancer is based on the woman's individual needs and, often, her preferences. Today, through breast examination, self-exams, and mammograms, breast cancer can be found at an early stage, when more surgical options are available. **Mastectomy** (removal of all or part of the breast tissue) and **lumpectomy** (removal of cancerous tumors only) are the two principal types of operations for the treatment of breast cancer. They are occasionally used for removing very large benign tumors. Both procedures may be followed by cosmetic or reconstructive surgery.

Treatment for breast cancer has become more conservative. Mastectomy once immediately followed a biopsy (performed under general anesthesia) that was positive for cancer.

However, this one-step process has been replaced by a two-step procedure that begins with a biopsy performed under local anesthesia. The test results are known within a few days. At that time, if cancer is present, the surgeon discusses treatment options with the woman. The two-step procedure gives the woman more informed control over her medical care. Treatment may include a mastectomy or a lumpectomy in conjunction with chemotherapy and/or radiation, supplemental chemical treatments that destroy or suppress cancer cells.

MASTECTOMY

Mastectomy is the surgical removal of all of the breast tissue including the nipple, areola (dark skin surrounding the nipple), and most of the overlying skin. The type of mastectomy performed is dependent on how far the disease has progressed and therefore the amount of tissue to be removed.

A **modified radical mastectomy** removes the breast, some fat, most of the axillary lymph nodes, and the lining of the chest muscle, but leaves the muscles intact. The modified radical mastectomy results in a more pleasing appearance and usually preserves normal arm and shoulder strength. It is the only radical surgery for cancer still performed, generally for women whose tumors are too large to be removed alone or who do not want long-term radiation therapy.

A **simple mastectomy** (or **total mastectomy**) involves the removal of only the breast tissue. This procedure is sometimes combined with **axillary dissection,** the removal of the lymph nodes closest to the breast. It is performed to determine the extent to which the disease has spread into the lymph nodes and if radiation and drug treatment are necessary. The combination of simple mastectomy and axillary dissection is usually recommended for women with Stage I cancer (small tumor without spread) and some women with Stage II cancer (cancer in some nodes but no spread elsewhere).

A **partial mastectomy** (or **segmental mastectomy** or **quadrantectomy**) is the removal of only the tumor and about one inch of surrounding tissue, including some of the overlying skin and part of the underlying muscle. While most of the breast is preserved, it is disfigured. Often it can be surgically restored at a later date, or even during the same surgery. The possibility that breast cancer may recur makes this procedure controversial. Partial mastectomy is always followed by radiation and/or chemotherapy in order to kill any cancer cells remaining in the breast. Some surgeons will also supplement the procedure by removing and examining a sampling of adjacent axillary lymph nodes in order to determine more accurately the progression of the disease.

A **subcutaneous mastectomy** is often performed prophylactically, meaning as a preventive surgery, for women with a high risk of developing breast cancer. It is most commonly done on women who have a strong family history of cancer, which means that two or more close blood relatives (especially the mother) had breast cancer at an earlier-than-usual age. A subcutaneous mastectomy involves removing about 95 percent of the internal breast tissue without disturbing the nipple. If after the removed tissue is examined, invasive cancer is found, both the remaining tissue and the axillary nodes are removed in a later operation.

Two types of mastectomy are no longer used. The Halsted radical mastectomy **(radical mastectomy)** involved the surgical removal of the breast and its skin, the underlying muscle of the chest wall, the lymph nodes in the adjacent armpit, and fat tissue. The **extended radical mastectomy** (or **extended thorough mastectomy** or **urban operation**) was identical to radical mastectomy except that it also involved the removal of the lymph nodes of the internal mammary chain, which usually meant removing a section of the rib cage. The physical results were a flattened, sunken chest, and the removal of the lymph vessels often resulted in chronic lymphedema, the accumulation of fluid and a resulting chronic swelling of the arm adjacent to the affected breast. The procedure usually left the adjacent arm and shoulder stiff and weak.

The Halsted mastectomy, which was first performed by Stewart Halsted in 1882, originated because of concern regarding the high rate of local breast cancer recurrence and metastasis (spreading of cancer to other parts of the body). There is no evidence, however, that the procedure improved survival rates. It has been replaced by less radical techniques. The extended radical mastectomy was popular for the removal of tumors located between the nipple and sternum (the breastbone), but since the 1960s the procedure has been abandoned.

LUMPECTOMY

Lumpectomy (or **segmented mastectomy**) differs from mastectomy in that it involves the removal of only the cancerous lump and a small margin of surrounding tissue. It is followed by radiation treatment of the breast and possibly chemotherapy. A recent study, part of the National Cancer Institute's National Surgical Adjuvant Breast Project, showed that women with early stages of cancer survive just as long with lumpectomy and radiation treatment as do

women treated by having their entire breast removed. Lumpectomy, in combination with chemotherapy and/or radiation, is part of the changed view regarding breast cancer therapy. The disease is now perceived as a systemic one that should be treated locally by removing the lump and administering radiation, chemotherapy, hormones, or other treatment. During a 20-year follow-up, the study showed that premenopausal women who had chemotherapy after surgery had significantly fewer deaths than those women treated only with mastectomy. However, the chemotherapy did not result in fewer deaths for postmenopausal women, especially those over age 60.

Though many lumpectomies are currently being performed, mastectomy is still the common treatment for breast cancer in the United States for several reasons. First, not every woman is a good candidate for lumpectomy. A woman with a large tumor and small breasts, multiple tumors, or cancer that has spread to the skin, lymph nodes, or nipple will not have good cosmetic results with lumpectomy. Some women, who don't want to have weeks of radiation therapy or to continue to check their breasts for a recurrence of cancer, prefer a mastectomy. Some doctors do not recommend lumpectomy because they are waiting to see if the procedure's long-term survival rates continue in further studies.

MAMMOPLASTY

Mammoplasty (which includes breast augmentation, breast reconstruction, and breast reduction) is a cosmetic or restorative surgical procedure done to increase or decrease the size of the breast or to restore the form of the breast following a mastectomy.

BREAST REDUCTION

Breast reduction, or **reduction mammoplasty,** may be performed for cosmetic or medical reasons. Extremely heavy breasts can cause chronic back pain, skin irritations from bra straps, and breathing problems.

There are two principal methods of breast reduction. In one technique the surgeon removes the nipple and areola, extracts extra tissue from the lower portion of the breast, and then replaces the nipple and areola. Reduction of nipple sensitivity and the inability to breast-feed are the disadvantages of this method. The other technique leaves the nipple and areola attached to the breast by a stalklike portion of tissue while the surgeon removes the excess breast tissue. This method preserves nipple sensitivity and in most cases, if enough of the tissue remains intact, makes breast-feeding possible.

BREAST AUGMENTATION

Breast augmentation, or **augmentation mammoplasty,** involves increasing the size of the breast for cosmetic reasons or restoring the form of the breast following a mastectomy. The breast may be enlarged or restored by surgically placing pouches of saline or silicone gel under the existing breast skin or, occasionally, under the pectoral (chest) muscle.

SILICONE GEL IMPLANTS

Silicone gel implants have been the center of much controversy because of their possible serious side effects. In 1988 it was announced that silicone implants caused cancer in rats, raising questions about their safety for humans. Around this time, many women began to report

WARNING SIGNS

If a woman with silicone or saline breast implants experiences any of the following symptoms, she should consult her surgeon and/or a rheumatologist or internist:

- Pain or hardening of the breast
- Body rash
- Extreme fatigue
- Fever
- Joint and/or muscle pain
- Burning or "electric" sensation within the breast or elsewhere in the body
- Skin "thickening" or hardening on the breast
- Other prolonged, unexplained, or undiagnosed body-wide physical symptoms

The most common complication of silicone gel and saline implant breast surgery is irregular and extensive scarring around an implant, especially if it leaks. Immediate complications of the surgery (which may occur with any surgery) include blood clots, hemorrhage, infection, and edema (fluid retention). The breast can also harden due to scar tissue forming around the implant.

problems with their implants that included infections, leaks, and excessive breast hardness.

Questions arose regarding the safety of the material encasing the implants as well. The silicone pouches causing the most concern were those made of polyurethane foam, which produces a cancer-causing agent, toluene diamine, or TDA. The manufacturer of the polyurethane-coated implants voluntarily withdrew them from the market in April 1991. In January 1992 the U.S. Food and Drug Administration (FDA) called for a moratorium on use of silicone-gel-filled implants, urging manufacturers to stop marketing them and surgeons to stop inserting them, but not forbidding them.

There is an intense controversy among medical professionals over whether or not silicone leaking into the body may trigger an autoimmune disorder marked by fatigue, muscle pain, weakness, dry eyes and mouth, and an array of other complaints. Studies have produced conflicting results. However, numerous women with silicone implants continue to report symptoms. The scientific issues surrounding the relationship between silicone leakage from breast implants and autoimmune response have not been resolved.

Women should be aware that, while symptoms are usually attributed to an implant that has ruptured, even an intact implant has a small amount of "gel bleed." A ruptured implant should be removed along with the capsule of scar tissue surrounding it, since the silicone will migrate to the surrounding tissues and lymph nodes.

Silicone gel implants have a "body life" of about 10 years, meaning that replacement surgery may be needed, even if the implants do not produce adverse symptoms. Generally, the removal of a nonproblematic implant that has not expired is not recommended. However, the decision is ultimately the woman's.

IMPLANTS AND MAMMOGRAPHY

Breast implants are visible on mammograms and may interfere with the diagnostic test's ability to detect breast lumps. If a woman has silicone gel or saline implants, she should inform the technician performing her mammography, so he or she will use the appropriate pressure to flatten the breast and take the best views.

Unfortunately, even the best mammogram may not detect the rupture of an implant. In response, a number of laboratories have developed a diagnostic blood test to determine if existing implants are leaking.

The FDA approved testing of implants filled with soybean oil in 1994. This material is thought to be safer because it uses triglycerides, a natural body fat. Early studies show that if the implants leaked, the woman would metabolize and excrete it just as she would if she ate fat. Further, the material is not likely to block the view of tissue during mammography.

SALINE-FILLED IMPLANTS

While no breast implant has been proved safe by FDA standards, experts consider saline-filled implants safer than silicone gel implants because saline (salt water) is harmless. However, the shell of a saline implant is made from a silicone product. Some women with saline implants have reported symptoms and complications similar to those of women with silicone gel implants. Another disadvantage is that saline implants cannot be cosmetically shaped and may not feel right.

If a women is considering having implants, she should ask her surgeon for information, available on package inserts and through the FDA. By reading all available information, the woman can make an informed decision.

MASTOPEXY

This procedure corrects the natural sagging of the breast. The incisions and surgical procedure are similar to those of breast reduction. Because the skin over the breast will once again lose its elasticity, the results are not permanent. Some surgeons advocate performing breast augmentation at the same time to increase the long-term effects of the operation.

BREAST RECONSTRUCTION

An option for women who desire breast reconstruction after a mastectomy is complex surgery through which the breast is reconstructed using tissue from the abdomen, back, or buttocks. Only women with usable tissue to spare are candidates for this operation. In the abdominal operation, the surgeon makes an abdominal incision and then tunnels the fat and flesh under the skin to the area of the missing breast. Because the tissue is not cut and reattached, it retains its own blood supply.

An alternative operation uses a portion of the broad back muscle and its overlying skin. This procedure maintains the shifted tissue's blood supply as well but makes a smaller breast. Another variation uses tissue from the buttocks. In this operation, the blood vessels are cut and then reconnected to blood vessels in the chest wall. Whatever the method of breast reconstruction, a nipple and areola may be created by skin grafting and tattooing in a later procedure.

All of these breast reconstruction procedures represent major surgery and have the potential for complications, including infection and uncontrolled bleeding. Women with chronic health conditions may be at greater risk of complications and should consult with their health providers about potential problems.

Some physicians recommend waiting three months after a mastectomy before performing reconstruction surgery; others offer immediate reconstruction at the time of the mastectomy. There is no time limit as to when the procedure can be performed after a mastectomy.

SEE breast biopsy; cancer, breast; chemotherapy; cosmetic and reconstructive surgery; mammography; radiation therapy; second opinion.

For more information on breast surgery, contact:

Reach to Recovery Program
American Cancer Society
1599 Clifton Rd., N.E.
Atlanta, GA 30329
800-ACS-2345
404-320-3333
http://www.cancer.org

Y-Me Breast Cancer Support Program
212 W. Van Buren St., 4th Floor
Chicago, IL 60607-3908
800-221-2141
312-986-8228
http://www.y-me.org

American Society of Plastic and Reconstructive Surgeons
444 E. Algonquin Rd.
Arlington Heights, IL 60005
800-635-0635
http://www.plasticsurgery.org

Breast Implant Information Line
Office of Consumer Affairs, HFF-88
Parklawn Building
5600 Fishers Ln.
Rockville, MD 20857
800-532-4440
http://www.fda.gov

CANCER

Cancer is an uncontrolled growth and spread of abnormal cells. When cells divide over and over, a tumor results. Tumors can be either benign or malignant. Benign tumors are not cancerous; malignant ones are.

Healthy, noncancerous cells of the body grow, divide, and replace themselves in an orderly process, which keeps the body in a healthy state and good repair. When cells become cancerous, they lose their ability to perform their particular function; they invade nearby tissues and take over the blood supply intended for normal cells. Cancer can affect any body organ or tissue. Cancerous cells can spread to other parts of the body, carried through the lymphatic or circulatory system. Cancer's ability to spread to different parts of the body is called **metastasis.** Most cancers form solid tumors.

TYPES OF CANCER CELLS

The two types of tissue cancers are carcinoma and sarcoma. **Carcinomas** are made up of the epithelial cells that line tissues; they are usually found in organs that secrete bodily fluids—for example, milk, mucus, and digestive juices. The breasts, lungs, skin, and the colon as well as the ovaries, cervix, and endometrium are all common sites for carcinoma.

Sarcomas are cancer cells that are made up of connective tissue cells, such as those in bones and muscle. Sarcomas can affect organs such as the uterus. Although sarcomas account for 2 percent of all human cancers, they are more aggressive than carcinomas.

There are tumors that contain both kinds of cells.

CAUSES OF CANCER

Cancer is caused by mutation, or changes, in genes; these mutations are brought about by internal and external environmental factors, including exposure to viruses, chemicals, and radiation. (There may need to be a defect in the gene for the factors to have an effect.) When these factors enter cells, they can harm the cell's DNA, its reproductive material, by either breaking or tangling the DNA molecules. Other factors can change the chemical composition of the DNA molecule. If a mutation causes the cell to become cancerous, the factor involved is known as a **carcinogen.**

MOST COMMON CANCERS AMONG WOMEN

In 1995 the American Cancer Society reported the following forms of cancer with the highest annual incidence and mortality for women:

Cancer Type	Incidence	Mortality
Breast	182,000	46,000
Lung	73,900	62,000
Colon and rectal	67,500	28,100
Cervix and uterus	48,600	10,700
Ovary	26,600	14,500
Lymphoma	24,700	11,330
Melanoma of skin	15,400	2,700

Family history appears to play an important role in certain forms of cancer. This may help explain why some heavy smokers develop lung cancer, while others do not. More than 100 distinct forms of cancer exist, and the cause of each may be different. However, research shows that the role of heredity is irrefutable in 5 to 7 percent of all cancer patients. Moreover, recent advances in genetics have identified genetic markers that predispose individuals to a particular cancer.

STAGING OF CANCER

Practitioners classify cancer according to stages. These stages indicate how large a tumor has grown or how far the cancer has spread. Staging is used to predict the outcome of the disease and to determine the best course of treatment. Each form of cancer has its own unique staging system that has been tailored to its progression.

In general, the earliest stage of cancer is stage 0 (carcinoma-in-situ), followed by stages I (local cancer) through IV (metastatic cancer, cancer that has spread to distant organs), indicating, progressively, how far the cancer has spread from its original site. These are followed by the recurrent cancer stage, indicating that the cancer has reappeared, even though there was no evidence of cancer when the original treatment was completed.

CANCER TREATMENTS

Cancer treatments vary according to the type of cancer, how far it has spread, and the health of the woman. Often a combination of treatments will be used to combat the disease. The most

conventional therapies for cancer are **surgery** (removal of a tumor), **radiation therapy** (the use of x-rays to kill cancer cells), and **chemotherapy** (the use of cell-destroying chemicals to kill cancer cells).

Another medical treatment is **hormone therapy,** the use of hormones or antihormones to halt the growth of cancer cells. Hormone therapy changes the hormonal environment to discourage further growth but does not kill cells directly. **Immunotherapy,** or **biotherapy,** is the introduction of a natural substance (such as the protein interferon) into the body to enhance disease-fighting systems.

A **bone marrow transplant,** the replacement of damaged bone marrow of a cancer patient with healthy marrow, may also be used to treat cancer. The transplant may be **autologous,** meaning the individual's own healthy marrow is removed and then reintroduced after the person has undergone radiation and chemotherapy. Bone marrow may also be donated by a relative or an unrelated person if it is genetically compatible.

In addition, research is being done into new areas of cancer control. These include work on **monoclonal antibodies** (using antibodies to deliver anticancer drugs directly to tumor cells, sparing healthy cells); **hyperthermia** (using heat to stimulate white blood cells to attack cancer cells); and **laser treatment** (directing a laser beam onto a tumor to destroy cancer cells).

ALTERNATIVE TREATMENTS

Alternative cancer treatments, also called unconventional, complementary, or unproven treatments, are not considered mainstream medicine. Rather than treating the symptoms of cancer—the tumors—many of these therapies attempt to treat the cause, whether it is poor physical health or spiritual well-being. Popular therapies may be categorized as follows:

■ Psychological approaches. Therapies, including psychotherapy and imagery, are used to enhance the quality of life, relieve pain and discomfort, reduce stress, and promote acceptance of treatment.

■ Diet and nutritional-metabolic approaches. Dietary regimens and supplement programs, such as the Hoxsie diet and the cartilage diet (which uses shark and bovine cartilage), are used to promote health.

■ Health-promoting lifestyles. This approach suggests that a healthful way of life can heal damaged cells. Therapies include yoga, aerobic exercise, relaxation exercises, detoxification, and an emphasis on harmony with nature.

■ Spiritual approaches. These methods emphasize transcendent methods of healing, such as faith healing and therapeutic touch.

■ Alternative immune stimulating therapies. Such programs are used to bolster the immune system. They include acupuncture, herbal remedies, and Chinese medicine.

■ Experimental medical therapies. These involve unconventional use of high-dose chemotherapy, radiation, and hyperthermia.

SEE biopsy; breast biopsy; chemotherapy; radiation therapy; specific cancers.

For more information on cancer, contact:

American Cancer Society
1599 Clifton Rd., N.E.
Atlanta, GA 30329-4251
800-ACS-2345
404-320-3333
http://www.cancer.org

National Cancer Institute
Cancer Information Service
9000 Rockville Pike
Bldg. 31, Room 10A31
Bethesda, MD 20892
800-4-CANCER
800-638-1234 (Alaska)
800-524-1234 (Hawaii)
http://wwwicic.nci.nih.gov

For information on alternative cancer treatments, contact:

Cancer Control Society
2043 N. Berendo St.
Los Angeles, CA 90027
213-663-7801

Committee for Freedom of Choice in Cancer Therapy
1180 Walnut Ave.
Chula Vista, CA 91911
619-429-8200

International Association of Cancer Victors and Friends
7740 W. Manchester Ave., Suite 203
Playa del Ray, CA 90293
310-822-5032

People Against Cancer
604 East St.
P.O. Box 10
Otho, IA 50569-0010
515-972-4444
http://www.dodgenet.com/nocancer

CANCER, BREAST

There are at least 15 different types of breast cancer, each classified according to where it develops, how far it has spread, and the appearance of the cancer cells. According to the American Cancer Society, breast cancer accounts for more than 30 percent of all cancers in women and strikes 182,000 women in the United States each year. Some 46,000 women (and about 240 men) die from breast cancer annually.

Breast cancer can develop in the milk ducts, between the ducts, in fat, in lymph or blood vessels, in the nipple, and in the lobes where milk is produced. The most common type of breast cancer is invasive ductal carcinoma, accounting for 70 to 80 percent of all breast cancers. The five-year survival rate for women with localized breast cancer is 94 percent, according to the American Cancer Society. For a diagnosis of regional breast cancer, the rate is 73 percent. If the cancer has spread, or **metastasized,** before diagnosis, the survival rate is only 18 percent.

RISK

The following factors contribute to an increased risk of breast cancer in women:
- An age of 50 or more
- A family history of breast cancer (a parent or sibling who had the disease)

UNDERSTANDING BREAST CANCER

Breast cancer terminology describes the type of breast cancer and its origins. If the cancer developed in a glandular tissue, the prefix "adeno," which means "glands," is attached to "carcinoma." So "adenocarcinoma" means that cancer cells are coming from glandular tissues.

To be even more specific, the terms "lobular" and "ductal" identify where in the glandular tissue the carcinoma developed. Ductal carcinoma is cancer that originated in the breast ducts, while lobular carcinoma is cancer that originated in the breast lobules. Therefore, cancer that develops, for example, in the breast lobules is called lobular adenocarcinoma. Often, the prefix "adeno" is not used with the terms "ductal" or "lobular" since these terms also refer to glands.

The terms "in situ" and "invasive" are used to identify whether a cancer has spread. **In situ carcinoma** is cancer that is contained within the tissue layer where it originated. **Invasive carcinoma** is cancer that has spread into surrounding tissues, other organs, or the lymph nodes. Putting all these terms together, ductal adenocarcinoma-in-situ, for example, means that cancer cells originated in the breast ducts and are contained in breast duct tissue only.

■ Late menopause

■ A first child born after age 30, or having never given birth

■ A diet with high levels of animal fat

■ Obesity

■ Exposure to diethylstilbestrol (DES) during pregnancy. Women who took DES while pregnant have shown a small but scientifically significant increased risk of breast cancer.

■ Exposure to certain chemicals, especially pesticides

SYMPTOMS

Breast cancer often begins as a painless growth or thickening that may not be able to be felt by hand. It can occur anywhere in the breast, including the nipple. A palpable lump or thickening does not necessarily mean breast cancer. Many women have benign, harmless lumps in the breast caused by a variety of conditions, such as a fibrocystic condition. Some 80 percent of biopsies on breast abnormalities show noncancerous conditions.

Additional symptoms of breast cancer are nipple discharge, scaling or bleeding of the nipple, change in nipple direction, change in breast contour, and skin dimpling. Pain is rare. However, many of these symptoms do not appear in the earliest stages of breast cancer. As a result, the cancer is often not detected until it has already spread beyond the site of origin.

To ensure early detection of breast cancer, women should perform monthly breast self-examinations and have yearly exams by a practitioner. Mammograms, or x-rays of the breast, are valuable tools in detecting breast cancer because they can locate suspicious areas too small to be felt by hand. Recommendations about the timing of mammograms are controversial. The National

BREAST CANCER: WHAT IS YOUR RISK?

You've heard or read the numbers: a woman has a one in eight chance of developing breast cancer—a statistic that has driven fear into the hearts of many women. The problem is, most women probably don't have the full story. When statistics say that there is a one in eight risk, it is the risk a woman has of developing cancer at the end of her lifetime. At different ages, women have different risks for developing breast cancer. The National Cancer Institute breaks it down as follows:

A Healthy, Cancer-Free Woman	Risk of Breast Cancer
By age 25	1 in 19,608
By age 30	1 in 2,525
By age 40	1 in 217
By age 50	1 in 50
By age 60	1 in 24
By age 70	1 in 14
By age 80	1 in 10
By age 85	1 in 9
Ever	1 in 8

As you can see, the risk of developing breast cancer is far from negligible. But in the absence of other risk factors, your risk rises to a significant level only as you age.

Cancer Institute (NCI) recommends annual mammograms for all women who are at high risk and those over the age of 50, but many experts believe these yearly screening mammograms should begin at age 40. The NCI is considering revising its guidelines. Women who have a

ESTROGEN AND BREAST CANCER

There has been a great deal of controversy about the role estrogen (present in oral contraceptives and hormone replacement therapy) plays in an increased risk of breast cancer.

To date, scientific research has found no conclusive link between breast cancer and estrogen. However, many experts suspect a link for several reasons: breast cancer is more prevalent in women than in men; estrogen may influence breast tissue by encouraging abnormal cell growth and the development of benign cysts in the breasts; and some forms of breast cancer are estrogen-dependent, meaning they grow in the presence of estrogen. In addition, a few studies show slight increases in cancer risks with the use of long-term estrogen supplements.

While the studies remain speculative, the American College of Obstetricians and Gynecologists' most recent technical bulletin reports that women who use estrogen replacement therapy for 15 or more years have a .5 percent increase in the risk of breast cancer over the course of a lifetime. The bulletin adds, "Whether the increased risk with long-term use that is observed in some studies is real must await clarification by future research."

The final vote on oral contraceptives is also not yet in. While again there is no scientific evidence of a link between oral contraceptives and breast cancer, there may be a slight increase in risk for women who have a history of breast cancer and take certain oral contraceptives for long periods of time.

mother, father, brother, or sister with a history of breast cancer will need to be screened earlier and more often.

SCREENING AND DIAGNOSIS OF BREAST CANCER

Suspicious (or abnormal) areas in the breast may be detected by hand, by mammogram, or by MRI (magnetic resonance imaging), a procedure that uses a magnetic field to create an image of the breast tissue. While these procedures can locate abnormalities, only a biopsy can determine if a suspicious area is cancerous or benign. A biopsy is the removal of a sample of tissue, which is then examined under a microscope for the presence of cancerous cells. (See "Breast Biopsy" for additional information.)

TYPES OF TREATMENT

SURGICAL TREATMENTS

The treatment of breast cancer is based on its type, the stage it is in, and the general health of the woman. Surgery is the primary method of treating breast cancer, although radiation therapy may be used as an alternative. Procedures for breast cancer include **lumpectomy** (removal of the lump and surrounding tissue); **partial** or **total mastectomy** (in which part or all of the breast is removed); and **radical mastectomy** (in which the entire breast, lymph nodes, and some chest muscles are removed). (See "Breast Surgery" for more information on surgical options.)

For early-stage breast cancer, a 10-year study by the National Cancer Institute reported that breast-conserving surgery, such as lumpectomy, when done with radiation, is just as effective in eradicating cancer as the more extensive mastectomy.

ADJUVANT THERAPIES

Breast cancer may also be treated with adjuvant, or supplemental, therapies after surgery to increase the chance that cancer is completely eliminated from the body. Adjuvant therapies include chemotherapy, radiation, treatment with the drug tamoxifen, hormone therapy, and immunotherapy.

In **chemotherapy,** anticancer drugs are administered orally or through injection. Chemotherapy is most often used along with surgery and radiation. If the cancer is widespread and the other treatment methods are not considered useful, it can be used alone. Side effects include vomiting, nausea, fatigue, and hair loss.

Radiation therapy, recommended less frequently than chemotherapy, uses radiation to destroy the cancer cells and prevent them from reproducing. It is most often used in conjunction with a lumpectomy or partial mastectomy or after chemotherapy to destroy any remaining cells. For women with more advanced cancer, radiation therapy is sometimes used to help shrink cancerous growths to make their surgical removal easier. Side effects include a sunburn-like rash, vomiting, nausea, and fatigue.

Tamoxifen is a newer breast cancer drug that blocks the action of estrogen, which can increase the risk of recurrence of some breast cancers. In a 1992 study of 30,000 women, the drug was shown to reduce the risk of recurring cancer by nearly 40 percent. Tamoxifen is currently being evaluated to see if it will prevent breast cancer in women at high risk of developing breast cancer. However, tamoxifen carries

---

TIPS FOR BREAST CANCER PREVENTION

- Maintain a normal weight.
- Cut back on fat in your diet. Some experts say a low-fat diet slows the progression of tumors and may help prevent cancer.
- Eat more fresh fruits, vegetables, and fiber. There's evidence that foods containing vitamin A and carotenoids offer protection against breast cancer.
- Breast-feed. There is some evidence that women who breast-feed their children reduce their risk of premenopausal cancers. Recent studies published in the *New England Journal of Medicine* and the *American Journal of Epidemiology* show that the risks decrease slightly with as little as two to three months of breast-feeding and continue to fall the longer breast-feeding is continued.
- Be aware that prolonged hormone replacement therapy (HRT) may carry a very slight increased risk of breast cancer.
- Increase fiber content to prevent constipation. Experts believe that an increased risk of breast cancer is more closely related to constipation than it is to HRT.

---

with it an increased risk of uterine cancer—up to three times more for women on the drug. Tamoxifen may cause hot flashes, menstrual irregularities, depression, and blood clots.

Hormone therapy uses drugs to counter the body's hormones that help the cancer grow. It is an adjuvant therapy that is used only to treat breast cancer. **Immunotherapy** uses drugs to boost the body's immune system, helping it fight the cancerous cells.

SEE breast biopsy; breast—fibrocystic conditions; breast lumps, benign; breast self-examination; breast surgery; cancer; chemotherapy; mammography; radiation therapy.

For more information on breast cancer, contact:

Breast Cancer Hotline
Physicians Committee for Responsible
   Medicine
P.O. Box 6322
Washington, DC 20015
800-875-4837

National Alliance of Breast Cancer
   Organizations (NABCO)
9 E. 37th St., 10th Floor
New York, NY 10016
212-889-0606
http://www.nabco.org

National Breast Cancer Coalition
1707 L St., N.W., Suite 1060
Washington, DC 20036
202-296-7477
http://www.natlbcc.org

Susan G. Komen Breast Cancer Foundation
5005 LBJ Freeway, Suite 370
Dallas, TX 75244
800-IM-AWARE
http://www.komen.com

Y-Me Breast Cancer Support Program
212 W. Van Buren St., 4th Floor
Chicago, IL 60607-3908
800-221-2141
312-986-8228
http://www.y-me.org

CANCER, CERVICAL

Cancer of the cervix, the opening of the uterus that connects to the vagina, is one of the most common cancers. The American Cancer Society reports that 15,800 cases of invasive cervical cancer are diagnosed annually.

Cervical cancer is one of the most preventable cancers, since routine Pap tests can detect many precancerous conditions early, decreasing health risks. The National Cancer Institute reports that 8.6 women out of every 100,000 will be diagnosed with cervical cancer. However, the rate of cervical cancer among women who do not have routine Pap tests is 50 to 60 per 100,000. If cervical cancer is diagnosed early, the five-year survival rate is 90 per-

cent. If the cancer is diagnosed in later stages, the rate drops to 67 percent.

RISK

Experts believe that certain risk factors increase a woman's chance of developing **dysplasia** (abnormal cell growth that may lead to cancer) or cancer of the cervix. These risk factors include:

- Sexual intercourse before age 18
- Multiple sex partners
- Sex partners who began having sexual intercourse at a young age, or who have had

many sex partners, or who had vaginal intercourse with women who had cervical cancer

■ More than five pregnancies

■ A history of syphilis and gonorrhea

■ Exposure in utero to diethylstilbestrol (DES), a drug that was prescribed for pregnant women between 1941 and 1971 for the prevention of miscarriage

■ Smoking or being exposed to heavy smoke for at least three hours a day

■ Exposure to some sexually transmitted viruses. Some types of the human papilloma virus (HPV) that do not cause genital warts have been linked to the cervical cell changes that may eventually become cancer.

SYMPTOMS

Cells on the surface of the cervix sometimes appear abnormal but are not cancerous. These changes may include inflammation, normal changes caused by cervical eversion, and intraepithelial lesions, also called dysplasia. Most cancers arise in women who have had dysplasia, even though most women with dysplasia never develop cancer. Precancerous changes in the cervix do not cause pain. In the early stages, a Pap test is the only way a woman would know she has dysplasia. Redness, inflammation, or sores on the cervix may be seen during a pelvic examination as the condition progresses.

Once cancer develops, the most common symptom is abnormal bleeding, unusually heavy and long menstrual bleeding, and bleeding after menopause. Increased vaginal discharge is also a symptom.

DIAGNOSIS

Tests include **colposcopy** (viewing the cervix through a specially designed microscope), a **cervical biopsy** (removal of a small sample of tissue from the cervix), **conization** (taking a cone-shaped sample of the tissue of the cervix for analysis), **loop electrosurgical excision procedures (LEEP)** (using a low-voltage radio wave to remove a tissue sample for analysis), and **endocervical curettage (ECC)** (scraping tissue from inside the cervical opening with a spoonlike instrument, called a curette). When tissue samples are taken, they are examined under a microscope for abnormal cells.

TO PREVENT CERVICAL CANCER:

■ Have routine Pap tests. These can detect most abnormal cell growth and alert you to the possibility of the presence of the human papilloma virus (HPV).

■ Don't smoke.

■ Practice safer sex. Using barrier contraceptives, such as the condom or female pouch, can reduce the risk of cervical cancer associated with sexually transmitted infections.

TREATMENT

Caught in its earliest stage, carcinoma-in-situ is 99 percent curable. If the cancer is only on the surface of the cervix, a practitioner may remove the cancerous cells through a variety of procedures. In **cryosurgery,** the lesions are frozen and the tissue sloughs away. **Laser surgery** uses a concentrated beam of light to cut away part of the cervix. A new treatment, called **loop electrosurgical excision procedures (LEEP),** uses a low-voltage radio wave to remove cancerous tissue in one piece. **Conization,** removal of a cone-shaped piece of tissue, may also be

BENIGN CONDITIONS OF THE CERVIX

There are a number of noncancerous conditions that may affect the cervix. **Cervicitis** is an inflammation of the cervix usually caused by chemical irritation, an infection (such as yeast or gardnerella), or a foreign body (such as a tampon or an IUD string). Symptoms may include heavy discharge, painful intercourse, and bleeding. The inflammation can be treated with creams and suppositories or antibiotics, depending on the cause. More serious infections may require cauterization (burning) or cryosurgery (freezing) to remove abnormal cells and allow for healing.

Cervical eversion occurs when the type of tissue found farther up the cervical canal replaces the normal tissue of the cervix. This condition, marked by increased cervical mucus production, usually occurs during pregnancy or puberty, when hormone levels are high. While most practitioners feel eversion does not require treatment, it may lead to an increased susceptibility of inflammation.

Polyps are noncancerous, fleshy tumors that grow in the cervix near the mouth of the body of the uterus. They usually have no symptoms but may cause spotting between periods. Large polyps may cause cramping. Polyps can be easily seen during a pelvic examination and can usually be removed in a practitioner's office.

used to remove the entire surface of the cervix.

Radiation therapy may be chosen instead of surgery, depending on the size of the cancer and the health of the woman. However, if the cancer has invaded deeper into the layers of the cervix but is still very small, surgical removal of the uterus and the cervix has been the main treatment. In more advanced cases, a **radical hysterectomy** (removal of the uterus and the cervix, along with the upper one-third of the vagina and lymph nodes in the groin area) may be necessary. If needed, either procedure may also involve a **bilateral salpingo-oophorectomy,** removal of the ovaries and fallopian tubes. Treatment after cervical cancer has progressed to this point is estimated to be 80 percent effective.

To ensure the cancer has been completely destroyed, several adjuvant, or supporting, therapies can also be used. **Chemotherapy** involves the use of strong drugs that travel through the body's blood and lymph system and destroy cancer cells. **Radiation therapy,** a treatment designed to inhibit a cancerous cell's ability to reproduce by destroying its DNA, is sometimes used alone to treat cervical cancer.

Cervical cancer is slow-growing, and many women who have not been cured through treatment live for several years without a cure.

SEE biopsy; cancer; chemotherapy; colposcopy; hysterectomy; oophorectomy; Pap test; radiation therapy.

For more information on cervical cancer, contact:

American Cancer Society
1599 Clifton Rd., N. E.
Atlanta, GA 30329-4251
800-ACS-2345
404-320-3333
http://www.cancer.org

Society of Gynecologic Oncologists
401 N. Michigan Ave., Suite 2200
Chicago, IL 60611
312-644-6610
http://www.sgo.org

CANCER,
COLON AND RECTAL

olon and rectal cancer is the growth of abnormal cells, or tumors, in the large intestine. The six-foot large intestine consists of the **cecum** (the pouch where the small intestine meets the large intestine), the **colon** (the main section) and the **rectum** (the last eight to 10 inches of the colon). Rectal cancer and colon cancer is often referred to as colorectal cancer because the rectum is part of the colon.

Colon and rectal cancer is the second most common cancer and the third leading cause of cancer deaths among women in the United States. According to the American Cancer Society, there are an estimated 67,500 new cases of colon and rectal cancer, and 28,100 deaths, for women each year. Colon cancer is slightly more common in women than in men, while rectal cancer affects more men than women. The disease is more prevalent in densely populated, industrialized regions than in rural areas.

The majority of cases occur in people over age 50; the average age at the time of diagnosis is 60. The five-year survival rates when the cancer is detected early are 93 percent for colon cancer and 87 percent for rectal cancer. If the cancer has spread to nearby organs, the rates decrease to 63 and 53 percent respectively. The survival rate is less than 7 percent for those diagnosed with widespread colon and rectal cancer.

PREVENTING COLON AND RECTAL CANCER

Cut down on red meat and high-fat foods. Studies show that people who ate fish or chicken, or no meat at all, had a lower incidence of colon and rectal cancer.

Eat foods high in fiber. Dietary fiber, found in fruits, vegetables, and whole grains, aids digestion and helps reduce the amount of time the lining of the intestines is exposed to carcinogens.

Those at risk for colon and rectal cancer should follow screening recommendations. Like most cancers, colon and rectal cancer is best treated when diagnosed early. The American Cancer Society recommends a digital rectal examination, occult blood test, and sigmoidoscopy to detect colon or rectal cancer in patients who have no symptoms. If you have symptoms, see your practitioner before your annual exam. The American Cancer Society guidelines advise:

■ After age 40, you should have an annual digital examination performed by your practitioner.

■ After age 50, you should have an occult stool blood test once a year and a sigmoidoscopy every three to five years.

RISK

The risk factors for colon and rectal cancer include:

■ A personal or family history of cancer or polyps (small growths on the mucous membrane of the colon). Polyps are usually not cancerous, but they may develop into colon cancer and should be monitored by a practitioner.

■ A history of inflammatory bowel disease (Crohn's disease)

■ A history of breast, endometrial, or ovarian cancer

■ A low-fiber, high-fat diet. Scientists think that dietary fat is associated with sluggish bowel transport and that it increases the amount of bile acids in the colon. The bile acids may damage the lining or may be converted to secondary bile acids, which are known to cause tumors in animals. Fat in the diet may also increase the amount of damaging chemicals in the bowel, which may result in changes in the cell membrane and/or affect hormone regulation. The National Cancer Institute is investigating what role—if any—vitamins A, C, and E, beta carotene, and calcium may play in preventing colon cancer in humans.

SYMPTOMS

The symptoms of colon and rectal cancer may include:

■ Diarrhea or constipation

■ Blood in or on the stool. The stool may be bright red or black in color.

■ Stools that are narrower than usual

■ Frequent gas pains

■ A feeling that the bowel doesn't empty completely

■ Loss of weight with no reason

■ Constant fatigue

■ Anemia

While other problems may cause these symptoms, if any persist for longer than two weeks, a practitioner should be seen.

DIAGNOSIS

Diagnostic procedures for colon and rectal cancer may include the following:

■ Digital rectal exam. An examination in which the practitioner inserts a gloved and lubricated finger into the lowest four inches of the rectum, checking the rectal wall surface for lesions

■ Sigmoidoscopy. An examination of the first 10 to 12 inches of the rectum. The practitioner inserts a sigmoidoscope (a thin, lighted tube) in the rectum to view the lower interior portion of the colon.

■ Occult blood stool test. A laboratory analysis of the stools for blood not detected by the naked eye

■ Colonoscopy. An examination in which the practitioner inserts a flexible colonoscope (a lighted tube) into the rectum to view the upper portions of the colon.

■ Lower gastrointestinal (GI) series. An examination of the colon by x-ray after administration of barium (a contrast dye)

■ CAT scans (computerized axial tomography scans) or MRI (magnetic resonance imaging). These imaging procedures may also be used to create an image of the abdominal contents.

■ Biopsy. The surgical removal of a portion of tissue for microscopic examination to determine if cancer cells are present. A practitioner may perform a biopsy during a colonoscopy or sigmoidoscopy.

TREATMENT

Treatment of colon and rectal cancer depends on the stage of the disease and the general health of the patient. Surgical removal of the cancer and some of the surrounding tissue, at times combined with radiation therapy, is the most effective method of treating colon and rectal cancer. If the cancer is confined to a polyp, the surgical procedure is known as a **polypectomy.** If the cancer is larger and more tissue must be removed, the procedure is known as a **wedge resection.** If nearby lymph nodes are also removed, the procedure is called a **bowel resection.**

For widespread cancer, a **colostomy** may be done, a procedure in which an opening is created in the abdominal wall allowing the elimination of waste from the body into a bag. Patients with colon and rectal cancer seldom need a colostomy. While most colostomies are temporary while the colon and rectum heal, an estimated 10 to 15 percent of colostomies are permanent.

Scientists are currently studying the role of chemotherapy in treating advanced cases.

SEE cancer; medical testing (appendix B); radiation therapy.

For more information on colon and rectal cancer, contact:

American Cancer Society
1599 Clifton Rd., N.E.
Atlanta, GA 30329-4251
800-ACS-2345
404-320-3333
http://www.cancer.org

United Ostomy Association, Inc.
36 Executive Park, Suite 120
Irvine, CA 92614
800-826-0826
714-660-8624
http://www.gulf.net/civic/org/uoa

CANCER, ENDOMETRIAL

Also called cancer of the lining of the uterus, endometrial cancer is the most common form of pelvic cancer in women. According to the National Cancer Institute, endometrial cancer affects 32,800 women each year.

Endometrial cancer attacks the uterine lining, or endometrium, and most often occurs in women over 50 years of age. According to the National Cancer Institute, 21.1 women out of 100,000 are diagnosed with endometrial cancer each year.

Endometrial cancer usually occurs after the onset of menopause. Seventy-five percent of endometrial cancer cases are diagnosed in the early stage, when the five-year survival rate is 94 percent. If the cancer becomes more widespread, the survival rate drops to 67 percent.

RISK

Factors that put women at higher risk for endometrial cancer include:

- An age of 55 or more
- Obesity
- History of infertility
- Anovulation (lack of ovulation)
- Few or no biological children
- Prolonged use of estrogen therapy without **progestin** (a synthetic form of progesterone, a hormone produced by the body that regulates menstruation). Postmenopausal women who are using estrogen without a balancing progestin are four to eight times more likely to develop endometrial cancer. However, these cancers are usually very nonaggressive and have a very high cure rate.
- A history of diabetes and high blood pressure
- Cirrhosis of the liver

Research indicates that the growth of abnormal or cancerous cells in the endometrium is related to hormones, especially unopposed estrogen (estrogen taken without progestin). Research also shows that fatty tissue converts certain hormones into estrone, a form of estrogen, part of the reason obesity is a major risk factor. Obese people are also less likely to ovulate and produce protective progesterone.

SYMPTOMS

The most common symptom of endometrial cancer is abnormal bleeding, especially after menopause. Bleeding does not necessarily indicate cancer, but it should not be considered a normal part of menopause and should be reported to a practitioner. For women who are still menstruating, grossly irregular periods and/or bleeding between periods should also be reported to a practitioner. Weight loss and pain occur as the cancer progresses.

DIAGNOSIS

To diagnose endometrial cancer, a practitioner may perform a number of tests. The cancer, if advanced, may be detected by a **pelvic exam,** or a woman may have a tissue sample removed and analyzed. A woman may have an **endometrial aspiration,** where tissue from the uterus is collected for analysis by means of a special vacuum apparatus. **Dilation and curettage (D&C),** in which tissue is removed by scraping the lining of the uterus with an instrument known as a curette, may also be used to diagnose cancer. Once the tissue is collected, it is examined under a microscope for evidence of abnormal cells. The collection of tissue for analysis is called a **biopsy.**

An **ultrasound,** a noninvasive procedure in which sound waves are used to create an image of the pelvic cavity, may also detect cancer. A **hysteroscopy,** a procedure in which a fiberoptic viewing scope is inserted into the uterus through the cervix, may also be used.

A **Pap test** is generally not sensitive enough to diagnose endometrial cancer, since the abnormal cells shed by the endometrium degenerate before reaching the vagina; it may be used in detecting, or perhaps ruling out, cancer of the cervix.

TREATMENT

Treatment depends on the stage of the cancer, the growth rate of the cancer, and the age and general health of the woman. Endometrial cancer is most often treated with surgery, radiation therapy, and chemotherapy. Rapid cell growth, or atypical hyperplasia, is precancerous and may develop into cancer. It can be treated with a progestin for three to six months. However, if the condition persists, removal of the cervix and the uterus may be recommended.

An adjuvant, or supplemental, therapy is often used in addition to primary treatment (usually surgery) to ensure that the cancer has been completely eliminated.

Chemotherapy involves the use of strong drugs that travel through the body's blood and lymph system and destroy cancer cells. Chemotherapy is most often used with surgery and radiation. If the cancer is widespread and the other treatment methods are not considered useful, it can be used alone. High-dose progestins are the most common form of chemotherapy.

Radiation therapy is designed to inhibit the cancerous cell's ability to divide by destroying its DNA with radiation, thereby preventing it from reproducing.

The cancer is usually treated with surgery. A **hysterectomy** (removal of the uterus and cervix) and a **salpingo-oophorectomy** (removal of the fallopian tubes and ovaries) may be recommended.

SEE biopsy; cancer; chemotherapy; dilation and curettage (D&C); hysterectomy; hysteroscopy; oophorectomy; radiation therapy.

For more information on endometrial cancer, contact:

American Cancer Society
1599 Clifton Rd., N.E.
Atlanta, GA 30329-4251
800-ACS-2345
404-320-3333
http://www.cancer.org

Society of Gynecologic Oncologists
401 N. Michigan Ave., Suite 2200
Chicago, IL 60611
312-644-6610
http://www.sgo.org

CANCER, LUNG

In the mid-1980s lung cancer passed breast cancer to become the leading cause of death from cancer among women. The American Cancer Society estimates that 74,000 American women are diagnosed with lung cancer annually and that 62,000 die of it each year. The greatest risk factor for lung cancer is smoking. According to the American Lung Association, 87 percent of lung cancer deaths are directly caused by smoking.

Lung cancer is particularly difficult to diagnose in its early stages, when treatment is most effective, because its symptoms do not appear until the disease has **metastasized,** or spread. As a result, only 13 percent of all patients survive five or more years after diagnosis, regardless of the stage the cancer has reached when it is discovered.

There are two types of lung cancer: **small cell** lung cancer (also called **undifferentiated small cell** or **oat cell**) and **nonsmall cell** lung cancer, which is also broken down into **squa-**

mous cell lung cancer (also called **epidermoid carcinoma**) and **adenocarcinoma.** Small cell lung cancer accounts for 20 to 25 percent of all lung cancers, and nonsmall cell lung cancer accounts for 75 to 80 percent of all lung cancers.

RISK

The National Cancer Institute estimates that 42 out of every 100,000 women will develop lung cancer. People who are at the greatest risk of developing lung cancer have smoked one or more packs of cigarettes a day for 20 years or longer, began smoking before the age of 20, or do not smoke but are exposed regularly to secondhand smoke.

The American Lung Association estimates that 12.5 percent of those with lung cancer are

PREVENTING LUNG CANCER

Lung cancer is highly preventable. The most important thing an individual can do to prevent lung cancer is not to smoke.

To find out more about how to stop smoking, contact:

Action on Smoking and Health
2013 H St., N.W.
Washington, DC 20006
202-659-4310
http://ash.org/

Smokenders
4455 E. Camelback Rd., Suite D150
Phoenix, AZ 85018
602-840-7414
smokenders@aol.com

nonsmokers. Some 10 percent of lung cancer cases may be attributed to radon, an odorless gas found in rock, soil, and water that breaks down into radioactive products. Radon is known to leak into homes and contaminate water and natural gas supplies used by people. There is a one in 300 chance that a resident of the United States will develop lung cancer from indoor radon. The National Safety Council offers a radon hotline at 800-SOS-RADON.

Exposure to industrial materials such as asbestos, uranium, nickel, arsenic, coal dust, and chromates also puts individuals at increased risk of lung cancer. Risks due to these materials are even higher for smokers.

SYMPTOMS

The most common symptoms of lung cancer are:

■ A persistent cough, usually caused by the tumor blocking the airway as it grows

■ Chest pain

■ Shortness of breath

■ Repeated episodes of pneumonia or bronchitis

■ Coughing up blood

■ Hoarseness

■ Swelling of the neck and face

DIAGNOSIS

To diagnose lung cancer, a practitioner may take a chest x-ray, the most reliable diagnostic procedure, and follow it up with one or several procedures, including a CAT scan, MRI, bronchoscopy, percutaneous needle biopsy, mediastinoscopy, and thoracotomy. In addition, if sputum is being coughed up, it can be studied—as a Pap test would be—for abnormal cells.

A **CAT scan** (computerized axial tomography scan) is a noninvasive diagnostic procedure that takes a series of cross-sectional x-rays, then uses a computer to create detailed images of the lungs. **MRI,** or **magnetic resonance imaging,** uses a magnetic field to create an image of the chest.

A **bronchoscopy** is an examination of the bronchi, trachea (windpipe), and the lungs. The procedure uses a bronchoscope, a flexible viewing instrument, which is inserted through the mouth or nose, down the throat, and into a lung, to examine the interior tissues. A sample of the tissue may also be taken for a microscopic examination through a procedure known as a **biopsy.**

A **percutaneous needle biopsy** involves inserting a thin needle through the chest and extracting a sample of the lung tissue through the needle. It is then examined under a microscope for the presence of cancer cells. This is a frequently performed procedure.

A **mediastinoscopy** is an examination of the mediastinum, the space in the chest between the lungs, breastbone, and spine. The procedure uses a mediastinoscope, a thin viewing instrument that is inserted through an incision above the collarbone, to view the lymph nodes and other structures. During this process, practitioners may also remove lymph nodes for biopsy.

A **thoracotomy** is a surgical opening of the chest and is used only when all other diagnostic methods have failed to produce a diagnosis. During this procedure, a small part of the lung containing the tumor is removed. This procedure is performed only if the surgeons believe it is possible to remove the mass; this cannot always be determined before surgery. The opening of the chest and the surgical removal of the cancer in the lung are the most likely treatments to result in a cure if the cancer is in its early stage and has not spread.

TREATMENT

Like all cancer, the treatment of lung cancer depends on its stage and the general health of the individual. If the disease is in its early stage, surgery, such as a thoracotomy and surgical removal of the cancer in the lung, may be performed. Sometimes these procedures are used in combination with **chemotherapy,** in which chemicals are injected into the body to destroy cancer cells, and external **radiation,** where cancer cells are destroyed with radiation. In small cell cancer, chemotherapy and radiation have replaced surgery as the primary treatment. The treatment has led to remission in many cases.

SEE cancer; chemotherapy; medical testing (appendix B); radiation therapy; smoking.

For more information on lung cancer, contact:

American Cancer Society
1599 Clifton Rd., N.E.
Atlanta, GA 30329-4251
800-ACS-2345
404-320-3333
http://www.cancer.org

American Lung Association
1740 Broadway
New York, NY 10019
800-LUNG-USA
212-315-8700
http://www.lungusa.org

CANCER—LYMPHOMA

Lymphoma is a general term for cancers developing in the lymph system, the part of the circulatory system that helps fight disease and infection.

The two principal types of lymphoma are Hodgkin's disease and non-Hodgkin's lymphoma.

HODGKIN'S DISEASE

Hodgkin's disease is relatively rare. According to the American Cancer Society, there were an estimated 7,800 new cases of Hodgkin's disease in the United States in 1995. These cases account for fewer than 1 percent of all cancers in the United States. Since 1970, the incidence of Hodgkin's disease has declined, especially among the elderly.

Medical experts do not know the cause or risk factors of Hodgkin's disease, but contributing factors may include reduced immune function and exposure to certain infectious agents. Study findings have shown a higher rate among woodworkers and chemists. Additional research has indicated a higher incidence among the brothers and sisters of people with Hodgkin's.

SYMPTOMS

Symptoms of Hodgkin's disease include:
- Enlarged lymph nodes or abdominal masses
- Itching
- Fever
- Night sweats
- Weight loss
- Fatigue, weakness

DIAGNOSIS

Diagnostic procedures for Hodgkin's disease may include blood tests; x-rays of the chest, bones, liver, and spleen; and a biopsy (microscopic examination) of tissue from an enlarged lymph node. A major factor that distinguishes Hodgkin's disease from other lymphomas is the presence of the Reed-Sternberg cell, a giant, abnormal cell with several nuclei. This cell type is almost always present in Hodgkin's disease, and medical experts rarely make a diagnosis of Hodgkin's disease unless they detect the Reed-Sternberg cell.

In addition, the **CAT scan** (computerized axial tomography scan), which creates a three-dimensional x-ray of the chest, and **MRI,** or **magnetic resonance imaging,** which uses a magnetic field to create an image of the chest, may both be used to locate and determine the extent of the disease.

TREATMENT

The two principal treatments that the medical community prescribes for Hodgkin's disease are radiation therapy and chemotherapy. Bone marrow transplantation, a fairly new treatment, is becoming more widespread.

Survival rates vary according to the stage of the disease and the types of cells present. The overall five-year survival rate for Hodgkin's disease is 79 percent.

NON-HODGKIN'S LYMPHOMA

Non-Hodgkin's lymphoma is the sixth most common cancer in the United States. According to the American Cancer Society, in 1995 there were an estimated 50,900 new cases of non-Hodgkin's lymphoma in the United States. Since the 1970s, the incidence rates for non-Hodgkin's lymphoma have increased more than 65 percent.

Non-Hodgkin's is slightly more common in men than in women, and there is a greater incidence in the white population than in the black population.

As with Hodgkin's disease, the causes of non-Hodgkin's lymphoma are unclear. However, exposure to environmental toxins and a decreased immune system appear to be two significant risk factors. Human immunodeficiency virus (HIV) and human T-cell leukemia/lymphoma virus I (HTLV-I) are associated with increased risk of the disease. Organ transplant patients taking immunosuppressive drugs are 40 to 100 percent more likely to develop non-Hodgkin's.

SYMPTOMS

Symptoms of non-Hodgkin's may include:
- Painless swelling of the lymph nodes in the neck, groin, or underarm
- Fever
- Night sweats
- Fatigue, weakness
- Weight loss
- Itching
- Nausea, vomiting, or abdominal pain

DIAGNOSIS

Diagnosis and evaluation of non-Hodgkin's lymphoma may include a thorough physical exam, x-rays, tomography (cross-sectional x-rays), CAT scan, MRI, blood test, urinalysis, bone marrow test, lymphangiography (an x-ray examination that follows the injection of dye into the lymphatic system), and a biopsy of tissue from an enlarged lymph node.

TREATMENT

Treatment depends on the stage of the disease, the general state of health of the individual, and other factors. Generally, treatment is radiation therapy and chemotherapy. Bone marrow transplantation is also an option.

Again, the survival rate varies according to the stage of the disease. The overall five-year survival for non-Hodgkin's lymphoma has steadily improved, increasing in the past 30 years from 31 to 52 percent.

SEE cancer; chemotherapy; radiation therapy.

For more information on lymphoma, contact:

American Cancer Society
1599 Clifton Rd., N.E.
Atlanta, GA 30329-4251
800-ACS-2345
404-320-3333
http://www.cancer.org

Lymphoma Research Foundation of America, Inc.
8800 Venice Blvd., Suite 207
Los Angeles, CA 90034
310-204-7040
http://www.lymphoma.org

CANCER, OVARIAN

A woman's ovaries are the two reproductive organs that produce estrogen and progesterone, the female hormones, and the ovum, the eggs released monthly for fertilization. Cancer of the ovaries accounts for 4 percent of all cancers in women and has a low overall five-year survival rate of only 41 percent. If the cancer is diagnosed while it is in an early stage, the five-year survival rate is 90 percent. However, once the cancer becomes invasive, the survival rate drops to 21 percent.

According to the American Cancer Society, 26,600 women develop ovarian cancer each year, and it is estimated that one in every 70 women will develop it in her lifetime. Ovarian cancer should not be confused with ovarian cysts, a common condition not associated with cancer.

Ovarian cancer is particularly difficult to diagnose in the early stages, when there are no symptoms. Because the disease spreads rapidly throughout the abdominal area, early detection is important but difficult. Though regular pelvic exams often cannot find ovarian cancer at the early stage, women who have regular exams still increase their chance of finding the cancer early, when treatment is most effective.

PREVENTING OVARIAN CANCER

Consider oral contraceptives. The Pill has been shown to reduce the risk of ovarian cancer in high-risk women when used for a period of five years. According to the National Cancer Institute, this may be because the Pill creates hormone levels in the body that mimic those during pregnancy—and pregnancy is known to lower the risk of ovarian cancer.

Be aware of the risks of fertility drugs. Medications such as Pergonal and Clomid stimulate the ovaries to produce more eggs and may or may not increase your risk of ovarian cancer.

RISK

According to the National Cancer Institute, researchers have found certain risk factors associated with developing ovarian cancer by studying large numbers of women all over the world. These factors include:

■ An age of 50 or more (though young women and even small children may also contract it)

■ A mother, sister, or daughter with the disease

■ No previous pregnancy. Each pregnancy reduces the risk of ovarian cancer by 10 percent.

■ No previous use of oral contraception. Oral contraceptives are shown to help prevent ovarian cancer.

■ A personal history of breast cancer

SYMPTOMS

Ovarian cancer may grow into its late stages before symptoms develop. Even then, the symptoms can be so vague they are easy to ignore or attribute to some other condition. In the late stages of ovarian cancer, pain, abdominal distension, and other problems may occur. As the tumors grow, a woman may experience a feeling of bloating or swelling, or general discomfort in her lower abdomen. She may also lose her appetite or otherwise feel full even after a light meal. Other symptoms include gas, indigestion, nausea, and weight loss. A larger tumor may put pressure on nearby organs, such as the bladder or bowel, causing diarrhea, constipation, or frequent urination. Bleeding may also be a symptom, but less often than other symptoms. (Bleeding and irregular periods are often symptoms of ovarian cysts.)

SCREENING AND DIAGNOSIS

Ovarian cancer often has no symptoms until the later stages, and there is no single reliable method for diagnosing it. Regular pelvic exams may show evidence of the cancer before it spreads and causes symptoms.

Enlarged ovaries are usually the first sign of ovarian cancer. A woman in a high-risk category may increase her chance of finding ovarian cancer in its early stages with a **Doppler ultrasound** (a procedure that uses sound waves to create images of the pelvic cavity) to measure the size of her ovaries and look for any abnormal blood flow to the ovaries.

In addition, tests for increased levels of the serum **CA 125** in the blood may indicate ovarian cancer, although CA 125 may be elevated in other, benign conditions. While neither of these procedures is very reliable on its own, ultrasound and CA 125 blood testing are slightly more effective in detecting cancer in women over the age of 50 when used in combination.

If ovarian cancer is suspected, several pro-cedures may be recommended to try to confirm the diagnosis: a **CAT scan** (computerized axial tomography scan), a three-dimensional x-ray; **MRI,** or **magnetic resonance imaging,** or an image created using a magnetic field; a **lymphangiography,** an **intravenous pyelogram,** or a **lower gastrointestinal (GI) series,** all of which involve injecting the body with a contrast material to make internal structures visible on x-rays; or an exploratory **laparoscopy,** in which a laparoscope, a thin viewing scope, is inserted into the abdomen through an incision. During laparoscopy, tissue may be collected and analyzed under a microscope in a procedure called a **biopsy.** A biopsy is the only way to definitively diagnose ovarian cancer.

TREATMENT

SURGERY

Most often, ovarian cancer is treated with surgery. A **prophylactic bilateral oophorectomy** (removal of both ovaries as a preventive measure) may be recommended to a woman who has a high risk of heredity ovarian cancer once she desires no more children and has reached the age of 35.

With certain kinds of cancer, if the cancer is still in its early stages and the woman is still of childbearing years and wants to have children, only the ovary that is affected may need to be removed. However, in almost all cases of diagnosed ovarian cancer, a **hysterectomy with a bilateral salpingo-oophorectomy** (the surgical removal of the ovaries, the uterus, and the fallopian tubes) is recommended. Additional surgery, called **cytoreductive surgery,** may also be done after supplementary treatments have been done to remove any remaining cancerous tissues or check for recurrence.

ADJUVANT THERAPIES

Ovarian cancer may also be treated with adjuvant, or supplemental, therapies after surgery to ensure that cancer is completely eliminated from the body. Adjuvant therapies include chemotherapy, radiation therapy, and drugs.

In **chemotherapy,** anticancer drugs are administered orally, through injection, or through a catheter that is inserted into the abdomen, in order to destroy remaining cancer cells. This last method is called **intraperitoneal chemotherapy** and allows the anticancer drug to reach the cancer directly. **Paclitaxol,** a well-known chemotherapy drug, may be used alone or in combination with other drugs.

Radiation therapy, recommended less frequently than chemotherapy, uses radiation to destroy the DNA of the cancer cells. Like chemotherapy, it can be administered directly to the cancer through a catheter in a procedure called **intraperitoneal irradiation.**

SEE cancer; chemotherapy; hysterectomy; laparoscopy; oophorectomy; ovarian cysts; radiation therapy.

For more information on ovarian cancer, contact:

Gilda Radner Familial Cancer Registry
Ovarian Cancer Hotline
Roswell Park Cancer Institute
Elm and Carlton Sts.
Buffalo, NY 14263
800-OVARIAN

Society of Gynecologic Oncologists
401 N. Michigan Ave., Suite 2200
Chicago, IL 60611
312-644-6610
http://www.sgo.org

CANCER, SKIN

Skin cancer is the most common cancer in the United States. According to the American Cancer Society, more than 800,000 cases are diagnosed in the United States each year. Most skin cancer can be attributed to exposure to ultraviolet radiation from the sun. An increase in the occurrence of skin cancer is due to several factors, including a depleting ozone layer, which protects the earth from the sun's ultraviolet rays. Pressures from a society that encourages outdoor activities and tanning may also contribute to the increase in skin cancer.

Being in the sun without protection is risky. It is important to begin protective measures in childhood, as 50 percent of all the sun exposure in one's lifetime is usually within the first 18 years. However, adults still need to take precautions as well.

While skin cancers are usually curable with early treatment, they can destroy the skin and the surrounding tissues if not treated, and could result in the loss of an ear, eye, or nose.

RISK

Risk factors for developing skin cancer include:

■ Fair complexion and light eye and hair color. However, dark skin color does not exempt you from risk.

■ A tendency to burn and/or freckle rather than tan

■ A family history of skin cancer

■ Prolonged exposure to sunlight related to working or vacationing; a history of vacations in sunny places

■ Precancers of the skin, such as **actinic keratoses,** dry, scaly patches often found on "weather-beaten" skin

■ Exposure to chemicals and substances such as coal tar, pitch, creosote, arsenic compounds, and radium

TYPES OF SKIN CANCER

The most common type of skin cancer is **basal cell carcinoma,** which rarely spreads and is highly curable. These carcinomas are raised, pearly nodules that may become open sores that bleed or crust. They are most often found on the face, by the eye or the nose, but they may be found anywhere on the body. Basal cell carcinomas grow deeper into the skin layers and may return after they are removed.

Squamous cell carcinoma is the second most common form of skin cancer. It begins as small, firm, painless lumps, or as flat, reddened areas, which grow slowly to resemble warts or ulcers. They are most often found on exposed areas of the body, such as the hands, but may appear anywhere. Squamous cell carcinoma is also very curable; however, if not treated, it may spread.

About 5 percent of all skin cancers are of the

PROTECTING YOURSELF FROM THE SUN

The best way to prevent skin cancer is to protect yourself from the sun's harmful rays. To do so:

■ Try to avoid the sun during its strongest hours, from 10 A.M. to 3 P.M.

■ Use a sunscreen or sunblock if you're going to be in the sun. Always choose a sunblock with a sun protection factor (SPF) of at least 15. The higher the lotion's SPF, the greater the protection.

■ Use a sunblock that is sweatproof and waterproof if you are physically active in the sun.

■ Apply the sunblock liberally and frequently.

■ Use sunblock on the hands and the face, as these are the areas that are exposed to the sun every day of every season and are targets for basal cell carcinoma. Cosmetic foundations with sunblock are also available; again, choose a foundation with an SPF of at least 15.

■ Wear tightly woven clothing to help protect your skin. A brimmed hat is also helpful.

■ Avoid tanning devices. Salon tanning beds and ultraviolet lamps are not safer than the sun; they expose you to the same ultraviolet radiation.

most dangerous type, **malignant melanoma,** which occurs in skin cells that produce the dark pigment melanin (the substance that produces a tan). The National Cancer Institute reports that 9.9 women out of every 100,000 will develop malignant melanoma. According to the American Cancer Society, it is diagnosed in 15,400 women in the United States annually, and 2,700 women die from it each year.

About 82 percent of malignant melanomas are diagnosed at an early stage, when the survival rate is 85 percent. If the melanoma becomes widespread, the survival rate drops to 15 percent.

Melanomas appear as small brown-black or larger multicolored patches that have an irregular outline. They usually grow from a preexisting mole that enlarges, changes colors, and bleeds or itches. They spread quickly and permeate all skin layers.

SYMPTOMS

The most common warning sign of skin cancer is a change in the skin. The signs of skin cancer, according to the Skin Cancer Foundation, include:

■ A skin growth that has increased in size and is pearly, translucent, tan, brown, black, or multicolored

■ A spot or growth that continues to itch, hurt, crust, scab, erode, or bleed

· ■ An open sore on the skin that does not heal or persists for more than four weeks, or heals and then reopens

■ A mole, birthmark, or beauty mark that changes color, increases in size or thickness, changes in texture, or is irregular in outline

DETECTING SKIN CANCER

The American Cancer Society recommends skin self-examinations on a monthly basis. It is important to check the entire body, using a mirror, for any changes, such as in a freckle's appearance or the shape of a mole. Children should also be examined regularly for skin changes. Regular visits to a dermatologist for an adult may aid in detecting skin cancer.

If a change is noted, a practitioner should be contacted. An examination and a biopsy, a tissue sample analyzed under a microscope, may be done to determine the type of growth and the appropriate treatment.

TREATMENT

Skin cancer is highly curable if caught at an early stage. The common treatments for skin cancer are **surgical excision** (where the skin layers containing the cancer are cut away), **radiation therapy, cauterization** (burning off the nodule), and **cryosurgery** (freezing off the nodule). **Chemosurgery,** in which toxic chemicals are used to remove cancerous tissue, and **chemotherapy,** the injection of toxins to kill cancer cells, may also be used. Reconstructive or cosmetic surgery may be necessary in some cases.

SEE chemotherapy; cryosurgery; radiation therapy; skin.

For more information on skin cancer, contact:

American Cancer Society
1599 Clifton Rd., N.E.
Atlanta, GA 30329-4251
800-ACS-2345
404-320-3333
http://www.cancer.org

Skin Cancer Foundation
245 Fifth Avenue, Suite 2402
New York, NY 10016
212-725-5176

CANCER, VAGINAL

Vaginal cancer accounts for less than 2 percent of all gynecological cancers. The most common form of vaginal cancer is **vaginal intraepithelial neoplasia (VAIN),** which develops on the surface of the lining of the vagina. This form of cancer has been linked to exposure to the **human papilloma virus (HPV),** which is thought to trigger abnormal growth of the cells lining the vagina. This cancer very rarely originates in the vagina. Generally, vaginal cancer is related to cancer of the vulva or the cervix. It is usually highly curable if detected early, although the prognosis depends on the age of the woman and the stage of the disease when it is diagnosed.

A type of vaginal cancer that begins in the vagina is the rare **clear cell adenocarcinoma,** a rapidly spreading cancer that is strongly linked to fetal exposure to the drug diethylstilbestrol, or DES, which was taken to prevent miscarriages. Daughters of women who took DES between 1941 and 1971 should have regular gynecological checkups for any signs of precancerous changes. In women at risk for adenocarcinoma, who have been closely monitored, the disease is highly curable.

RISK

Research suggests that the sexual practices of a woman and her partner are linked to the development of vaginal cancer because a type of HPV, which may trigger abnormal cell growth, is sexually transmitted. Factors that increase risk include:

- Sexual intercourse before age 18
- Multiple sex partners
- Sex partners who began having sexual intercourse at a young age, or who have had many sex partners, or who were previously partnered with women who had cervical cancer
- A history of syphilis and gonorrhea

Women whose mothers took DES while pregnant are at a higher risk for clear cell adenocarcinoma. This cancer of the vagina develops in fewer than one in every 1,000 DES daughters, most often in women aged 15 to 22.

SYMPTOMS

Symptoms of vaginal cancer include:

- Vaginal bleeding or spotting
- Foul-smelling discharge not associated with menstruation
- Difficult or painful urination
- Pain during sexual intercourse
- A feeling of pain, pressure, or fullness in the pelvic area

These may also be symptoms of other disorders. For example, vaginal discharge may be a symptom of an infection.

DIAGNOSIS

While a pelvic exam and a Pap test may detect signs of vaginal cancer, they do not provide reliable diagnosis. A **biopsy,** microscopic examination of a tissue sample, is the definitive test. A **colposcopy,** microscopic examination of

Clinical Trials

When laboratory research shows that a new treatment has promise, the method is used in clinical trials to answer questions regarding its safety and effectiveness. Any woman who has any form of cancer and is interested in participating in a clinical trial should discuss this option with her practitioner.

One way to learn about clinical trials is through Physicians Data Query (PDQ), a resource developed by the National Cancer Institute (NCI). PDQ contains an up-to-date list of trials all over the country. NCI can provide PDQ information to practitioners, patients, and the public. The National Cancer Institute can be reached at 800-4-CANCER.

The National Cancer Institute also provides a booklet, "What Are Clinical Trials All About?" also available through their toll-free number.

---

the vagina with a viewing scope, may be done to determine suspicious areas for biopsy.

Women who have been exposed to DES should have regular exams designed for DES daughters. The exam should include a Pap test and a **four-quadrant smear** of all of the walls of the vagina to determine if a biopsy is needed to check for cancer.

TREATMENT

The treatment of vaginal cancer depends on its stage and the health of the patient. If it occurs at the top of the vagina, it may be treated as cervical cancer; if it appears at the bottom, it may be treated as vulvar cancer.

Surgery is the most common treatment for all stages of vaginal cancer. The various treatments available are **laser surgery** (vaporization of lesions), **wide local excision** (surgical removal of the cancer and the tissue surrounding it), **partial** or **complete vaginectomy** (removal of the vagina), and **radical hysterectomy** (removal of the uterus, vagina, and lymph nodes in the groin). **Chemotherapy** and **radiation therapy** may also be used, perhaps in combination with surgery.

For very advanced cancer that has spread to other organs, it may be necessary to perform **pelvic exenteration,** the surgical removal of the uterus, fallopian tubes, ovaries, regional lymph nodes, part of the vagina, the bladder, and the rectum.

SEE biopsy; cancer; cancer, cervical; cancer, vulvar; chemotherapy; colposcopy; diethylstilbestrol (DES); radiation therapy.

For more information on vaginal cancer, contact:

American Cancer Society
1599 Clifton Rd., N.E.
Atlanta, GA 30329-4251
800-ACS-2345
404-320-3333
http://www.cancer.org

Society of Gynecologic Oncologists
401 N. Michigan Ave., Suite 2200
Chicago, IL 60611
312-644-6610
http://www.sgo.org

CANCER, VULVAR

Cancer of the vulva is almost always a type of skin cancer, known as **squamous cell carcinoma,** which has affected the labia, or lips, surrounding the vagina. It accounts for 3 to 5 percent of all gynecological cancers. The disease is 90 percent curable when it is diagnosed and treated early.

Vulvar cancer appears as a raised lump or sore on the vulva that can be readily seen or felt. Eighty percent of all vulvar cancers develop after exposure to the **human papilloma virus (HPV).** Different types of HPV are responsible for genital warts, but the strains associated with cancer are usually not associated with warts. Some experts believe that there is a direct link between HPV and vulvar cancer. Vulvar cancers may also develop after exposure to syphilis, chlamydia, and herpes, which are all sexually transmitted. A skin cancer known as **melanoma,** when present on the labia, is also considered vulvar cancer, although its appearance on the vulva is rare.

RISK

Women at high risk for vulvar cancer have had sexual intercourse before age 18 and have had multiple sex partners. Research often links such sexual practices to development of vulvar cancer because sexually transmitted infections frequently include HPV.

In the past, almost all cases of vulvar cancer were diagnosed in postmenopausal women. Today, however, 40 percent of all vulvar cancers are diagnosed in women under the age of 40.

SYMPTOMS AND DIAGNOSIS

Symptoms include lumps, open sores, itching, pain, burning, bleeding, and discharge. It is not uncommon for the cancer to go undiagnosed for more than six months after symptoms appear because the cancer may resemble other conditions, such as genital warts or a fungal infection, making it difficult for some women to identify. For diagnosis, the vulva can be washed with a blue dye known as **toluidine blue,** which is absorbed by precancerous cells to show signs of cancer, then examined through **colposcopy,** a diagnostic procedure in which a special viewing scope is used to magnify cells. Visible lesions are removed for **biopsy,** or microscopic analysis.

Regular genital self-examination can catch vulvar cancer early. A practitioner should be seen if a lump persists for more than two weeks.

TREATMENT

As with all cancer, treatment depends on the stage of the cancer and the general health of the woman. If precancerous lesions exist, they are removed using **laser surgery** (vaporization of the lesions), **cryosurgery** (freezing off the lesions), **radiation therapy,** or **chemotherapy.** Surgery is usually confined to the removal of precancerous warts or clustered tumors.

If cancer is present, treatment can entail a **vulvectomy,** the surgical removal of the labia, clitoris, underlying glands in the groin, about half of the vagina, and several inches of skin on each side of the vulva. For very advanced cancer that has spread to other organs, extreme surgery known as **pelvic exenteration** may also be necessary. This procedure is the surgical removal of the uterus, fallopian tubes, ovaries, regional lymph nodes, part of the vagina, the bladder, and the rectum. The rectum and bladder are replaced by openings in the abdomen.

SEE biopsy; cancer; cancer, skin; chemotherapy; colposcopy; cryosurgery; radiation therapy.

For more information on vulvar cancer, contact:

American Cancer Society
1599 Clifton Rd., N.E.
Atlanta, GA 30329-4251
800-ACS-2345
404-320-3333
http://www.cancer.org

Society of Gynecologic Oncologists
401 N. Michigan Ave., Suite 2200
Chicago, IL 60611
312-644-6610
http://www.sgo.org

CHEMOTHERAPY

Chemotherapy is the use of certain chemicals to treat illness. While chemotherapy is most often connected with the treatment of cancer, the drugs (which include antibiotics) may also be used to treat a variety of other conditions. Depending on the type of cancer being treated, the drugs may be administered orally or through a vein.

Anticancer chemotherapy drugs work by traveling through the body's blood and lymph system and destroying cancerous cells and preventing their reproduction. Chemotherapy is called a **systemic** method of treatment, since the drugs travel throughout the body and are not isolated to one area. It is also used as an **adjuvant** therapy; that is, it is used to assist the primary means of treatment, such as surgery or radiation therapy.

Before surgery, chemotherapy may be used to reduce the size of the tumor. After surgery, it is used to prevent any remaining cancerous cells from thriving, even when it is thought that all of the affected tissue has been surgically removed. Chemotherapy is most effective on small tumors. The larger the tumor, the greater the number of cancerous cells and the greater the possibility that some of the cells will become resistant to the anticancer drugs.

A woman undergoing chemotherapy may receive the treatment in a hospital's outpatient service, a clinic, a practitioner's office, or even at home. Depending on a woman's health, she may need to stay in the hospital during treatment. In whatever setting, chemotherapy is administered in cycles: a treatment period followed by a recovery period, then another treatment period, and so on.

There are a number of different types, or classes, of anticancer drugs used in chemotherapy, each designed to destroy a certain type of cancer cell in a certain phase of its cycle. Because some cancers are made up of more than one kind of cell, a combination of drugs may be used. The dosage a practitioner prescribes is carefully chosen so the drugs kill only the cancerous cells, but some healthy cells are also affected. Any cell that is dividing, cancerous or not, is most vulnerable to being destroyed.

The side effects of chemotherapy depend on the woman's health, the type of anticancer drugs she receives, and the dosage. Anticancer drugs affect cells that divide rapidly, such as those in hair roots and the lining of the digestive tract. They may also affect healthy cells that fight off infection, help the blood to clot, and carry oxygen to all parts of the body.

SIDE EFFECTS OF CHEMOTHERAPY

Side effects of chemotherapy include:
- Hair loss
- Nausea and vomiting
- Mouth sores
- Reduced immunity to infection
- Anemia
- Lowered white blood cell count
- Bone marrow depression, a condition in which the bone marrow loses some or all of its ability to make red and white blood cells and platelets
- Changes in smell and taste
- Loss of appetite
- Feelings of tiredness
- Body aches
- Bloating and weight gain
- Night sweats

Chemotherapy may also cause chemically induced depression and mood swings, as well as irregular periods, or it may cause periods to stop altogether (known as medical or nonsurgical menopause).

Most women who undergo chemotherapy do not experience more than a few of the side effects. Most of the side effects, such as nausea and vomiting, disappear a day or so after each cycle of treatment. Other effects, such as hair loss, will disappear after the treatment has ended.

SEE cancer; radiation therapy; specific cancers.

For more information on chemotherapy, contact:

American Cancer Society
1559 Clifton Rd., N.E.
Atlanta, GA 30329-4251
800-ACS-2345
404-320-3333
http://www.cancer.org

ChemoCare
231 North Ave., W.
Westfield, NJ 07090-1428
800-55-CHEMO
908-233-1103 (New Jersey)

Chemotherapy Foundation
183 Madison Avenue, Suite 403
New York, NY 10016
212-213-9292

CHILDBIRTH— CHOOSING A PRACTITIONER

Women have many options in the choice of birth practitioners. Skilled obstetricians, family practitioners, and midwives are available in most areas of the country. One woman may prefer traditional hospital care from an obstetrician, another may favor the intimacy of being attended by a midwife at home or in a birth center. Practitioners may have different approaches to such issues as routine ultrasound, amniocentesis, surgical intervention, and drugs during delivery.

Before choosing a practitioner, a woman should consider the wide range of birthing options and decide which ones she prefers. With her birth plan in mind, a woman can approach a practitioner with similar practices and beliefs.

OBSTETRICIANS AND GYNECOLOGISTS

A majority of women choose a specialist called an obstetrician-gynecologist for their birth practitioner. Obstetricians deliver four out of every five babies born in the United States, making them the most popular choice for birth practitioners.

Obstetrician-gynecologists are licensed physicians who have completed an approved program of specialty training (called a residency) in the area of the female reproductive system and

MATERNAL AND FETAL MEDICINE

A subspecialist of obstetrics and gynecology who handles high-risk pregnancies is a **maternal and fetal medicine specialist,** also called a **perinatologist.** If a woman has complications during pregnancy or is dealing with a chronic condition such as diabetes or cystic fibrosis, her regular practitioner may recommend such a specialist.

Perinatologists are usually board-certified by the American Board of Obstetrics and Gynecology (ABOG) or the American Osteopathic Board of Obstetrics and Gynecology; however, physicians can call themselves specialists without certification. Credentials can be verified by contacting the ABOG at 214-871-1619 for an M.D., and the American Osteopathic Board of Obstetrics and Gynecology at 312-947-4630 for a D.O., a doctor of osteopathy.

associated disorders. The training includes all aspects of medical and surgical care. Residency programs run from three to seven years, after which graduates go on to take a national certifying examination, administered by the American Board of Obstetrics and Gynecology.

To verify the credentials of any obstetrician or gynecologist, call the American Board of Medical Specialties (ABMS) at 800-776-CERT. If the obstetrician is a doctor of osteopathy (D.O.), contact the American Osteopathic Board of Obstetrics and Gynecology at 312-947-4630.

The public library or local hospital library may have a copy of the *American Medical Directory: Physicians in the United States* or *The Official ABMS Directory of Board Certified Medical Specialists*, which lists physicians and their credentials.

FAMILY PRACTITIONERS

Though a primary-care physician may not come to mind as an option when choosing a birth practitioner, some women receive their prenatal and obstetrics care from a family practice specialist.

Family practice is concerned with the total health care of the individual and the family and is not limited to any age, gender, organ system, or disease entity. The board-certified family practitioner (F.P.) has three years of training following medical school, including a minimum of three months of obstetrics and gynecology. Because the F.P. can provide comprehensive care to the entire family, many pregnant women like the continuity of care this practitioner offers. Not every family practitioner has obstetrical experience; it is important to ask what proportion of the F.P.'s practice is obstetrics.

To verify the credentials of an M.D. board-certified in family practice, contact the ABMS at 800-776-CERT, or, for a D.O., the American Osteopathic Board of General Practice at 847-640-8477.

MIDWIVES

Prior to the 20th century and into the 1920s, women having babies were attended, usually in their own homes, by other women. These attendants, known as midwives, monitored the natural birth process and aided the woman during her delivery. The option of midwifery began to be overshadowed in the early 1900s as states, with the encouragement of the American Medical Association, began to redefine childbirth as a medical event that must be overseen by a licensed physician. By the 1960s, birth had been moved almost entirely out of the home setting and into the hospital.

Today, the midwife is still an option for women choosing a birth practitioner. While the hospital setting is comforting to some, more and more women with low-risk pregnancies are turning to midwives in an effort to avoid high costs and possibly unnecessary medical intervention. Experts say that midwife-attended births have fewer complications than similar hospital births. A 1994 study published in the *British Medical Journal* reported that in low-risk births attended by midwives, the woman was more likely to be able to move around, less likely to be intensively monitored, and less likely to receive a spinal or epidural anesthesia, and the fetus was less likely to experience distress.

There are two main categories of midwives: certified nurse-midwives, who have a background in obstetrics and nursing and are licensed in many states; and lay midwives (also called direct-entry midwives), who have practical rather than academic training. A third classification, certified professional-midwives, is currently being organized; these practitioners have formal education and training, but no nursing credentials.

FINDING A MIDWIFE: REGULATIONS, RESOURCES, AND RECOMMENDATIONS

In most states, nurse-midwives work under the supervision of a physician or facility; however, specific laws on what a certified nurse-midwife can and cannot do (such as breech presentation, multiple pregnancies, and forceps deliveries) vary from state to state. Contact your state's nurse licensing board for more information on state laws.

To find a certified nurse-midwife, call a university near you to see whether it has a nurse-midwifery program, or contact certified childbirth education programs. For the name of a certified nurse-midwife in your area, or for more information on nurse-midwives, contact:

American College of Nurse-Midwives
818 Connecticut Ave., N.W., Suite 900
Washington, DC 20006
202-728-9860
http://www.acnm.org

State laws concerning the legal status and practice of lay midwifery are diverse. All states specify that midwives confine their practice to low-risk, or "normal and uncomplicated," pregnancies, and some require at least one prenatal examination by a physician even though the woman is working with a lay midwife.

Legislation is in such a state of flux that it is hard to make any certain pronouncements. To find the current legal status of the practice of lay midwifery in your state, contact your state health department. If you do not get the information you need there, you can try your state nurse licensing board or medical licensing board, but remember that in a number of states lay midwifery is frowned upon.

It is important to verify the training and credentials of any birth practitioner you are considering, and the same holds true for lay midwives—especially since their training and experience vary—and also their backup physicians. If you choose a lay midwife because you both agree that your pregnancy seems "normal and uncomplicated," be sure to have a medical backup for any problems that do come up.

Don't forget to ask for recommendations from friends and family. Again, certified childbirth education programs may be able to refer you to midwives in your community. Follow up your research with plenty of questions. You will want to know:

■ How long has the midwife been practicing?

■ Is the midwife certified by the American College of Nurse-Midwives?

■ Will the midwife deliver the baby at a home, hospital, or birth center? What settings are available?

■ Does the midwife have a medical backup in case of complications?

■ How much does maternity care cost?

■ What method of childbirth preparation is preferred by the midwife? What options are available?

CERTIFIED NURSE-MIDWIVES

A **certified nurse-midwife** is a registered nurse who has completed at least one year of obstetric training in an approved graduate midwifery program, demonstrated clinical experience, and passed the national certification examination given by the American College of Nurse-Midwives (ACNM). Like all nurses, nurse-midwives must then obtain a license or permit to practice in the state where they intend to work. Maine is the only state that does not recognize or require current ACNM certification for licensure.

According to the ACNM, there are 4,000 ACNM-certified nurse-midwives practicing in the United States today. The National Center for Health Statistics reports that, in 1992, 185,000 births were attended by a certified nurse-midwife, accounting for 4.5 percent of all births in the United States. The majority of births (85 percent, according to the American College of Nurse-Midwives) attended by nurse-midwives occur in hospitals, 11 percent in birthing centers, and 4 percent in homes.

Nurse-midwives manage the maternity care of women whose progress through pregnancy and labor and delivery is normal and uncomplicated. They provide postpartum care to both the mother and the newborn baby and can practice in a hospital setting, birthing center, or home. The certified nurse-midwife is trained to recognize the signs of an abnormal situation in either pregnancy or childbirth and to refer to a specialist, when necessary. If a serious complication occurs during labor, the woman is transported to a nearby hospital for care, or an on-call physician is brought in.

For many pregnant women, the enormous appeal of nurse-midwifery lies not only in its noninterventional approach to childbirth but also in its affirmation of psychological as well as medical support of the woman. Nurse-midwifery is an important alternative for women who have low-risk pregnancies.

LAY MIDWIVES

While few women use the services of lay midwives, they are an option for women seeking a birth practitioner. Unlike the nurse-midwife, the **lay midwife** is not a licensed nurse, does not have formal training in obstetrics, and practices in a home setting. In most cases, she has learned by doing; she has attended births, usually first as an apprentice to more experienced midwives, then as the primary birth attendant. Lay midwives are sometimes called empirical midwives because they acquire their skills through observation and experience. However, today, many lay midwives have adopted the more professional-sounding term "direct-entry midwife."

CERTIFIED PROFESSIONAL-MIDWIVES

Practitioners across the country have recently begun to organize in an attempt to create national standards of education and competency for practicing midwives who are not registered nurses. At this time there are no certification programs for lay or direct-entry midwives; however, there are several in development.

These programs would include formal academic training as well as apprenticeships and would culminate in a national examination. A graduate of such a course of study would be known as a **certified professional-midwife**.

Once they are developed, certified professional programs would be rated by outside

QUESTIONS TO HELP YOU CHOOSE YOUR BIRTH PRACTITIONER

To find out more about the attitudes of a practitioner, and the options available, a woman should ask:

■ How long have you been in practice? What are your credentials?

■ What is the cost of maternity care? Are there any payment plans available?

■ Will my insurance coverage be accepted?

■ Will the same practitioner who provided my prenatal care attend the birth? (This is especially important in a group practice where you may not have met all the practitioners in the group.)

■ What method of childbirth preparation do you prefer?

■ What prenatal tests/procedures do you recommend?

■ Do you encourage or allow the partner's presence, both in prenatal visits and during labor and birth? What about during a cesarean section?

■ Do you encourage or allow siblings to visit the baby in the setting where you practice?

■ Do you encourage breast-feeding? Do you allow the woman to breast-feed immediately following birth, while she's still in the delivery room (assuming both woman and baby are healthy)?

■ What is your cesarean-section rate? What indications or criteria do you follow?

What is your position on vaginal birth after a cesarean?

■ In what percentage of your patients do you induce labor? Are episiotomies routine in your practice? What about forceps delivery or vacuum extraction—what percentage of the births in your practice?

■ Do you routinely use drugs—analgesic or anesthetic—in the management of pain and labor? If so, what are the most common ones?

■ Do you encourage women to try different birthing positions? What options are available?

■ Is electronic fetal heart-rate monitoring a routine procedure in childbirths you attend?

To ensure your wishes are followed, the practitioner can be asked to sign a written agreement called a **birth plan.** This checklist of preferences and instructions really works best as a reminder to the practitioner of the important care issues discussed and treatment options agreed upon *long before* the labor and delivery, not the best time to be making important decisions. Ask the practitioner to keep a copy of the birth plan in your medical record at the office and send a copy to the hospital or birthing center where you expect to deliver. Take your copy with you when you go to the hospital.

organizations. The American College of Nurse-Midwives already has accreditation standards in place for evaluation of these upcoming pro-grams. Another organization, the Midwives Alliance of North America, is also working toward that goal.

SEE board certification; childbirth interventions; childbirth—methods and options; childbirth settings; practitioners, how to choose.

For more information on choosing a birth practitioner, contact:

American Board of Obstetrics and Gynecology
2915 Vine St.
Dallas, TX 75204
214-871-1619

American College of Nurse-Midwives
818 Connecticut Ave., N.W., Suite 900
Washington, DC 20006
202-728-9860
http://www.acnm.org

American Osteopathic Board of Obstetrics and Gynecology
5200 S. Ellis Ave.
Chicago, IL 60615
312-947-4630

Midwives Alliance of North America
P.O. Box 175
Newton, KS 67114

CHILDBIRTH INTERVENTIONS

While it is commonly believed that 90 percent of all women are capable of giving birth without medical assistance, there are several procedures commonly used by birth practitioners to monitor complications that may arise and to intervene when necessary. These medical interventions should be used for a sound medical reason, not merely for the sake of convenience. The woman and her practitioner should discuss the necessity, risks, and benefits of each procedure before the woman's due date.

ELECTRONIC FETAL MONITORING (EFM)

An electronic fetal monitor is an instrument that measures uterine contractions and fetal heart rate during labor. It is used to monitor how the fetus is tolerating labor and should alert the practitioner to signs of fetal distress. There are two ways to do this—externally and internally.

The external monitor, which generally uses a sensitive microphone to pick up the heartbeat, has wide straps or belts that go around the woman's abdomen. With an internal fetal heart-rate monitor, an electrode is attached to the fetus's presenting part, usually the scalp. The readings from the internal monitor are considered more accurate than the external device.

Reserved for high-risk pregnancies when first introduced, EFM is a widespread practice today, with approximately three-quarters of births electronically monitored. However, it has been shown that EFM is not necessary when dealing with low-risk pregnancy. Studies have shown that routine electronic fetal monitoring can lead to more cesarean-section deliveries, but not necessarily healthier babies. Studies have also found no benefit from EFM when compared with careful, periodic monitoring using a specialized stethoscope called a fetoscope or using ultrasound, a procedure that creates an image of the fetus using sound waves.

The American College of Obstetricians and Gynecologists (ACOG) recommends that women with high-risk pregnancies (including premature deliveries) have either continuous electronic fetal monitoring or intermittent checks with a stethoscope every 15 minutes early on and then every five minutes later. For normal pregnancies, the group recommends only periodic monitoring (every 30 minutes early on and every 15 minutes in later stages) by auscultation (listening with a stethoscope).

INDUCTION AND AUGMENTATION OF LABOR

Induction is the stimulation of labor before it begins spontaneously or naturally. Augmentation is used to further a labor that has slowed or stopped—usually with the use of drugs. The procedures should be used for medical reasons, not matters of convenience, because of possible risks to the woman and the fetus. Induction may be used when it is hazardous for the pregnancy to continue to term, such as in the event of maternal high blood pressure or kidney disease; preeclampsia, a toxic condition characterized by high blood pressure, edema, and protein in the urine; maternal diabetes; and Rh disease or isoimmunization (a blood incompatibility).

Although not necessarily a risk factor, postmaturity (a prolonged pregnancy) is another common reason given for induction, because of its association with placental insufficiency. In other words, labor is induced because the placenta has a limited life span and may not be able to sustain the fetus properly in an overly long pregnancy.

AUGMENTATION OF LABOR

Labor can be augmented or induced by intravenous administration of Pitocin, a synthetic version of the natural hormone **oxytocin.** Oxytocin is given intravenously, in gradually increasing doses, every 20 to 40 minutes. Continuous fetal monitoring should be employed to gauge the strength, duration, and frequency of the uterine contractions and the fetal response to labor (indicated by the fetal heart rate). Overstimulation of labor can produce harmful effects for both the fetus and the woman. Rapid contractions can decrease the ability of the fetus to get enough oxygen, and too much oxytocin can produce uterine rupture.

Oxytocin should only be used when there is no physical obstruction to vaginal delivery and when the fetus is healthy and positioned correctly in the womb. A woman should ask her provider to explain why oxytocin is necessary if it is recommended.

AMNIOTOMY

Amniotomy is the deliberate breaking of the **amniotic membranes,** or bag of waters, surrounding the fetus. It may be done to induce or start labor, to speed up labor already in progress, or to look for signs of fetal distress. The procedure is done by guiding an amniohook or other surgical instrument into the mouth of the cervix, then piercing the amniotic membranes to allow the fluid to escape.

After the procedure, labor usually starts within 12 hours; the faster the cervix dilates and softens, the more quickly labor will occur. If labor does not begin within 24 hours, it can be induced using drugs. One study by Roberto Caldeyro-Barcia, M.D., an expert in the effects of amniotomy, found that, at most, amniotomy cuts 30 to 40 minutes off labor, if any at all. Amniotomy also increases the woman's chance of infection during and after birth.

Certain conditions or problems may mandate artificial rupturing. For instance, the practitioner who suspects fetal distress may rupture the membranes to see if the amniotic fluid contains a greenish brown fluid indicating the presence of meconium (a fetal bowel movement), a sign of possible fetal distress. A practitioner may also rupture the membranes in order to begin internal electronic fetal monitoring if a suspicious fetal heart rate shows signs of fetal distress.

ANALGESICS AND ANESTHETICS

Pain relief for the woman is the prevailing reason for giving drugs during hospital birth. For the fetus, the drugs may mean depression of the central nervous system. At birth, antidotes to narcotics may be required for the newborn. For the woman, drugs may slow or prolong labor and blunt the experience of childbirth. However, if a woman is unable to tolerate her childbirth because of pain, medication may be helpful.

Drugs should be administered in the smallest dosage possible. A practitioner should explain well in advance of delivery the risks and effects of each drug that may be used.

Most commonly, the narcotic **meperidine** (Demerol) is the pain reliever used during childbirth to relax the woman and ease pain. Though it causes less vomiting and nausea for the woman than morphine, meperidine can slow or prolong labor or stop it entirely. Meperidine also depresses breathing, of both the woman and the fetus, and respiratory equipment may be necessary for the newborn. Naloxone hydrochloride (Narcan), a drug that counteracts the effects of narcotics, may be administered to the newborn to reverse respiratory depression.

Butorphanol (Stadol) is also used during childbirth. It is reported to depress breathing to a lesser degree than some other drugs. **Alphaprodine** and **nalbuphine** (Nubain) are two other narcotics commonly used for pain relief during labor.

Tranquilizers and **barbiturates** may also be used. The commonly used tranquilizer diazepam (Valium) is not recommended during labor because it may cause depression, feeding problems, and other problems in the newborn. Barbiturates enhance the sedative effect of narcotics and may be used as the cervix dilates during the first stage of labor.

The use of **local anesthesia** entails numbing medication injected into specific tissue. Two forms of it are **pudendal block,** usually given at the end of labor, which anesthetizes the vulva (external female organs), vagina, and muscles of the pelvic floor; and **paracervical block,** which anesthetizes the lower uterus, cervix, and upper vagina, but which is being used less and less because the site of injection is too close to the placenta. It may also be injected into the perineal tissue (the area between the vagina and the anus) to numb this region.

Regional anesthesia, in the obstetric context, causes loss of sensation in the lower half of the body. Probably the most widely used form is the **lumbar epidural,** also known as *continuous* regional anesthesia because the anesthetic can be continuously readministered during labor and delivery. Through a tiny catheter placed in the back, the medication is administered by injection into a hollow space in the spine. Some of the advantages are that it deadens pain without dulling mental faculties and only partially affects motor function; however, the woman may need more coaching on when to push, since she cannot feel the contractions as well.

Another kind of regional anesthetic, a type of spinal anesthetic called a **saddle block,** is injected directly into the spinal cord. The injection anesthetizes the area from the midabdomen to the toes and necessitates the use of forceps or vacuum extraction (a procedure where gentle suction is used) to deliver the baby.

A woman should discuss the risks and benefits of any type of anesthetic with her practitioner or anesthesiologist. Too much medication, or the use of drugs before active labor begins, may slow labor and increase the woman's risk of cesarean section. However, severe pain, particularly with prolonged labor, may also exhaust a woman, making it more difficult for her to push during the second stage of labor, which could also lead to a cesarean section. Again, it is important that you and your practitioner have a thorough discussion on the use of anesthetics prior to labor and delivery, and it should be an important part of the birth plan.

FORCEPS AND VACUUM EXTRACTOR

Obstetric **forceps** are metal blades used to grasp the sides of the fetus's head and help guide the fetus through the birth canal in difficult deliveries. In general, forceps are employed when anesthesia or the position of the fetus prevents the woman from pushing it out herself, when there is severe fetal distress, or when certain maternal conditions necessitate shortened labor and delivery.

Forceps should not be used in uncomplicated deliveries, when there is no medical need to hurry the delivery. Even with a skilled practitioner, the procedure is not without dangers to the woman—including lacerations, hemorrhage, and infection—and it may prompt the use of painkilling drugs and an episiotomy. Some of the risks for the fetus are hemorrhage and damage to the head and/or brain, nerve damage, and bruising.

Forceps deliveries are classified as low, mid, and high, according to how close the baby's head is to the opening of the pelvis. The majority of forceps deliveries are low. Mid-forceps deliveries are more difficult and are believed to carry potentially serious problems and pose greater dangers to the woman and fetus than low forceps. A high forceps delivery is considered too risky to be done except as an occasional last resort to deliver a fetus rapidly.

Another instrument for assisting delivery is the **vacuum extractor.** Considered less risky than forceps, vacuum extraction involves a small suction cup, which is placed on the fetus's head, and the creation of a vacuum to gently bring the fetus down through the birth canal.

EPISIOTOMY

An episiotomy is an incision made in a woman's perineal tissue—tissue that extends from the vagina to the anus—to enlarge the opening for birth, following which the incision is sewn up. It is done to aid the delivery, reduce compression of the baby's head (from battering against

✔ AVOIDING CESAREAN SECTION

Cesarean section is the most common major operation performed on American women. According to a 1993 Centers for Disease Control and Prevention National Hospital Discharge Survey, 22.8 percent of deliveries were by cesarean. Many groups, including the Centers for Disease Control and Prevention (CDC), consider this rate to be much too high, an indicator that the procedure may be being performed more often than needed.

In many cases, a cesarean section may be necessary or preferable to a trial of labor. However, if you have decided that you wish to deliver vaginally, the following questions may help you choose a practitioner who is willing to save the cesarean as a last resort:

■ Ask your practitioner what his or her C-section rate is, as well as the hospital's. The CDC considers 15 percent the desired rate.

■ Ask what the practitioner's definition of and indications for **dystocia** ("abnormal labor") are. Dystocia, a leading reason for cesareans, has been called a catchall term. Get a good sense of what your practitioner means by "abnormal labor," and if he or she says "failure to progress," find out what the reasoning is.

■ Ask, in the event of dystocia, what methods your practitioner would be willing to try as alternatives to a cesarean. A willingness to allow you to try different birth positions, walk around, rest or sleep, or just wait shows a supportive provider with your interests in mind.

■ Ask what your practitioner's training and experience are in vaginal breech deliveries, vaginal births after previous cesareans, premature rupture of membranes, and large-baby and multiple births.

■ Ask whether your practitioner will accept a flat fee for delivery, regardless of whether it is vaginal or cesarean. Some professionals do have procedure-neutral fees for deliveries. That way, the economic incentive to perform a cesarean is eliminated.

the perineum, the wall that separates the vagina from the rectum), and prevent tearing of the tissue, specifically tears to the anal sphincter and through the rectum.

Proponents of episiotomy believe that a surgical cut is preferable to a jagged tear and that episiotomy prevents excessive stretching of the perineum and subsequent enlargement of the vagina and loss of muscle tone.

Critics of the procedure, however, say the benefits are debatable, except in certain cases of fetal distress, and that episiotomy increases postpartum pain and discomfort. In addition,

episiotomy can cause numbness where muscles and nerves were cut, increase the risk of postpartum infections, and expose the fetus to the dangers of the anesthetic used in the procedure.

Furthermore, some experts point out that the lithotomy position for birth, where the woman lies flat on her back with her knees bent and feet in stirrups, creates a tension in the perineum that may cause tears or lead to episiotomy. The perineal tissue normally stretches at the vaginal opening to allow the fetus's head to come out, and is resilient.

Some believe that employing midwifery techniques reduces the need for an episiotomy. These techniques include changing the traditional hospital birth position to an upright, sitting, or squatting one; massaging the perineal tissue with oils and wet compresses; helping the delivering woman relax with breathing and other techniques; and coaching properly so that the fetus can be eased out without damage to either the woman or the baby.

VBAC: VAGINAL BIRTH AFTER CESAREAN

Practitioners used to believe that if a cesarean section was performed, all future deliveries must be done by cesarean to avoid rupturing previous scars. However, the American College of Obstetricians and Gynecologists (ACOG) now recommends vaginal birth after cesarean in most circumstances, as improved methods of cesarean incisions have reduced the risk of rupture during subsequent labor.

Be sure to find a practitioner who advocates VBAC. Much of the nation's high cesarean section rate can be attributed to the long-standing practice of automatically delivering by cesarean if the woman has previously delivered a child that way. Even though ACOG issued strong guidelines some years back stating that repeat cesarean deliveries should no longer be routine, some physicians have been slow in their movement away from the "Once a cesarean, always a cesarean" dictum.

ACOG estimates that between 50 and 80 percent of women who have low transverse uterine incisions can deliver vaginally unless specific complications arise. But the group's guidelines still recommend against vaginal birth for women with the classical uterine incision, an incision rarely used these days. If there are complications during a trial of labor and a cesarean becomes necessary, ACOG guidelines call for hospitals to be able to perform the operation within 30 minutes.

If you wish to have a vaginal birth after a previous cesarean delivery, you can do a number of things to ensure that you get a trial of labor. First off, don't wait for your practitioner to recommend it. Long before your delivery day, make sure your health-care provider is up-to-date on the most current recommendations by the American College of Obstetricians and Gynecologists—which encourages efforts to lower the overall cesarean rate and attempt labor and VBAC. And take advantage of groups providing support and information about VBAC, two of the more prominent of which are:

Cesarean/Support, Education and Concern, Inc. (C/SEC, Inc.)
22 Forest Rd.
Framingham, MA 01701
508-877-8266

International Childbirth Education Association, Inc.
P.O. Box 20048
Minneapolis, MN 55420
612-854-8660
http://www.icea.org

CESAREAN SECTION

A cesarean section is a major surgical operation in which the practitioner makes an incision into the abdomen and uterus to remove the fetus when it cannot be delivered vaginally. This may occur if the fetus is not in a head-down position or if there are other complications. Most commonly, a **low transverse uterine incision** (across the lower part of the uterus) is made. Less commonly, a **classical incision** (an incision made vertically into the body of the uterus) is made. The low transverse uterine incision means less blood loss, less postoperative infection, and easier repair, but its use depends on the fetus's size and position. The classical section allows the practitioner more freedom in the abdominal area and is generally only used for premature or malpositioned fetuses.

Traditionally, cesarean section has been considered necessary and safer than vaginal birth in a number of high-risk situations, including:

■ Multiple birth (twins, triplets, etc.), in which the first baby is not positioned head-first

■ Delivery of an infant that is too large to pass through the woman's pelvis

■ *Abruptio placentae,* separation of the placenta from the uterine wall. This condition may cause severe bleeding and may necessitate a quick delivery.

■ *Placenta previa,* extension of the placenta over the opening of the cervix, preventing the birth of the fetus. Like *abruptio placentae,* this condition may cause life-threatening bleeding and necessitates a quick delivery.

■ Prolapse of the umbilical cord (delivery of the cord before the rest of the fetus or alongside it)

■ Breech or transverse presentation. Rather than the usual head-first presentation, the fetus presents bottom-first ("frank breech") or feet-first ("footling breech"), or lies sideways in the uterus.

■ Fetal distress, as indicated by fetal monitoring, of prolonged, accelerated heart rate, a slowed heart rate, or sudden, rapid slowing of heart rate

SEE childbirth—choosing a practitioner; childbirth—labor and delivery; childbirth—methods and options; childbirth settings; pregnancy—prenatal concerns.

CHILDBIRTH—
LABOR AND DELIVERY

Labor is the process of giving birth to a baby, with the actual birth called the delivery. Labor—also known as accouchement, childbirth, confinement, or parturition—usually begins spontaneously at the end of gestation, the period of fetal development that on average lasts 40 weeks. At this time, the fetus is mature enough to survive on its own outside the uterus.

SIGNS OF LABOR

In the days or weeks before it begins, the woman may experience several signs that labor may start soon. These signs include:

■ A sudden burst of energy or inability to sleep

■ More frequent contractions. These irregular contractions usually consist of a dull ache or pressure in the lower back.

■ Feelings of pressure, dropping, or movement on the upper abdomen, which occur as the fetus moves into the birth position in the pelvis. The movement is called **lightening** because it becomes easier for the woman to breathe; however, it may cause increased pressure on the bladder.

■ Expulsion of the **mucous plug**, the barrier of the cervix that protects the fetus from infection. When this occurs, the vaginal discharge becomes thicker and tinged with blood and is known as the **show,** or **bloody show.**

■ The breaking of the protective **amniotic membranes,** or bag of waters, that surrounds the fetus. About two pints of watery fluid leak from the vagina. For most women, the water does not break until labor begins, but in 20 percent it occurs before labor begins. If the water breaks before labor, a woman should contact her practitioner for instructions as soon as possible,

FALSE AND TRUE LABOR

Many women experience **Braxton-Hicks contractions,** or false labor, during their pregnancies, most commonly as they approach their due dates. False labor differs from actual labor because the contractions of the uterine muscles are mild and intermittent, do not increase in intensity as they progress, and do not dilate the cervix.

True contractions are strong, occur at regular intervals, and become increasingly more intense and frequent. A woman experiencing contractions should monitor them to be sure they are growing in intensity and are occurring at regular intervals. Ask your practitioner beforehand how far apart the contractions should be before he or she is contacted, and when you should go to the hospital or birth center for labor and delivery.

PRETERM LABOR

Labor is considered preterm when it begins before week 37 of pregnancy. According to the American College of Obstetricians and Gynecologists, preterm deliveries represent 8 to 10 percent of births in the United States, but more than 60 percent of the perinatal complications and death.

The factors associated with the risk of preterm labor include:

■ Prior preterm delivery

■ Multiple gestation (twins, triplets, etc.)

■ Three or more first-trimester abortions or a single second-trimester abortion

■ Cervical incompetence (a weakened cervix)

■ Maternal conditions such as infections, bleeding, *abruptio placentae* (a condition in which the placenta separates from the wall of the uterus), congenital abnormalities of the uterus, and heavy smoking

■ Lack of prenatal care or poor prenatal care

■ Use of drugs and alcohol by the woman

If you are at risk for preterm delivery, there are steps you can take to prevent the premature birth of your baby. You should have proper prenatal care and avoid smoking and drinking during pregnancy. While most women may continue working, some may be asked to refrain from heavy lifting, strenuous tasks, and some exercises. Ask your practitioner about what activities (including sexual activities) you should avoid. Various levels of bed rest may be prescribed for women with previous preterm labor and birth. Some women may engage in limited activity, while others must stay in bed all of the time.

Your practitioner should be contacted immediately if you are at risk of preterm labor and any of the following symptoms occur:

■ Regular uterine contractions, with or without pain, continuing for one hour

■ Dull, lower back ache, pressure, or pain

---

since the fetus is no longer protected by the sac. If labor does not begin within 24 hours, labor may be induced using the drug oxytocin, which causes uterine contractions.

There may also be some emotional changes as the time of birth approaches. A woman nearing delivery may become more anxious, thinking of the changes and uncertainties the new baby may bring. Some women become very active, working to prepare the home for the arrival of the child. Insomnia and increased anxiety are normal during late pregnancy.

FIRST STAGE

The first stage of labor begins when the first regular, timable uterine contractions occur, and ends with full dilation of the cervix. It lasts, on average, 12 hours for the delivery of the woman's first baby. The contractions consist of a shortening of the muscles of the uterus.

Throughout the pregnancy, changes in hormones have caused the cervix to **efface,** or soften or thin out. This is also known as the **ripening** of the cervix. During the first stage,

■ Intermittent lower abdominal or thigh pain

■ Intestinal cramping

■ Rupture of amniotic membrane (breaking of the waters)

■ A change in vaginal discharge

If preterm labor does occur, it may be stopped or suppressed with drugs until the fetus is ready to be born. In some cases, the labor may be too advanced, or it may be safer to deliver the baby prematurely than to allow the pregnancy to continue. Premature babies are more often born via cesarean sections, especially if they are in a breech presentation.

If the baby is too small and fragile, it may be cared for in a neonatal intensive-care unit (NICU) until it is able to survive on its own. Premature babies usually have a low birth weight and may have organs—such as the lungs—that have not developed fully. A premature baby may be put on a respirator to aid breathing or may be fed through a tube if there are problems swallowing. A low-birth-weight baby may also have trouble maintaining body temperature. Very premature, low-birth-weight babies should be delivered and cared for at hospitals experienced in such care, if possible. Such babies have increased risk for some conditions, such as cerebral palsy and conditions associated with birth trauma.

The following table details the chances of survival according to the age and weight of a premature baby. The lower the chances of survival, the more likely it is that the fetus will suffer brain damage or other complications.

Gestational Age (*weeks*)	% Chance of Survival
23	0–8
24	15–20
25	50–60
26–28	85
29	90 or greater

the contractions of the uterus and the pressure of the head of the fetus cause the softened cervix to continue to efface and to widen, or **dilate.** Full dilation is about ten centimeters, or four inches.

Labor may also be induced in order to begin labor or to speed delivery. It may be induced when the woman suffers high blood pressure, kidney disease, preeclampsia (a serious condition marked by development of high blood pressure, edema, and protein in the urine during pregnancy), or prolonged pregnancy (postmaturity), which endangers the health of the fetus. Postmaturity is a common reason for induced labor; it is done because the placenta, which nourishes the fetus, has a limited life span and may not sustain the fetus until labor begins naturally.

Labor is most often induced by rupturing the amniotic sac, which sometimes prompts labor. Labor can also be augmented by administering a drug, usually the hormone oxytocin (Pitocin), which increases the intensity of the contractions.

SECOND STAGE

The second stage of labor begins with a full dilation of the cervix and ends with delivery, the expulsion of the fetus. This stage lasts on average two hours (although it may be longer) for a first baby and generally is less with subsequent babies. In a normal delivery, the fetus is pushed downward by the uterine muscles, which are aided by the abdominal muscles and the diaphragm. While pressure from above expels the fetus, the pelvic floor muscles cause the fetus's head to rotate and extend, allowing for its passage by molding and directing the head. The head delivers slowly, while the body and legs follow quickly. If the amniotic membranes have not yet ruptured, they will during this stage.

TYPES OF PRESENTATION

In a common, or head-first (also called cephalic), delivery, the fetus's head distends the vagina and vulva, eventually appearing at the vaginal opening. This appearance is called **crowning.**

Any other type of presentation of the fetus is called an **abnormal presentation.** This includes **breech presentation,** where the feet or the buttocks are the first to arrive and are followed by the trunk, shoulders, and head. When the feet are extended straight up along the body, the position is known as a **frank breech presentation.** A breech birth may slow the flow of oxygen to the fetus by compressing the umbilical cord between the body of the fetus and the wall of the vagina. Because the body of the fetus does not widen the cervix as the head would have, the delivery may become difficult. In many cases a breech presentation

can be delivered vaginally if the practitioner is experienced in the technique and believes the woman to be a good candidate. A woman should discuss this option with the practitioner before labor begins.

Other abnormal presentations are:

■ Brow presentation, when the forehead leads the descent into the vagina

■ Face presentation, when the face leads

■ Shoulder, or transverse, presentation, when one of the fetus's shoulders leads; this occurs when the fetus is in a sideways position.

■ Posterior presentation, when the fetus descends head-first, but with the face toward the woman's abdomen rather than her back

If the fetus cannot be delivered naturally, the practitioner may perform an emergency **cesarean section,** in which the fetus is surgically removed from the uterus through the abdomen.

THIRD STAGE

In the third stage of labor, the **placenta,** or **afterbirth,** which provided the fetus with nourishment during the pregnancy, is separated from the uterine wall and expelled. The uterus shrinks after the baby is born, putting pressure on the placenta until it separates from the uterine wall and is expelled. Remaining amniotic membranes are also expelled by uterine contractions. This stage usually takes about five minutes.

Labor tends to be faster in women who have given birth previously because the cervix supplies less resistance after it has been dilated once, and the pelvic floor is more relaxed. Labor also occurs more quickly when the amniotic sac ruptures before labor has begun.

AFTER DELIVERY

Fatigue is a common symptom after delivery. After labor has ended, a woman should try to get as much rest as possible, then return to normal activity gradually over the course of a few weeks. Pain associated with an episiotomy generally subsides within five days, and analgesics may be used to relieve discomfort. Women who are breast-feeding should ask their practitioners about the safety of taking pain relievers.

During this period, the uterus begins to return to its normal size, and cramps are common during the first week following delivery. The uterus returns to normal more quickly in women who breast-feed. Some women may feel mildly depressed after delivery, a common condition known as the baby blues. If depression worsens or does not disappear within two weeks, a practitioner should be contacted. (See "Depression" for more information on the baby blues and postpartum depression.)

Vaginal intercourse should be avoided for six weeks after delivery to prevent infection and allow the vagina to heal. Some discomfort during intercourse is normal after delivery. Kegel exercises, which involve tightening the muscles that control the flow of urine, can help to strengthen and tone the vagina after childbirth (see page 228).

SEE childbirth interventions; childbirth—methods and options; childbirth settings; depression; miscarriage.

CHILDBIRTH—
METHODS AND OPTIONS

There are many different ways for a pregnant woman to prepare for labor and delivery. Prepared childbirth is a system of preparation that fully educates women on the birthing process in order to reduce pain with minimal use of drugs or other interventions. These systems are designed to ease the pain and tension of labor by educating the woman about what to expect during childbirth. In addition, a woman may be taught breathing and relaxation techniques, and other exercises, which she can use to actively participate in the childbirth process.

These methods were once known as natural childbirth; however, the term took on a negative connotation and was thought of as primitive and full of suffering. As a result, "prepared childbirth" is used today to describe these systems.

In addition to the childbirth method, the woman also has options in birth position and other aspects of the birth.

CHILDBIRTH METHODS

Dick-Read method. Pioneering the earliest theories of natural childbirth was a British physician named Grantly Dick-Read. His work in the 1930s led him to conclude that women are culturally conditioned to fear childbirth; this fear in turn creates a tension, which then produces pain, thus causing even more tension and pain.

With the Dick-Read method, education and knowledge, in combination with physical awareness, breathing control, and relaxation techniques, help to eliminate fear and enable most women to deliver comfortably without anesthesia. This birthing method avoids medications and medical intervention as much as possible. This method also involves visualization techniques, where the woman pictures in her mind the internal stages of birth. Dick-Read was the first physician to encourage men to go into the delivery room and act as birth partners. It is taught by the Read Natural Childbirth Foundation.

Bradley method. In the Bradley method, or partner-coached childbirth, the partner provides the woman with support with his or her presence, encouragement, and coaching. The Bradley method of childbirth involves mimicking the six conditions found in the animal world that a woman requires to give birth naturally in the hospital: darkness and solitude; quiet; physical comfort; physical relaxation; controlled breathing; and closed eyes and the appearance of sleep. This method is taught and used early in pregnancy. It emphasizes good nutrition, is completely medication-free, and uses relax-

CHOOSING A CHILDBIRTH METHOD

Women should discuss prepared childbirth options with their practitioners. The method of childbirth preparation preferred by the practitioner should be known in advance. Some practitioners may disapprove of a nontraditional birth position. There are several steps that women should take when deciding what sort of birth to have:

■ Decide on delivery type. Women should choose the method and labor position that will prepare them specifically for the type of childbirth experience they want to have. Some may want to avoid any pain-relief medication and thus should look for a program that advocates the use of medication only as a last resort. Different educational classes should be examined beyond their name; many actually combine approaches or use a term (such as Lamaze) only for its name recognition.

■ Be flexible in your approach to birth positions. Shifting positions and experimenting during childbirth may speed labor, though some women may labor better in the same position.

■ Gather information. The childbirth course itself should be examined. The factors that women need to address when choosing a class include whether a strongly couple-oriented program or a woman-centered approach is desired; whether they want to begin childbirth education classes earlier or later in pregnancy; and whether they want hospital-sponsored or private

ation techniques for all of the body's muscle groups, normal diaphragmatic breathing, and different birthing positions.

Lamaze method. The Lamaze method of childbirth teaches women the physiology of childbirth and exercises to be used during labor, including different types of breathing for the various stages of labor. This method works on the theory of conditioned reflexes; feelings of pain are blocked, because contractions serve as the stimulus to relax certain muscles through the use of particular breathing techniques.

This method is also called psychoprophylaxis because of the psychological prevention of pain through controlled breathing and concentration on specific distracting stimuli (for example, staring at a focal point, or "spot") to block sensations of pain. It also encourages the idea of labor support or coaching. While the method advocates unmedicated hospital childbirth, the use of drugs is not forbidden in the practice of Lamaze in this country.

LeBoyer Method. The LeBoyer method, which is also called birth without violence or gentle birth, aims at reducing the trauma of birth for the baby. This method was developed in the 1970s by French obstetrician Frederick LeBoyer. The highlights of the LeBoyer method are:

■ Delivery is in a darkened, quiet room. The fetus is delivered with as little intervention, such as pulling, as possible.

■ Immediately after birth, the baby is placed on the woman's abdomen and massaged. LeBoyer advised this procedure to encourage bonding between the woman and her newborn baby.

classes. Early-pregnancy classes focus on the ongoing physical and emotional changes being experienced rather than covering only labor and delivery, as late-pregnancy classes do.

■ Know your options. Both hospital-sponsored and private classes are available. Practitioners usually recommend the course given by the hospital where the delivery will be, or they may have a childbirth educator in the office. Hospital courses are often larger and may limit women's options by focusing on that particular hospital's routine and regulations. Advantages are that hospital classes may be conducted by obstetric nurses, and women are able to familiarize themselves with the surroundings in which they will deliver. Private classes tend to be more informal than hospital classes.

Usually, the woman's partner serves as her assistant during childbirth classes and throughout the actual delivery. If her partner does not attend, the woman may choose to have someone else, such as a friend or relative, be her partner and act as a support throughout the pregnancy as well as during labor and delivery.

In order to get complete, accurate information about a program, women should ask for a syllabus or copies of the materials used in the class. They may also request to sit in on one of the sessions. Cost information and methods of payment should be secured as well.

■ The partner then washes the infant in warm water, to mimic its previous environment of amniotic fluid.

■ Finally, the baby is dried and wrapped.

BIRTHING POSITIONS

Women have several options in birthing positions to choose from. The most common position during labor is the **lithotomy position,** a horizontal position in which the woman lies flat on a birthing bed with her legs apart and her feet set in stirrups. The lithotomy position has become the standard position for childbirth. It allows the practitioner full access to the woman's genital area and the coming fetus, and fetal monitors and other equipment are easily connected.

However, some experts believe the lithotomy position prolongs labor, thus making more pain-killing drugs and labor-augmenting drugs necessary. It may also interfere with blood circulation and cause a drop in blood pressure that could lower oxygen supply to the baby. Some women feel the position creates a sense of helplessness and infirmity during the childbirth process.

Critics of this position also contend that the lithotomy position requires the woman to work against the natural force of gravity. They also point out that the IV apparatus and the fetal monitor constrict movement and restrict experimentation with different birth positions. The horizontal position is also believed to be easier for the birth attendant—no bending down or squatting—than it is for the laboring woman.

Research has found that an **upright position** actually reduces the length of labor by more than an hour and reduces maternal trauma, such as vaginal tears, during delivery. Surveys have indicated that during labor most women would prefer to stand, sit, or walk.

A woman can give birth in a variety of positions: squatting, sitting, on her side, or kneeling. Some recommend birthing under water, a method supporters say is useful in restarting stalled labor. Should a woman be interested in an alternative position, she should discuss it with her practitioner as soon as possible. The squatting method, for example, requires special training, since a great deal of strength and experience is needed to maintain it without support. Midwives and birth centers are more likely to promote the use of different birthing positions than are obstetricians and hospitals.

CHILDBIRTH AIDS

An aid to the squatting method is the **birth cushion.** Developed in Britain, it is a U-shaped foam plastic cushion that supports the woman's thighs and has handles on both sides to help her push out the baby. Some British practitioners say that it reduces the need for forceps deliveries and cuts time spent in the second stage of labor, which begins when the cervix is fully dilated and ends with the birth of the baby.

Birthing stools are backless seats that allow the mother to be in a sitting position during labor and delivery. In this position, the pelvis is shortened and widened, and gravity helps to expel the baby. It is useful in preventing back labor, the pain felt in the lower back during labor, and is especially effective close to the time of delivery. **Birthing chairs,** which allow the woman to sit upright or recline, are also available.

SEE childbirth—choosing a practitioner; childbirth interventions; childbirth—labor and delivery; childbirth settings.

For more information about childbirth methods, contact:

American Society for Psychoprophylaxis in Obstetrics/Lamaze
1200 19th St., N.W., Suite 300
Washington, DC 20036
800-368-4404
202-857-1128
http://www.lamaze-childbirth.com/

Bradley Method Pregnancy Hotline
P.O. Box 5224
Sherman Oaks, CA 91413
800- 423-2397
800- 4-A-BIRTH
818-788-6662

International Childbirth Education Association, Inc.
P.O. Box 20048
Minneapolis, MN 55420
612-854-8660
http://www.icea.org

National Association of Parents and Professionals for Safe Alternatives in Childbirth
Rte. 1, Box 646
Marble Hill, MO 63764
314-238-2010

Read Natural Childbirth Foundation, Inc.
P.O. Box 150956
San Rafael, CA 94915
415-456-8462

CHILDBIRTH SETTINGS

The decision of where to deliver her child is one of the most important choices an expectant mother must make. Some women prefer a familiar setting, as similar to their own homes as possible. For others, the traditional medical environment is a comfort. The choices for birth settings include the hospital, a freestanding birth center, and the home.

THE HOSPITAL SETTING

Many hospitals offer two birth settings, a standard delivery room and a birthing room. The **standard delivery room,** a suite that includes a labor room, a delivery room, and a recovery room, is a sterile setting, much like an operating room. Women who have a high risk of complications during delivery, such as women over age 35 or women with diabetes, often choose the delivery room to guarantee the presence of medical equipment if any complications arise. Other women find themselves in the delivery room if an emergency cesarean or other intervention is needed.

Unlike the more clinical environment of the delivery room, a hospital **birthing room** is usually decorated to look as homelike as possible, complete with wall hangings, quilts, and comfortable chairs. The setting allows the woman and her partner to stay in the same room for labor, delivery, and recovery. Though the rooms

QUESTIONS TO ASK: THE HOSPITAL SETTING

To ensure that the hospital setting is compatible with your plan for the birth of your baby, the following questions can be asked:

■ What is the hospital's rate of nosocomial infections (infections acquired during hospitalization)? The newborn nursery's infection rate? There is no national standard on acceptable rates. A Centers for Disease Control and Prevention study estimates that 5 to 10 percent of patients in a hospital acquire a nosocomial infection. Of course, the closer the hospital's rate is to zero, the better.

■ What is the hospital's rate of cesarean section? Although the rate in the United States in 1993 was 22.8 percent, suggested figures range from 7.6 to 12 percent.

■ Will the hospital staff attempt to follow your birth plan?

■ What childbirth preparation method is the staff familiar with? Does the hospital offer any childbirth classes? Are partners welcome to attend?

■ Can the partner attend a birth? What about another coach, such as a friend or a midwife?

■ Does the hospital provide for any alternative birth positions? If so, which ones?

■ Is a woman guaranteed a birthing room, if she wishes, on her delivery day?

■ Can the partner be present in the operating room if a cesarean section is necessary?

■ Can the baby stay with the mother at all times (an arrangement called rooming-in), if the mother wishes? How soon after birth can rooming-in start?

■ Is breast-feeding immediately after birth encouraged (assuming both the mother and baby are healthy)?

■ Is there open visiting for partners after the birth? Can young siblings visit the mother in the hospital?

---

appear homelike, medical monitoring equipment is nearby if necessary.

Visiting or touring the hospital labor and delivery area is an important part of choosing the setting for birth. Most hospitals regularly schedule tours and answer questions.

THE BIRTH CENTER

A birth center, also called a childbearing center, is a facility located outside of a hospital that offers a homelike setting for childbirth. Most freestanding birth centers are owned by physicians or certified nurse-midwives, with most of the care provided by certified nurse-midwives working in consultation with obstetric and pediatric specialists on 24-hour call. Some centers operate under the aegis of hospitals, and others are operated by community health centers or nonprofit groups. Birth centers are designed for women with low-risk pregnancies and may refer women with complications to a hospital before or during delivery.

The use of birth centers is not encouraged by the American Academy of Pediatrics and the American College of Obstetricians and Gynecologists because large-scale scientific studies are not available to evaluate the safety and out-

QUESTIONS TO ASK: THE BIRTH CENTER

To find out more about the procedures and operations of a birth center, ask the following questions:

■ Does the center provide prenatal, childbirth, and postpartum care and education?

■ Are the primary-care providers certified nurse-midwives? Is there a physician backup?

■ What emergency and essential life-support equipment does the center have on-site? What is the emergency transfer capability and protocol to a hospital with maternity services?

■ Which are the backup hospitals?

■ Is the birth center accredited by any national organizations? An accredited birth center can be found by contacting:

National Association of Childbearing Centers
3123 Gottschall Rd.
Perkiomenville, PA 18074
215-234-8068
birthctr@midwives.org

come of births in freestanding clinics. However, many obstetricians and midwives believe birth centers are a safe, lower cost alternative to a hospital birth. Available studies show birth centers have a similar rate of maternal and infant mortality and a lower rate of cesarean sections.

THE HOME SETTING

A home setting for delivery may be the choice of a woman seeking a family-centered birth in an intimate setting. Rare in the United States, home births require much preparation and are recommended only for women with normal pregnancies with few risks for complications. A prepared childbirth method must be chosen by a woman early in the pregnancy and mastered before the delivery day, and any self-training and medical techniques should be discussed with the birth practitioner.

Many physicians will not attend home births; a certified nurse-midwife or lay midwife is more likely to accept the assignment. In addition, some states' laws restrict home birth and the use of lay midwives. Current state laws can be obtained by contacting the state health department or state nurse licensing board. For more information on how to have a safe home birth, contact:

National Association of Parents and Professionals for Safe Alternatives in Childbirth
Rte. 1, Box 646
Marble Hill, MO 63764
314-238-2010

Homebirth Options, Midwifery Independence (HOME)
P.O. Box 336
New Hampton, NY 10958
914-355-3529

SEE childbirth—choosing a practitioner; childbirth interventions; childbirth—labor and delivery; childbirth—methods and options.

CHINESE MEDICINE

Traditional Chinese medicine practitioners use acupuncture, massage, and herbal treatments to harmonize a person's life energy, or Qi (pronounced *chee*), and to maintain balance between the dualities of yin and yang, which roughly correspond to Western concepts of female and male, light and dark, and positive and negative. The Qi flows along paths known as meridians, sets of invisible pathways that cover the body in set patterns.

Practitioners of Chinese medicine rely upon looking, listening, smelling, asking, and touching to make their diagnosis. A theory of Chinese medicine, one basic to determining a particular illness and the prescribed treatment, is called Five Elements. The five elements—fire, wood, earth, metal, and water—are used to evaluate bodily functions, organs, acupuncture meridians, emotions, and external influences. Practitioners seek to discover some disturbance in the flow of Qi throughout the body.

By carefully taking the pulse, the practitioner can detect slight imbalances that may indicate a condition or disease. The practitioner detects various components in the pulse as it flows along the meridians of the body, and since the meridians connect to every organ system, it is possible to determine which organ or body part is affected.

When diagnosis is complete, the practitioner decides upon a treatment. Acupuncture, massage therapy, and herbal treatments are used alone or in combination to restore the body's balance.

SEE acupuncture; herbal medicine; massage therapy.

For more information on traditional Chinese medicine, contact:

American Association of Acupuncture and Oriental Medicine
433 Front St.
Catasauqua, PA 18032
610-433-2448
aaaom1@aol.com

American Foundation of Traditional Chinese Medicine
505 Beach St.
San Francisco, CA 94133
415-776-0502

American Oriental Bodywork Association
Glendale Executive Campus, Suite 510
1000 White Horse Rd.
Voorhees, NJ 08043
609-782-1616
shinnaobta@aol.com

CHOLESTEROL

Cholesterol is a soft, fatlike, waxy substance found in all the body's cells. Technically, cholesterol is not a fat but a closely related substance. It belongs to a class of compounds called sterols. The body uses cholesterol to form cell membranes, certain hormones, and other necessary substances. **Serum cholesterol,** or **blood cholesterol,** is the name for the level of cholesterol in the blood. Most medical experts agree that high blood cholesterol levels are linked to the formation of atherosclerosis (a condition in which layers of artery walls become thick and irregular due to deposits of fat, cholesterol, and other substances) and coronary heart disease.

Most people are probably more familiar with **dietary cholesterol.** It is a substance present in all animal foods, especially egg yolks, meat, fish, poultry, whole-milk products (such as cheeses, yogurt, sour cream, ice cream, and butter), and organ meats. The majority of studies have shown that dietary cholesterol, as well as saturated fat, raises blood cholesterol levels in many people. However, two 1995 Columbia University studies revealed that consuming added cholesterol within a low-saturated-fat diet resulted in only modest increases in the blood cholesterol levels. Studies are continuing on the effects of dietary cholesterol in the body.

LIPOPROTEINS

Because cholesterol doesn't dissolve in water (the major component of blood) and cannot move through the blood on its own accord, it attaches to protein, forming lipoproteins. ("Lipo" means "fat," and cholesterol is a fatlike substance.) The principal lipoproteins are high-density lipoproteins (HDLs) and low-density lipoproteins (LDLs).

High-density lipoproteins (HDLs) are manufactured in the small intestine and liver and then released into the bloodstream. HDLs then carry cholesterol back to the liver to be processed and disposed. Because these lipoproteins escort excess cholesterol from the body and help to eliminate it, HDLs are sometimes called good cholesterol.

Low-density lipoproteins (LDLs) carry cholesterol to cells in the body where it is used to form cell membranes and hormones. However, if there is more cholesterol available than cells can take up and use, LDL ends up circulating in the bloodstream until, eventually, it sticks to artery walls; hence it's called bad cholesterol.

Several medical studies have associated high levels of blood serum to heart disease, but recent research suggests that it is the proportion of HDL and LDL to total cholesterol that provides a more accurate indication of risk. In other words, the problem is not how much cholesterol there is, but how it circulates and what company it keeps, especially among women, for whom low HDL and high triglycerides (another type of fat in the blood) are more important in determining risk for heart disease than total cholesterol levels.

CHOLESTEROL LEVELS

In the past, cholesterol-level guidelines have focused on total cholesterol levels. The conservative recommendation for minimum heart disease risk is a total cholesterol level under 200 mg/dl (milligrams per deciliter of blood), preferably in the 160 to 180 range. But recent studies suggest that tests for total cholesterol are a crude measurement and inaccurate indicator of health risks.

Most experts now favor tests that read the proportion of HDL and LDL to total cholesterol. (All cholesterol screenings involve a blood test.) The real danger does not seem to lie in the total cholesterol level, but rather in a low HDL and a high LDL level. If total cholesterol is high because of a high LDL level, then risk factors are likely; however, if total cholesterol is high because of high HDL, then there usually is not a need for concern. Most experts recommend that women aim for LDL levels below 130 and HDL levels above 55. But the American Heart Association suggests that heart disease patients drop their LDL levels to below 100 mg/dl. Dropping cholesterol levels does not clean out existing plaque from arteries, but new studies show it appears to prevent the formation of clots that cause heart attacks.

Because the test that isolates LDL levels is costly, some practitioners may simply test for the ratio of HDL to total cholesterol, then determine the LDL level by subtracting the level of HDL and the level of triglycerides divided by 5 from total cholesterol.

Medical guidelines suggest a ratio of less than 4.5 (total cholesterol divided by HDL) as desirable. Anything over 7.0 is considered dangerous.

On the other hand, cholesterol that drops to noteworthy lows sometimes indicates the presence of a disease, often pernicious anemia or hyperthyroidism, a condition in which the thyroid gland malfunctions.

WOMEN AND CHOLESTEROL

Generally, women have higher total cholesterol levels than men. But in many women the high total number is attributed to high HDL levels. Women's beneficial HDL levels peak during the childbearing years. After menopause their HDL tends to fall and total cholesterol rises, yet they still maintain an edge in HDL over men. Nevertheless, high cholesterol may still pose a problem for some women.

Estrogen, found in oral contraceptives, helps to reduce the risk of heart disease by raising levels of HDL and lowering levels of LDL. However, women who have high cholesterol levels should take the Pill only under close medical supervision and may consider having a complete lipoprotein workup performed before going on the Pill. In extremely rare cases, heart attack or stroke associated with the Pill can occur in women who have high cholesterol or triglycerides. However, the benefits of the Pill usually outweigh the risks of heart disease for these women.

During pregnancy many women's cholesterol levels rise by as much as 30 percent but return to normal by about 20 weeks after delivery. In fact, many practitioners will recommend cholesterol-rich foods during pregnancy because cholesterol is needed for new cell development and proper fetal growth. However, if a woman begins a pregnancy with a cholesterol level 240 or higher, she should discuss a modified diet with her practitioner.

CONTROLLING CHOLESTEROL LEVELS

Although scientists disagree on methods aimed at lowering blood serum cholesterol levels and whether or not a low-cholesterol diet is effective to any large degree, they do agree that people who already have heart disease ought to be on a low-cholesterol diet. And many practitioners tell the majority of their patients that it is probably wise and generally healthier to eat a low-fat, low cholesterol diet, just in case.

CHOLESTEROL-LOWERING DRUGS

There are drugs that lower serum cholesterol levels, although (as with nearly everything else associated with the study of and research into cholesterol, atherosclerosis, and heart disease) results have been mixed.

Estrogen is the most effective cholesterol-lowering drug, as it raises levels of HDL and lowers levels of LDL. Premenopausal women have the benefit of natural estrogen; after menopause, when the ovaries stop functioning, hormone replacement therapy (HRT) may be used to restore levels of estrogen in the body and therefore lower the risk of heart disease. A woman considering HRT should discuss the benefits and risks of the regimen with her practitioner.

In July 1995 the Food and Drug Administration approved the marketing of simvastatin (Zocor), a statin drug, as the first anticholesterol drug that reduces deaths. The approval is based on a five-year study of 4,400 coronary patients in which simvastatin lowered deaths from heart disease by 42 percent and also significantly reduced nonfatal heart attacks and the need for rehospitalization. Currently, simvastatin is prescribed for heart disease patients exclusively; studies have not yet indicated that the drug is suitable for people with high cholesterol but without coronary disease. The statin

 LOWERING YOUR CHOLESTEROL

While studies on the effectiveness of dietary cholesterol reduction in lowering total cholesterol—and the role of diet in heart disease altogether—conflict, here are some things that might help:

■ Eat fewer calories because losing weight helps. It isn't as important as other risk factors, but it shouldn't be ignored.

■ Cut your intake of saturated fats.

■ Eat foods rich in fiber, such as carrots, celery, breads, and cereals.

■ Eat more fruits and vegetables and replace animal fats—especially those that are solid at room temperature—with vegetable oils, such as corn, olive, safflower, soybean, and sesame. A vegetarian diet may be protective.

■ Get yourself a chart of foods and their dietary cholesterol content and place a ceiling of 300 mg a day on your meals.

■ Cut down on coffee. Caffeine can elevate heart rate and cause arrhythmias, irregular heartbeats.

■ Drink one ounce of water for every two pounds of body weight per day.

■ Try soy proteins, found in tofu and soy milk. These have been found to lower cholesterol levels in those who eat 30 to 40 g a day.

drugs generally have mild side effects. Simvastatin is not for use by people with liver disease and women who are pregnant or breast-feeding, and it occasionally can cause muscle disease.

Other drugs used to reduce serum cholesterol levels are colestipol hydrochloride, lovastatin, nicotinic acid, gemfibrozil, and sodium dextrothyroxine.

For many years, experts believed that drugs should not be used as the first treatment of choice, but instead only when a long-term regimen of diet and exercise failed—and only in dire emergencies. However, new research shows that it is critical to aggressively fight cholesterol in heart disease patients by dropping cholesterol quickly and to ultra-low levels.

TRIGLYCERIDES

Triglycerides are another form of fat in the body. Having a high serum triglyceride reading is as risky as having a high serum cholesterol level. According to the American Heart Association, triglyceride levels normally range from about 50 to 250 mg/dl, depending on age and gender. More conservative guidelines define 30 to 175 mg/dl as normal. As people get older (or heavier or both), their triglyceride and cholesterol levels tend to rise. Women also tend to have higher triglyceride levels than do men.

Several clinical studies have shown that an unusually large number of people with coronary heart disease also have high levels of triglycerides in the blood. However, some people with this problem seem remarkably free from atherosclerosis. Thus, elevated triglycerides, which are often measured along with HDL and LDL, may not directly cause atherosclerosis but may accompany other abnormalities that speed its development.

SEE heart disease; nutrition.

CHRONIC FATIGUE SYNDROME

Chronic fatigue syndrome (CFS) is a condition characterized by long-term, constant exhaustion and muscle pain. CFS is a serious, debilitating condition that is difficult to diagnose because of its wide range of symptoms and is often confused with fibromyalgia. It generally occurs suddenly, coming on over a few hours or a few days, usually after a viral infection. An estimated 200 per 100,000 people are said to have the condition, which usually affects young adults, and women twice as often as men. It is also known as chronic fatigue immune dysfunction syndrome (CFIDS) and has also been called yuppie flu because of the myth that it occurs more often in young, upper-class professionals and because it frequently follows a flulike illness.

CONDITIONS FOR WHICH CFS IS COMMONLY MISTAKEN

Condition Mistakenly Diagnosed	Symptoms Similar to CFS
Alzheimer's disease	Disorientation
Emphysema	Fatigue, difficulty exhaling
Enteric candidiasis (intestinal fungal infection)	Fatigue, abdominal pain
Hodgkin's disease	Swollen glands
Hypoglycemia	Episodic fatigue and weakness
Hypothyroidism	Fatigue
Leukemia	Lymph node swelling
Lupus	Confusion, rash
Multiple sclerosis	Fatigue, muscle weakness
Fibromyalgia	Fatigue, muscle pain
Lyme disease	Fatigue, arthralgia (nerve pain in one or more joints)

SYMPTOMS

According to the Centers for Disease Control and Prevention, the condition involves an unexplained, persistent, or recurring fatigue that has lasted for longer than six months. The fatigue interferes with daily activities, does not result from exertion, and does not improve with rest. In addition, four of the following symptoms must be present:

■ Impaired memory or concentration
■ Recurrent sore throat
■ Tender lymph nodes
■ Muscle or joint pain
■ Exceptional fatigue after usually tolerable exercise, which persists for more than 24 hours
■ Severe headache
■ Unrefreshing sleep

Minor symptoms include fever and chills, sudden mood changes, loss of appetite, cravings for strange foods, and visual problems or fear of light.

DIAGNOSIS

Diagnosing CFS is difficult, and there are no tests that can confirm its presence. Many practitioners interpret the symptoms as the sign of another condition, or believe the problem to be psychological or imagined. A woman who suspects she has CFS should find a practitioner who takes the condition seriously. She can do so by seeking a referral from a CFS support group or by asking local health-care providers about their beliefs concerning the condition.

To diagnose CFS, a practitioner must first rule out a number of other disorders (see box above.) A person may also undergo tests such as a complete blood count (CBC), adrenal and thyroid function tests (which monitor the functions of hormone-producing glands), blood sedimentation rate tests, chest x-rays, or a urinalysis. Blood may also be analyzed for the amounts of different substances, such as alpha-interferon and different types of lymphocytes, which may indicate CFS.

✓ SELF-CARE FOR CHRONIC FATIGUE

Several lifestyle changes can be made to help reduce the debilitation caused by CFS. A person with CFS should:

■ Get plenty of bed rest, offset by a scheduled program of regular exercise. Activity helps to alleviate fatigue.

■ Eat a well-balanced diet. Vitamin regimens have been shown to be effective in treating the syndrome, and maintaining proper nutrition is important to keep energy levels up and to stay healthy. Persons with CFS may suffer loss of appetite or feel strong cravings for strange foods, and they often do not eat properly. In addition, those with CFS should be careful to drink enough water every day.

■ Eliminate from his or her diet foods and chemicals that trigger allergic or sensitive reactions.

■ Try alternative therapies. While there is no cure for CFS, acupuncture, Chinese medicine, homeopathy, and herbal therapies may provide relief from symptoms by raising energy levels, reducing stress, and alleviating headaches and muscle pain.

CFS is difficult to diagnose mainly because its cause is unknown. At one time, CFS was thought to be associated with the Epstein-Barr virus, the herpes virus that causes infectious mononucleosis, and was known as chronic Epstein-Barr virus syndrome. Some experts believe CFS to be an autoimmune disease (a disease in which the body produces an immune response to attack its own tissues), while others link it to fibromyalgia, another unexplained condition of muscle pain and disease. It has also been linked to Lyme disease, a tick-borne illness.

TREATMENT

There presently are no definitive drugs that can cure or even alleviate the symptoms of CFS. Individual complaints may be treated. For example, antidepressants may be prescribed for depression and analgesics for headaches. Some experimental drugs, such as the drug ampligen, are being developed for use against CFS. A person may be detoxified; nutritional support and plenty of water are also recommended.

While the condition cannot be cured, it does not get worse over time and often improves over the course of several years. Individuals affected by CFS live with the condition and often rearrange their lives around the limitations of CFS.

SEE fibromyalgia.

For more information on CFS, contact:

Chronic Fatigue Immune Dysfunction Syndrome (CFIDS) Association
P.O. Box 220398
Charlotte, NC 28222
800-442-3437
704-362-CFID
http://cfids.org/cfids

COLPOSCOPY

Colposcopy is an explorative procedure used to examine the surface cells of the vaginal walls and cervix. It is also used to examine external sores or other abnormalities on the vulva. Colposcopy is usually the first procedure done after abnormal cells show up on a Pap test.

Colposcopy is less invasive than other diagnostic procedures because no incision is necessary, and it is virtually painless (though it may be uncomfortable) and risk-free. The procedure is more accurate than a Pap test in diagnosing cervical cancer, since it can identify the specific suspicious areas for a biopsy, a microscopic examination of the tissue.

REASONS FOR COLPOSCOPY

Colposcopy is done to diagnose abnormal bleeding and to locate the abnormal cells that a Pap test indicates are present for biopsy.

Colposcopy can also help the practitioner determine the next stage of treatment. For example, information provided by the examination can help determine if yet another procedure, such as a cone biopsy (in which a cone-shaped sample of the cervix is taken for analysis), is necessary. On the other hand, if inflammation of the cervix is discovered as the cause of the abnormality, then no further explorative procedure is necessary.

Frequent colposcopy exams are recommended for all DES daughters. These are women whose mothers took the drug diethylstilbestrol (DES) during pregnancy to prevent miscarriage. Exposure to this drug, which was widely used between 1941 and 1971, can cause clear cell adenocarcinoma, a rare vaginal cancer. Regular colposcopy exams can help physicians find abnormal cells in the early stages when the condition is most successfully treated.

PROCEDURE

Colposcopy is a simple, nearly painless procedure. The entire procedure takes about 15 minutes to perform and, because it does not require an anesthetic, can be done in a practitioner's

BEFORE COLPOSCOPY

Before you agree to have a colposcopy done, ask your practitioner the following questions:

■ Is this the most appropriate procedure for my condition?

■ How much time will the procedure require?

■ What are the most common complications resulting from the procedure?

■ Are these complications self-limiting (meaning they resolve on their own), or do they require further medical intervention?

■ Are there any alternatives to the procedure you recommended?

■ What could happen if I decline the procedure?

office. The procedure is performed by either a gynecologist or another practitioner with special training in colposcopy.

As with Pap tests, a metal or plastic instrument called a **speculum** is inserted into the vagina in order to separate the vaginal walls for optimal viewing. Then the physician swabs the vaginal walls with a vinegar-like solution to remove the mucus. In addition, the same solution may be applied to reveal certain types of abnormalities.

The physician examines the cervix, vagina, and vulva with the **colposcope,** an instrument that looks like binoculars on a tripod. The colposcope, which allows the practitioner to magnify six to 40 times, is placed at the opening of the vagina. The instrument never enters the vagina. In fact, it doesn't even touch the body.

During the procedure, the practitioner usu-ally takes a sample from any suspicious areas where abnormal cells may be located. This is done by scraping away cells from the areas in question with a metal loop called a **curette.** A plug of tissue, called a **punch biopsy,** may be taken from the cervix or vulva with an instrument similar to a paper punch. The samples are then taken to a laboratory for diagnosis.

RISKS AND SIDE EFFECTS

There may be some slight bleeding afterward if a sample is taken for biopsy. Some pain and cramping may occur after a biopsy of the cervix is done. Women are recommended to avoid intercourse, douching, and using tampons for a week after a cervical biopsy to allow the cervix to heal.

SEE biopsy; medical testing (appendix B).

CONTRACEPTION

A contraceptive is a device, substance, or method used to prevent pregnancy. Some 85 percent of women who do not use contraceptives during vaginal intercourse become pregnant each year. While the only guarantee against pregnancy is to not have vaginal intercourse, contraceptives can significantly reduce the risk of unwanted pregnancy. Some contraceptives also help to protect against sexually transmitted infections (STIs).

Contraceptive methods work by:

■ Destroying or making sperm inactive
■ Introducing a physical or chemical barrier that prevents sperm from entering the cervix
■ Suppressing ovulation and/or the production of sperm through the use of hormone medication
■ Making the uterine lining unreceptive to fertilized eggs

Most contraceptive methods are temporary, or reversible. Some methods, such as sterilization, are permanent and intended to be irreversible.

The effectiveness of contraceptives is measured according to perfect use and typical use.

Typical use refers to the rate for women and men whose use is not consistent or always correct. **Perfect use** refers to the rate for those whose use is consistent and always correct.

ABSTINENCE

Continuous abstinence, the only way to guarantee against pregnancy, is refraining from any vaginal intercourse. **Periodic abstinence** is not having vaginal intercourse during the fertile period of the woman's menstrual cycle, which lasts from about five days before ovulation to three days after.

Effectiveness: Continual abstinence is 100 percent effective in preventing pregnancy as long as it is practiced without fail. In typical use, periodic abstinence is 80 percent effective.

Advantages: There are no medical or hormonal side effects. Religious groups may endorse abstinence for unmarried people. Some

TO PRACTICE PERIODIC ABSTINENCE: FERTILITY AWARENESS METHODS (FAMs)

There are several ways you can determine your fertile period. By refraining from intercourse or using another form of contraception during the fertile period, you can avoid pregnancy. Many women use fertility awareness methods when trying to conceive as well. Methods include:

Basal body temperature method: Take your temperature every morning before getting out of bed. The temperature will rise between 4° and 8°F the day ovulation occurs and will stay at that level until your next period. You are fertile during the first three full days after ovulation. This method is 80 percent effective with typical use and 97 percent effective when always used consistently and correctly.

Cervical mucus method: Observe the changes in your cervical mucus. Seven to eight days before predicted ovulation, normally cloudy, tacky mucus becomes clear and slippery and will stretch between the fingers. At that time, you are in your most fertile phase and should abstain from vaginal intercourse or use a barrier contraceptive. In typical use, this method is 80 percent effective. It is 97 percent effective with perfect use.

Calendar, or "rhythm," method: By charting your menstrual cycles on a calendar, you may be able to predict ovulation if your periods occur at the same time each month. To prevent pregnancy, abstain or use a barrier contraceptive during the "unsafe" days. It will be more difficult to predict ovulation if your cycle is irregular. This method is 80 percent effective in typical use. With perfect use, it is 91 percent effective.

Symptothermal method: This method combines the basal body temperature, cervical mucus, and calendar methods. It is 80 percent effective in typical use and 98 percent effective with perfect use.

Postovulation method: Abstain or use a barrier method from the beginning of your period through the morning of the fourth day following your predicted ovulation. This method is 80 percent effective with typical use. With perfect use, it is 99 percent effective.

promote periodic abstinence during marriage.

Disadvantages: Many find it difficult to refrain from having sex, or end their abstinence without preparing themselves against unwanted pregnancy. Periodic abstinence is not effective against STIs. Care is needed in keeping records and interpreting signs.

WITHDRAWAL

The withdrawal method is the removal of the penis from the vagina during intercourse before the man ejaculates.

Effectiveness: It is 82 percent effective with typical use and 96 percent effective with perfect use.

Advantages: It may be used if no other method of birth control is available.

Disadvantages: It requires self-control, experience, and trust. It does not protect against STIs. In addition, the small amount of fluid that is released before ejaculation contains sperm.

SPERMICIDES

Contraceptive creams, jellies, films, foams, and suppositories are liquids or solids that are inserted into the vagina before intercourse and dissolve into a thick liquid that spreads throughout the vagina. They block the cervix and contain spermicides that inactivate sperm.

Effectiveness: With typical use, contraceptive creams, jellies, films, foams, and suppositories are 79 percent effective. With perfect use, they are 97 percent effective. Using a condom in conjunction with these methods increases contraceptive effectiveness and helps protect against STIs.

Advantages: Spermicides are available

without a prescription and are easy to use.

Disadvantages: They must be inserted 10 minutes before intercourse and therefore can interfere with spontaneity. Side effects include possible irritation to the penis or vagina. Some women and men complain of messiness or leakage.

CONDOMS

Condoms, also called "rubbers" or "jimmy hats," are sheaths of thin rubber, plastic, or animal tissue worn over the penis during intercourse. They prevent semen from entering the vagina, collecting the ejaculate in the tip of the condom. They are available dry or lubricated. Condoms are also prophylactic—they prevent the spread of some sexually transmitted infections. Each condom packet contains a manufacture date or an expiration date. Condoms properly stored can be used up to five years past the manufacture date. If the date is an expiration date, it should be marked as such.

Effectiveness: Condoms are 88 percent

USING SPERMICIDES

The instructions on the package insert should be followed, as each method and brand may vary. Most spermicides must be inserted 10 minutes before intercourse; effectiveness lasts about an hour after insertion. A woman can lie down or sit on her heels, then insert the spermicide deep into the vagina. More spermicide must be inserted each time sex is repeated. Douching should be avoided for six to eight hours following intercourse with these methods.

effective with typical use and 98 percent effective with perfect use. Protection is increased when a spermicide is used in addition to the condom.

Advantages: Condoms are available without a prescription and are inexpensive. They have no side effects, though 1 to 3 percent of women and men are allergic to latex. Latex condoms offer good protection against STIs, including HIV. They can be put on as part of sex play.

Disadvantages: Condoms may break, especially if they are not worn correctly. Animal-tissue condoms may not provide the same protection against sexually transmitted infec-

USING A CONDOM

The condom should be put on the erect penis before it has any contact with the vagina. Pull back the foreskin and place the rolled condom on the tip of the erect penis. Pinch the air out of the half inch at the end of the condom and roll the condom down over the erect penis. Do not used oil-based lubricants, such as petroleum jellies or mineral oils, on a latex condom because they can cause the latex to deteriorate. Use only water-based lubricants, such as K-Y jelly, with a latex condom.

After climax, hold the rim of the condom against the penis as it is withdrawn from the vagina to avoid spilling semen. Use a fresh condom each time you have intercourse. If the condom breaks, withdraw the penis and condom immediately, then remove the condom and replace with a new one. Spermicide can be tried as an emergency measure if a condom breaks, though its effectiveness is unknown.

USING THE VAGINAL POUCH

Lubricate the closed end of the vaginal pouch with a water-based lubricant. Squeeze together the sides of the inner ring and insert into the vagina like a tampon. The ring should be pushed into the vagina as far as it can go. Let the outer ring hang about an inch outside the vagina. Be careful of sharp nails or rings when inserting the pouch.

During intercourse, the pouch normally moves from side to side. If the outer ring of the pouch slips into the vagina, or if the penis slips between the pouch and the vaginal wall, stop intercourse. Remove the pouch from the vagina and reinsert.

After intercourse, squeeze and twist the outer ring of the vaginal pouch to prevent semen from leaking. Then pull the pouch out of the vagina and discard. Do not flush the vaginal pouches down the toilet.

tions as latex condoms. Condoms can interfere with spontaneity, and some men feel they dull sensation during intercourse. They can, however, help relieve premature ejaculation.

VAGINAL POUCH

One of the latest developments in birth control is the vaginal pouch, also called the female condom. The pouch is a sheath of soft polyurethane with a ring at each end. It is inserted into the vagina, with one ring against the cervix and the other outside the vagina. The pouch collects semen before, during, and after ejaculation. It provides some protection against STIs and may be purchased over-the-counter.

Effectiveness: The vaginal pouch is 76 percent effective with typical use and 90 percent effective with perfect use.

Advantages: The pouch gives women a contraceptive option that helps prevent against STIs and allows her control over her own health.

Disadvantages: The pouch may slip in the vagina during intercourse, and the rings may irritate the penis and the vulva. Some say sensation is reduced.

DIAPHRAGMS AND CERVICAL CAPS

The diaphragm and cervical cap are barrier methods of contraception available only by seeing a health-care provider because they must be fitted to the individual woman. The diaphragm is a shallow, dome-shaped soft rubber cup with a flexible rim that fits securely in the vagina to cover the cervix.

The cervical cap, also made of rubber, is smaller than the diaphragm and is thimble-shaped to fit snugly over the cervix itself. Both methods are used with spermicide jelly or cream, blocking the cervical entrance and immobilizing the sperm.

Diaphragms and cervical caps can be used by most women when they are not menstruating.

Effectiveness: With typical use, diaphragms and cervical caps are 82 percent effective in preventing pregnancy; with perfect use, they are 94 percent effective. The spermicide used with diaphragms and cervical caps offers some protection against certain STIs, including gonorrhea and chlamydia.

Advantages: Insertion is easy once it is

USING A DIAPHRAGM OR CERVICAL CAP

Diaphragms or cervical caps are inserted into the vagina, along with a spermicide, before intercourse to cover the cervix. The practitioner who prescribes the diaphragm or cap will show you how to insert it. The device must be in place each time you have sex and must remain in place for eight hours after the last intercourse. Because the cap may become dislodged, you should check its position before and after intercourse.

Women who wish to return to the use of a diaphragm after a pregnancy should visit a practitioner to have the diaphragm checked to be sure it is still the right size. A woman should also have the size of her diaphragm checked when there is an increase in sexual activity. The diaphragm and cervical cap should be checked periodically for weak spots or pinholes by holding it up to a light.

learned, and it can be shared by both partners during sex play. If properly placed, these devices cannot be felt by either partner during intercourse.

Disadvantages: Diaphragms are not recommended for women with poor vaginal muscle tone or a sagging uterus; cervical caps can be used by women whose pelvic muscles are too relaxed for diaphragms. It may be impossible to fit a cap or a diaphragm in a woman who has an irregularly shaped cervix. While most women have no side effects with either diaphragms or cervical caps, some are prone to frequent bladder infections when using a diaphragm. When cervical caps are worn for more than two days, an unpleasant odor may result.

INTRAUTERINE DEVICES (IUDs)

Intrauterine devices, or IUDs, are reversible methods of birth control available by prescription. They are devices made of plastic containing either copper or a natural hormone that are placed in the uterus. They work primarily by preventing fertilization of the egg and also affect the uterine lining in such a way as to prevent implantation. There are only two IUDs currently available in the United States. The woman's practitioner will determine which type is right for the woman. The copper IUD Para-Gard may be left in place in the uterus for 10 years, while the hormone IUD Progestasert must be replaced every year. Insertion and removal of IUDs are done by practitioners. A string attached to the IUD hangs down through the cervix and into the vagina. This string should be checked occasionally, such as after menstruation, to be sure the IUD is in place.

Effectiveness: With typical use, ParaGard is 99.2 percent effective. With perfect use, it is 99.4 percent effective. Progestasert is 97.4 percent effective with typical use and 99.9 percent with perfect use.

Advantages: An IUD is a completely reversible, long-term form of contraception. It does not interfere with spontaneity during sex, and it is also not necessary to remember to take a pill every day.

WHO CAN USE IUDs?

IUDs are the most popular form of reversible birth control in the world. More than 85 million women use them. An IUD may be right for you if:

■ You have only one sex partner who has sex only with you.

■ You have had a baby.

You should *not* use the IUD if you have:

■ More than one sex partner, or if your partner has more than one sex partner

■ A recent history of pelvic infection

■ Postpartum endometriosis or infectious abortion in the past three months

■ Untreated acute cervicitis or vaginitis, including bacterial vaginosis, until infection is controlled

■ Unexplained abnormal vaginal bleeding

■ Pregnancy or suspicion of pregnancy

■ Abnormality of the uterus that results in distortion of the uterine cavity

■ Any disease that decreases your ability to fight infections, such as leukemia or HIV, the human immunodeficiency virus that can cause AIDS

■ Had an abnormal Pap test recently

■ Actinomycosis (a type of bacterium) in the reproductive tract

■ A previously inserted IUD that has not been removed

Copper IUDs should *not* be used if you are allergic to copper, have Wilson's disease, or if you are having diathermy (heat) treatments.

Do not have an IUD inserted if there is a chance that you are pregnant. Be sure to tell your practitioner if you think there is any chance that you are. A special evaluation must be done if you have a history of heart disease or certain other medical conditions.

Disadvantages: Possible side effects of IUDs include greater cramping (usually for a short time following insertion), bleeding between periods, and heavier and longer-lasting periods. Antibiotics given during insertion can reduce the chances of infection. Infection of fallopian tubes is a risk with IUD users who have more than one sexual partner, or with a user whose partner has other partners. Such infection can increase the risk of ectopic pregnancy, cause sterility, and in rare cases require the removal of reproductive organs. Also, rarely, the IUD may pierce the wall of the uterus, usually during insertion.

The IUD is recognized by the World Health Organization and the American Medical Association as one of the safest and most effective temporary forms of birth control for women. However, several years of negative publicity in the 1970s brought on by the sale and use of a faulty IUD—the Dalkon Shield—raised questions about the safety of all IUDs, and most types (even the ones considered safe) were removed from the market. Because of this speculation, the variety of IUDs available in the United States is limited.

IUDs are also used as an emergency contraceptive when inserted within five days of unprotected intercourse, because they keep the fertilized egg from implanting.

ORAL CONTRACEPTIVES

Oral contraceptives (called the Pill) are monthly series of pills taken daily to prevent pregnancy. **Combination pills** contain the synthetic hormones estrogen and progestin and work by preventing the eggs from ripening and ovulation from occurring. Combination pills are packaged in either 21-day or 28-day packs.

USING THE PILL

Correct and consistent use of the Pill increases your protection against pregnancy. It is very important not to skip pills, even if you have spotting or bleeding between periods or if you do not have vaginal intercourse very often. The Pill should be taken at the same time every day to increase effectiveness.

Be sure to follow the instructions on the package. Your practitioner will explain how to use the Pill, on what day you should start taking the series, and what you should do in the event that you miss a pill.

Women taking the Pill or minipill should consult their practitioner if they experience any of the following symptoms:

■ Unusual swelling or pain in the legs

■ Sudden abdominal, chest, or arm pain

■ Sudden shortness of breath

■ Severe headaches

■ Sudden blurred or double vision, or loss of vision in one eye

■ Yellowing of the eyes or skin

■ Severe depression

In a 21-day pack, one pill is taken each day for 21 days and none taken for the following seven days, regulating a 28-day cycle in which menstruation takes place. With a 28-day pack, there are 21 active pills followed by seven inactive pills, or placebos. Menstruation occurs during the fourth week of the pack.

Minipills contain only progestin and work

mainly by thickening cervical mucus, preventing sperm from joining with the egg. They may also prevent implantation of fertilized eggs. Minipills are taken every day.

Effectiveness: The Pill and minipill are 97 percent effective in preventing pregnancy with typical use and more than 99 percent effective with perfect use. Neither the combined nor the progestin-only pill provide protection against STIs.

Advantages: Women who use the Pill have more regular periods, less menstrual flow, and less cramping. There are fewer cases of iron-deficiency anemia, fewer ectopic pregnancies, and less pelvic inflammatory disease. Women may also have less acne, less premenstrual tension, and less rheumatoid arthritis. The Pill offers significant protection against ovarian and endometrial cancer, noncancerous breast tumors, and ovarian cysts.

Disadvantages: Women must remember to take the Pill every day, at about the same time. Side effects of the Pill and minipill that usually subside after two or three months of use include spotting between periods, breast tenderness, nausea, vomiting, weight gain or loss, and depression.

Pill users have a slightly greater chance than nonusers of developing certain serious problems that can be fatal in rare cases. These include heart attack, stroke, blood clots in the veins, and liver tumors. The chance of developing some of these problems increases with age—especially when certain other health problems are present. Risks are increased by smoking more than 15 cigarettes a day, and by diabetes, high blood pressure, and high cholesterol levels. These risks are vastly reduced if a woman uses a progestin-only pill.

Women with liver disease, high blood pressure, or high cholesterol levels or who have had gestational diabetes may need special tests before going on the Pill or minipill. Women should *not* take oral contraceptives if they:

- Are over 35 years old and smoke heavily (over 15 cigarettes per day)
- Have unexplained vaginal bleeding
- Have had blood clots in the veins
- Have breast or uterine cancer
- Have malignant melanoma (a type of skin cancer) that has spread to another part of the body
- Have cystic fibrosis
- Have sickle-cell anemia

Women should discuss the risks of oral contraceptives with their practitioners. Women who suspect they may be pregnant or who are breast-feeding should not take combination pills.

NORPLANT

Norplant is a reversible form of birth control available by prescription. Six soft capsules (each about the size of a cardboard matchstick) are inserted under the skin of the upper arm. The capsules contain the synthetic hormone levonorgestrel, similar to the hormone that regulates the body's menstrual cycle. The hormone is constantly released, preventing the ovaries from releasing eggs, and thickening cervical mucus to prevent sperm from joining with the egg. Norplant is effective against pregnancy for five years.

Effectiveness: Norplant is over 99 percent effective; out of 10,000 women using Norplant, only four become pregnant. Norplant offers no protection against STIs.

Advantages: Norplant provides continuous, long-term, reversible birth control. There is no pill that a woman needs to remember to take every day. Norplant contains no estrogen and can be used while breast-feeding anytime after six weeks following delivery.

USING NORPLANT

Women using Norplant should contact their practitioner if they experience:

■ Vaginal bleeding that is much heavier and lasts longer than their regular periods

■ A late period following a long interval of regular cycles

■ Severe abdominal pain

■ Pain, bleeding, or pus at the implant site

■ An implant that seems to be coming dislodged

Women should *not* use Norplant if they:

■ Are pregnant

■ Have unexplained vaginal bleeding

■ Are breast-feeding during the first six weeks after delivery

■ Have blood clots or inflammation of the veins

■ Have serious liver disease

■ Cannot tolerate irregular bleeding

Women who have migraine headaches, diabetes, high cholesterol or blood pressure, heart disease, seizures that require medication, serious depression, or clotting or bleeding disorders may be able to use Norplant under medical supervision.

Disadvantages: One common side effect of Norplant, which is not serious, is irregular bleeding. This includes:

■ Irregular intervals between periods

■ Irregular bleeding or spotting between periods

■ Longer menstrual flow

■ No menstrual flow for months at a time

Other side effects some women may experience are:

■ Headaches

■ Nausea

■ Change in appetite

■ Weight loss or gain

■ Breast soreness

■ Acne

■ Hair loss

■ Depression

■ Vaginal dryness

■ Increased facial and body hair

■ Skin discoloration over the implants

■ Enlarged ovaries

There is a greater chance of ectopic pregnancy in the rare chance that Norplant fails.

Removal may be difficult if the rods were not well placed. Several attempts may be required. Excess scar growth may occur in women prone to scarring.

DEPO-PROVERA

Depo-Provera is a synthetic hormone that is injected into the arm or buttock every 12 weeks. It is a reversible form of birth control available through prescription. Depo-Provera works by preventing the ovaries from releasing eggs and by thickening cervical mucus to keep sperm from meeting the egg. It is effective in preventing pregnancy for 12 weeks.

Effectiveness: Depo-Provera is over 99 percent effective. Out of 1,000 women using this method, only three will become pregnant during the first year. It offers no protection against STIs.

Advantages: Depo-Provera prevents pregnancy for 12 weeks. It does not need to be taken daily, contains no estrogen, and doesn't require surgery. It reduces menstrual cramps and anemia and offers protection against endometrial and ovarian cancers. It can be used six weeks after delivery by women who are breast-feeding.

Disadvantages: The most common side effect of Depo-Provera is irregular bleeding, including:

- Irregular intervals between periods
- Spotting between periods
- Longer menstrual flow
- No menstrual flow for months at a time

The longer a woman is on Depo-Provera, the more likely these symptoms are to subside. However, over half of users have no periods after one year of use. Other possible side effects are:

- Headache
- Dizziness
- Nausea
- Change in appetite
- Weight gain
- Breast soreness
- Nervousness
- Hair loss
- Increased facial and body hair
- Acne, skin rashes, or spotty darkening of the skin
- Depression
- Vaginal dryness
- Increased or decreased sex drive

The effects of using Depo-Provera cannot be reversed immediately.

- It may take as long as 18 months to become pregnant after use is stopped.
- Side effects may continue for up to eight months until Depo-Provera is cleared from the body.
- It can take three months or longer before regular ovulation and menstruation resume, especially if cycles were irregular before Depo-Provera was initiated.

USING DEPO-PROVERA

Women using Depo-Provera should contact their practitioner immediately if they experience:

- Vaginal bleeding that is much heavier and lasts much longer than their regular periods
- Sudden, severe abdominal pain
- Severe headaches
- Major depression
- Frequent urination
- Yellowing of the skin or eyes

Although ectopic pregnancies occur much less frequently for Depo-Provera users than for women using no birth control method, some users have had ectopic pregnancies.

It is not advisable for women to use Depo-Provera without medical supervision if they have concerns about weight gain, diabetes, major depression, a recent history of liver disease (such as hepatitis), or recently had blood clots in the eyes, legs, or lungs.

Women should *not* use Depo-Provera if they:

- Are pregnant
- Have unexplained vaginal bleeding
- Have serious liver disease or growths of the liver
- Have a known or suspected breast cancer
- Have Cushing's syndrome and are being treated with Cytadren
- Are allergic to the hormone depotmedroxprogesterone acetate (DMPA)
- Cannot tolerate irregular bleeding or loss of menstrual periods

145

SEE contraception, emergency; contraception—sterilization; menstrual cycle and ovulation; safer sex.

For more information on contraceptives, contact:

Advocates for Youth
Center for Population Options
1025 Vermont Ave., N.W., Suite 200
Washington, DC 20005
202-347-5700
advocates@internetmci.com

National Family Planning and Reproductive Health Association
122 C St., N.W., Suite 380
Washington, DC 20001-2109
202-628-3535
judithdesamo@msn.com

National Organization of Adolescent Pregnancy and Parenting and Prevention
4421A East-West Hwy.
Bethesda, MD 20814
301-913-0378
noappp@aol.com

Planned Parenthood Federation of America, Inc.
810 Seventh Avenue
New York, NY 10019
For the Planned Parenthood nearest you, call:
   800-230-PLAN
http://www.ppfa.org/ppfa

CONTRACEPTION, EMERGENCY

Emergency contraception is designed to prevent a pregnancy after unprotected intercourse. Emergency hormonal contraception may also interfere with fertilization. It is also called postcoital contraception. It can be requested if a woman thinks her method of contraception has failed, if she was a victim of rape, or whenever no other method of contraception was being used.

Emergency contraception will not work when the woman is already pregnant.

Emergency contraception is provided in two ways. **Emergency IUD insertion** can be done by a practitioner within five days of unprotected intercourse. Of 100 women who use emergency IUD insertion, only one will become pregnant. **Emergency hormonal contraception**—"the morning-after pill"—is prescribed by a practitioner. It is a sequence of two doses of certain combined oral contraceptives taken 12 hours apart and within 72 hours of unprotected intercourse. Nausea, vomiting, and cramping are frequent side effects. Depending on the point in the cycle that emergency hormonal contraception is used, effectiveness ranges from 75 to 97 percent. The closer to ovulation a woman is, the less likely the method will succeed. Emergency hormonal contraception should *not* be used by women who are pregnant.

A woman who uses emergency contraception should schedule a follow-up visit with her practitioner if menstruation does not occur or if she has other symptoms of pregnancy. If pregnancy is suspected, a pregnancy test and pelvic exam should be performed.

SEE abortion.

For more information on emergency contraception, contact:

**Planned Parenthood Federation of
America, Inc.**
810 Seventh Avenue
New York, NY 10019
For the Planned Parenthood nearest you, call:
800-230-PLAN
http://www.ppfa.org/ppfa

CONTRACEPTION — STERILIZATION

Tubal sterilization is a surgical procedure that involves the cutting or blocking of the fallopian tubes in order to prevent eggs from entering the uterus. With the tubes blocked, there is no way the ovum (egg cell) and sperm can join in the fallopian tubes, thus effectively preventing pregnancy. Sterilization is intended to be a permanent form of birth control and is, in fact, the most widely used form of birth control in the United States. Surgical sterilization is 99.6 to 99.8 percent effective, with the small percentage of failure attributed to surgical error, regrowth of the fallopian tubes, or pregnancy before sterilization.

The advantages of permanent sterilization are freedom from birth control and pregnancy and a one-time cost. The procedure may be planned after a cesarean section or after abortion. However, women should keep in mind that sterilization does not protect against sexually transmitted infections and that reversal may be impossible.

CHOOSING STERILIZATION

Because surgical sterilization is a permanent form of birth control, it is usually the choice of women who already have children and do not want to have any more. For this reason, most women who undergo the procedure are usually past 30 years of age.

Sterilization is available to women of all ages, but because its effects are permanent, it is not recommended for young women, women without children, and women who are not absolutely sure they do not want more children. Women who are having marital or other problems should reconsider sterilization; the number one reason given by women wanting to reverse the surgery is remarriage and the desire for another child with the new partner.

PROCEDURE

There are several different procedures used to perform sterilization. The practitioner may use laparoscopy, mini-laparotomy, culdoscopy, colpotomy, or laparotomy to reach the site of the fallopian tubes, then clamp, clip, cut, or tie them off. The tubes can be blocked, or occluded, through cauterization (burning) or through the attachment of spring clips or elastic bands. Hysterectomy, surgical removal of the uterus, also results in sterilization. However, because of the risk of side effects and complications of hysterectomy, it should not be used for sterilization alone.

All of the procedures take 10 to 45 minutes and can be done under general or local anesthesia, usually in a hospital setting. Either an obstetrician-gynecologist or a specially trained general surgeon can perform surgical sterilization. A board-certified specialist, if available, is likely to give better results than a surgeon who is not certified.

Laparoscopy. In this procedure, which is the most commonly used technique, a long, slender, telescope-like instrument called a laparoscope is inserted through a small incision at the bottom edge of the navel. This instrument allows the surgeon to see the internal organs,

STERILIZATION FOR MEN

Vasectomy, sterilization for men, blocks the vasa deferentia, the small tubes on either side of the scrotum that carry sperm into the penis. The method is 99.8 percent effective and carries less risk of complications and less recovery time than any form of sterilization for women. Vasectomy also tends to be less expensive than sterilization for women.

In a vasectomy, the practitioner—usually a urologist—injects a local anesthetic. Each vas deferens is then located and tied off, cauterized (burned), or blocked. If an incision is made, it heals in a matter of days. There is little or no scarring in most cases. Masculinity and the ability to become erect are not affected by vasectomy.

After a vasectomy, sperm is still produced in the body, and the man will continue to have orgasms and ejaculate. However, the sperm (which makes up only 2 to 5 percent of the semen) is not ejaculated. Side effects, which occur rarely, include swelling, pain, infection at the wound site, and skin discoloration.

Because sperm are still contained in the semen in a man's reproductive tract at the time of the operation, other birth control methods should be used after vasectomy until all the sperm is gone from the ejaculate. Sperm are usually cleared from the seminal fluid after about 15 ejaculations. In rare cases, a vas deferens may reconnect. Follow-up sperm analyses are done by the practitioner to be sure the sperm count is zero.

including the fallopian tubes. To make viewing easier, gas is pumped into the abdomen to lift the skin and other tissues away from the organs.

Through another small incision the surgeon can insert a long, slender instrument specially designed for sterilization. It can be used to clamp and apply a ring to each of the tubes.

Culdoscopy or Colpotomy. In a culdoscopy, an incision is made in the vagina just below the cervix. An instrument called a culdoscope is used to view the internal organs. This instrument, which has a light on the end, is inserted through the incision. The tubes are located, then clipped, blocked, or tied and cut. No scar is visible, but because the vagina contains more bacteria, there is a greater risk of infection.

In a colpotomy, an incision is made in the vagina, and the tubes are located and closed off without the aid of a visualizing instrument.

Laparotomy. For this procedure, a longer incision is made in the abdomen. The surgeon cuts the muscle layers of the abdomen and finds and separates the fallopian tubes from the other organs. Each tube is then tied and cut. A laparotomy is performed only when previous surgery has left scars that could interfere with a simpler procedure. The operation requires general or spinal anesthesia.

Mini-Laparotomy. This procedure is similar to a laparotomy but does not involve a large abdominal incision. First, the surgeon inserts a slender surgical tool (called an elevator) into the vagina to locate the incision site. This is done by finding the top of the uterus and pushing it up toward the outside of the body. About a one-inch incision is made in the abdomen near the top of the uterus. Each fallopian tube is lifted out through the incision, is tied and cut, and is then replaced through the incision.

RISKS AND SIDE EFFECTS

Some women may experience vaginal bleeding and some discomfort in the incision for a day or two following the procedure. If the procedure involves an incision in the vagina, intercourse must be avoided for four to six weeks to prevent infection. Women undergoing laparoscopic sterilization may experience bloating or mild pain in the abdomen, shoulder, or rib cage area for a few days. This is from the carbon dioxide gas that is used in laparoscopic procedures.

Other rare complications are cardiac irregularity caused by injecting the carbon dioxide, injury to the intestines or connective tissue (during surgery), and bleeding. Laparoscopic sterilization may infrequently change some women's menstrual periods for the worse, possibly because a change in the blood supply to the ovaries during the surgery can cause impaired ovarian functions. Rarely, laparoscopic procedures may result in cardiac arrest due to gas embolism or an anesthetic problem.

Rarely, pregnancies occur after sterilization. Of pregnancies that occur after sterilization, about 50 percent are ectopic. An ectopic pregnancy is a life-threatening condition that occurs when a fertilized egg implants outside of the uterus. It can cause severe abdominal pain and bleeding, both vaginally and in the abdomen. Other possible complications of sterilization are pelvic inflammatory disease (PID) and infection, especially when the incision is made through the vagina.

REVERSAL

The surgery can be reversed in some cases through microsurgery (a process that uses a surgical microscope). The surgeon sutures the ends of the fallopian tubes, once again joining them together. The rate of pregnancy is highest during the first year following the reversal and decreases after that (for as-yet-unexplained reasons). Young women with a regular pattern of ovulation and menstruation have the greatest chance of successful reversal. The success of the operation depends more upon which procedure was used for sterilization than on how long it has been since the procedure was performed. Women who have been sterilized by cauterization have the lowest chance of having a successful reversal because this procedure destroys a portion of the tube, making it impossible to rejoin.

SEE colposcopy; contraception; hysterectomy; laparoscopy.

For more information on sterilization, contact:

Access to Voluntary and Safe Contraception International (AVSC International)
79 Madison Avenue, 7th floor
New York, NY 10016
212-561-8000
http://www.avsc.org

National Women's Health Network
514 10th St., N.W., Suite 400
Washington, DC 20004
202-347-1140

Planned Parenthood Federation of America, Inc.
810 Seventh Avenue
New York, NY 10019
For the Planned Parenthood nearest you, call:
800-230-PLAN
http://www.ppfa.org/ppfa

COSMETIC AND RECONSTRUCTIVE SURGERY

Plastic surgery is the alteration of a part of the body done in order to improve appearance or repair a disfigurement. When a procedure is done only for aesthetic reasons—for example, to improve appearance, minimize the effects of aging, or sculpt a facial or body feature—it is known as **cosmetic surgery.** If the procedure is being done in order to repair injuries or disfigurement, it is known as **reconstructive surgery.** According to a survey of the members of the American Society of Plastic and Reconstructive Surgery, 86 percent of all cosmetic procedures done in 1992 were performed on women.

Women often undergo cosmetic surgery in order to improve their own self-image. While it

QUESTIONS TO ASK

A plastic surgeon should answer all of your questions about the procedure and discuss with you your motivations and expectations. The surgeon should fully explain possible complications, alternatives to surgery, and potential outcomes. A high-pressure surgeon who assures you that nothing will go wrong should be avoided. A second opinion can be obtained before undergoing a procedure. Since most insurance plans do not cover cosmetic surgery (though they may cover reconstructive surgery), costs and payment methods should also be explained.

Questions to ask your surgeon include:

■ What training do you have in the procedure I want? How many of these types of procedures do you perform in a year?

■ Are you board-certified in surgery?

■ How safe is the operation? What are the possible side effects and complications?

■ How long will the effects of the treatment last?

■ What are the risks and benefits of the surgery?

■ Where can the operation take place? In the office? In a hospital?

■ What will happen to me before, during, and after the procedure? Are my expectations of the surgery realistic?

■ What are your fees? In what ways can I pay?

■ Will my insurance cover all or part of the costs of the procedure?

■ Can I contact your former patients to learn more?

can be helpful in increasing self-confidence and can produce radical changes in appearance, such surgery is not a solution to deeper emotional and psychological problems. When considering plastic surgery, it is important to think not only about desired looks, risks, costs, and proper medical care but also about personal motives. A woman should also consider the social issues of cosmetic surgery. While it is a widely accepted practice in the United States, most women do not admit to having the procedures done and try to hide postoperative effects, such as swelling and bruising. In addition, cosmetic surgery does not stop the aging process, and in many cases, its effects are not permanent.

A board-certified plastic surgeon can be found by consulting the *Official ABMS Directory of Board Certified Medical Specialists,* published by Marquis Who's Who, which is available in most libraries. Board certification can be verified by calling the American Board of Medical Specialties at 800-776-CERT. Friends and a regular practitioner are also good sources for recommendations.

For the best results, a woman contemplating cosmetic surgery should be in good physical condition and close to her desired weight. Women who smoke or who have hypertension are more likely to develop **hematomas** (swellings containing blood) after surgery.

The most common types of plastic surgery, along with descriptions of the procedures and possible complications, are listed below.

Cheek implants (malar augmentation). This procedure is performed to alter the cheekbones, adding "high cheekbones," which give definition to the face. Incision is usually made between the upper gums and the cheek. The soft cheek tissue is elevated and a pocket created over the cheekbone. The implant is slipped through the incision. Implants are made of medical-grade plastic.

Possible complications: Infection; implant may slip; implant may be visible in thin individuals; scars may be visible.

Chin augmentation or reduction (mentoplasty). Surgery done to alter the appearance of the chin. A small incision is made inside the mouth, between the lower lip and gum, or in the small crease under the chin. The bone and cartilage are shaved off, or an implant made from semisolid, spongelike, or mesh synthetic material is put in place. Augmentation can be done at the time of nose surgery, using an implant of removed nasal cartilage.

Possible complications: Facial paralysis or loss of sensitivity; inserted material may slip; nerve damage to the lower lip.

Collagen or fat injections. Wrinkles can be reduced and lips can be made fuller by injecting collagen or fat. Liquid silicone is also sometimes offered; however, it has not been approved by the Food and Drug Administration and should not be used. Injections must be repeated every six months. Side effects include temporary swelling and redness, which may take up to 10 days to subside.

Possible complications: Allergic reaction; excessive fullness; irregular appearance. Wrinkles recur as aging process continues.

Ear surgery (otoplasty). This procedure is usually done to alter protruding ears. An incision is made in back of the ear, in the crease where the ear joins the back of the head, and a small amount of skin and cartilage is removed.

The ideal age for the procedure is five to six, after the ear has stopped forming, though it can be performed at any later time.

Possible complications: Hematomas (swellings containing blood); infection; scarring; recurrence or reappearance of protrusion, causing the need for further surgery.

Eyelid lift (blepharoplasty). This procedure removes excess skin from the upper eyelid or protruding fatty tissue from the lower eyelid. Excess skin in the upper lid is removed through an incision in the natural crease above the eye. Fatty tissue in the lower lid is removed through an incision just below the lower eyelid. The bruising can last for several weeks.

Possible complications: Temporary blurred vision; visible scar; constant dry eyes; excessive tear production; eye injury; an increase in small blood vessels; hematomas (swellings containing blood).

Face-lift (rhytidectomy). Sagging skin and underlying facial muscles are lifted and repositioned. Excess skin and fat are removed. Incisions usually begin in temple hair above and in front of the ear, and extend down in front of the ear, around the ear lobe, up behind the ear, and backward into the hair of the scalp. Bruising and swelling are visible for several weeks after surgery, and surgical drains are sometimes inserted to remove blood and fluid that collect under the skin.

Possible complications: Hematomas (swellings containing blood); hair loss around the incision; heavy scarring; paralysis or loss of sensation in the face; loss of a mass of dead skin caused by lack of blood to the surgical site.

Forehead lift (coronal lift). This procedure improves drooping or heavy eyebrows and permanently furrowed brow. The incision is made across the hairline. The forehead and brows are lifted and redraped upward, and the resulting excess skin is removed. Surgical drains may be inserted to remove blood and other fluid.

Possible complications: Hematomas (swellings containing blood); development of excess scar tissue; infection; permanent patches of numbness.

Liposuction (suction-assisted lipectomy). The procedure is done to remove pockets of fat. The deposits are sucked out of small incisions through plastic tubing into collection bottles. This method is used for removing fat from thigh, buttock, hip, abdomen, upper arm, and chin.

Possible complications: Rippling, dimpling, or sagging skin; embolism (blockage of a blood vessel caused by a blood clot carried through the bloodstream); infection. Fat may be regained. Very rarely, embolism may cause death.

Nose surgery (rhinoplasty). The size or shape (appearance) of the nose is changed by removing or inserting bone and cartilage through inci-sions hidden inside the rim of the nostrils. The procedure is done under local or general anesthesia and can result in swollen, bruised eyelids, and some numbness for several weeks. The ideal age for the procedure is over 15 for girls, if bone growth is complete.

Possible complications: Bleeding from the nose; formation of excessive scar tissue; poor cosmetic result; difficulty breathing through nose.

Tummy tuck (abdominoplasty). A procedure to remove excess skin from the abdomen. Under general anesthesia, an incision is made in the shape of a "W" running from side to side and across the lower part of the abdomen. Excess fat and skin are removed, and a drain may be inserted to remove blood and liquefied fat. A girdle is worn for six weeks after the operation until healing takes place. Scars can be significant.

Possible complications: Bleeding and hematomas (swellings containing blood); loss of a mass of dead skin or tissue because of infection.

SEE aging; board certification; breast surgery; second opinion; skin.

For more information on cosmetic and reconstructive surgery, contact:

American Society of Plastic and Reconstructive Surgeons
444 E. Algonquin Rd.
Arlington Heights, IL 60005
800-635-0635
http://www.plasticsurgery.org

Facial Plastic Surgery Information Service
1110 Vermont Ave., N.W., Suite 220
Washington, DC 20005
800-332-3223

CRYOSURGERY

Cryosurgery, sometimes called cryotherapy, is the destruction of abnormal cells through freezing. It is commonly used to remove warts on the vulva as well as abnormal cells in the cervix or vagina. It is also used for the removal of warts, moles, lesions on the skin, and hemorrhoids (varicose veins on the anus). During brain and eye surgery, it may be used for delicate procedures.

The technique uses liquid nitrogen or carbon dioxide to freeze the abnormal cells. Cryosurgery is easier, less painful, and causes much less damage to tissue than the more traditional procedure of cauterization, which burns away abnormal tissue. However, for cervical disease, cryosurgery may be more destructive than electrosurgery, a procedure that uses an electric current to cut and seal tissue.

REASONS FOR CRYOSURGERY

Cryosurgery is used to treat:
- Benign growths of the cervix
- Warts and moles, including precancerous and cancerous lesions, and those warts located on the vulva and vagina
- Hemorrhoids
- Endometriosis involving the cervix or vagina
- Severe cervical infections

PROCEDURE

The procedure takes only about five minutes and can be done in a practitioner's office. If the cryosurgery is to be done on the cervix, vagina, or vulva, it should be scheduled shortly after the menstrual period so that healing can take place before menstruation begins again.

A handheld, metal-tipped instrument called a cryoprobe is used to freeze any abnormal tissue. The probe, which is cooled with liquid nitrogen or carbon dioxide, is held against the affected area for about two minutes. Once the tissue is thoroughly frozen, the probe is removed. Mild cramping as well as a cold sensation in the vagina may occur during such procedures.

RISKS AND SIDE EFFECTS

Complications are rare, but bleeding and infection can occur. Side effects from cryosurgery performed on the cervix or vagina include spotting, cramping, swelling, and tenderness. Some women also experience a persistent watery discharge and temporary changes in the cervical mucus.

After cervical cryosurgery, it is recommended a woman not douche, use tampons, or have sexual intercourse for two to three weeks to allow the cervix to heal and to minimize the risk of infection. Pap tests will be inaccurate and difficult to interpret until the cervix is healed and the surface cells have regrown.

DES daughters (women whose mothers took diethylstilbestrol, a drug widely prescribed to pregnant women between 1941 and 1971 to prevent miscarriage) sometimes experience serious after effects from cervical cryosurgery, including narrowing of the cervical canal. This can cause problems during menstruation and childbirth.

DEATH AND DYING

Death and dying are no longer issues that are faced only by the elderly and their families. With the increase in cases of AIDS and cancer, the issues of dying with dignity, the right to die, and the stress of losing a loved one have become important to young and old alike. When a person's quality of life has greatly diminished and medical treatment only delays death, the question of how far medical treatment should go arises. Women, who are traditionally in the role of caretaker, must often be responsible for difficult decisions made on behalf of dying family members. How does one legally guarantee that his or her wishes about medical treatment will be followed? How do family members provide a comfortable environment for their loved one? And, finally, how do family members face the grief of their loss?

THE DEFINITION OF DEATH

Thirty years ago, death seemed simple to define. When the heart stopped, breathing stopped, and the eyes dilated, a person was considered dead.

Today, the definition of death involves four specific points: lack of movement; inability to breathe without a respirator; unresponsiveness to stimuli; and absence of reflexes. This means there must be an irreversible loss of brain functions, including the functions of the **brain stem,** a part of the brain where no communication or thought processes exist. By this definition, a person with brain damage that has diminished cognitive thought and awareness may still be considered alive if the brain stem (which controls reflex functions such as breathing) is still working. This state, called persistent vegetative state, or PVS, is also called cognitive death, yet it does not fall under the legal definition of death.

The revolution of intensive care has also changed the definition of death. Technology enables artificial ventilation, artificial circulation, and intravenous feeding. Dialysis machines allow the elimination of waste products. In other words, the machines used in the intensive-care unit can keep a body alive by performing its usual, basic functions.

RIGHT-TO-DIE ISSUES

As the definition of death becomes more encompassing and complicated, many people fear they will lose control over the quality of their lives. Right-to-die issues center around the legal right to reject mechanical life support and the right to define the limits of medical treatment. In other words, these issues are concerned with the right to refuse treatment and the right to be allowed to die. A woman can protect her right to die with documents called **advance directives.**

Generally, advance directives are written statements or documents that state how a person would want medical decisions to be made should she become incapacitated. The two most common forms of advance directives are a living will and durable power of attorney for health care.

LIVING WILL

A living will is a directive or declaration that expresses a person's desires and wishes as to the type of medical care she wants (or doesn't want) if she becomes unable to make her own decisions. Preprinted forms may be filled out, or the statement of preferences can simply be written down. Each state has its own laws regarding living wills. A woman should ask her attorney or practitioner any specific questions.

The living will should illustrate an understanding of the technology and medical treatment a person would or would not want to use to sustain her life. The woman should also make clear what treatments she wants or does not want under any circumstances. In other words, the intent must be made perfectly clear. For example, a woman could decide whether or not to be put on a respirator, receive emergency resuscitation, intravenous feeding, or dialysis. Although a person cannot predict every possible circumstance, it is important that she define her boundaries and what outside limits she wants to place on medical treatment.

While a living will can help express intentions regarding health care, it still has its shortcomings. It can leave room for legal, ethical, medical, and personal-value uncertainties; and it is limited by the laws that govern it in each state. In addition to drawing a living will, it is a good idea to also consider appointing someone durable power of attorney.

On the next page is an example of a living will for the state of Florida. (Contact Choice in Dying at 800-989-WILL to receive a free copy of the appropriate advance directives for a particular state.)

THE PATIENT SELF-DETERMINATION ACT

The Patient Self-Determination Act, a federal law that went into effect December 1991, requires workers at all federally funded institutions, including hospitals, health maintenance organizations, hospices, skilled nursing facilities, or facilities accepting Medicare or Medicaid, to inform patients of their right to establish an advance directive. No state agency presides over advance directives, but the institution itself should be able to explain your state's provisions. Institutions with their own ethical or moral codes, however, may impose restrictions on your treatment and your advance directive. Before admission, ask about the institution's policies.

DURABLE POWER OF ATTORNEY FOR HEALTH CARE

The durable power of attorney is a document by which a person can transfer certain legal authority to someone else. Unlike the power of attorney, it has no time limit. Therefore, if a woman becomes incompetent due to sudden illness or injury, the person to whom she has assigned the durable power of attorney can make health-care decisions for her.

On pages 159-160 is an example of a form used to designate a health-care agent in the state of Florida. (Contact Choice in Dying at 800-989-WILL to receive a free copy of appropriate advance directives for a particular state.)

These types of health-care decisions are not limited to life-sustaining treatments. The person who makes the decision is known as an agent. He or she communicates directly with a health-

(continued on page 161)

FLORIDA LIVING WILL

Instructions	

Print the date.

Print your name.

Declaration made this _____ day of _____, 19____. I,

_____, willfully
and voluntarily make known any desire that my dying not be artificially
prolonged under the circumstances set forth below, and I do hereby
declare:

If at any time I have a terminal condition and if my attending or treating
physician and another consulting physician have determined that there is
no medical probability of my recovery from such condition, I direct that
life-prolonging procedures be withheld or withdrawn when the application
of such procedures would serve only to prolong artificially the process of
dying, and that I be permitted to die naturally with only the administration
of medication or the performance of any medical procedure deemed necessary to provide me with comfort care or to alleviate pain.

It is my intention that this declaration be honored by my family and physician as the final expression of my legal right to refuse medical or surgical
treatment and to accept the consequences for such refusal.

In the event that I have been determined to be unable to provide express
and informed consent regarding the withholding, withdrawal, or continua-
tion of life-prolonging procedures, I wish to designate, as my surrogate to
carry out the provisions of this declaration:

**Print the name,
home address, and
telephone number
of your surrogate.**

Name: _____

Address:_____

_____ Zip Code: _____

Phone: _____

© 1995
Choice in Dying, Inc.

(continued on page 158)

(continued from page 157)

Print the name, home address, and telephone number of your alternate surrogate.	I wish to designate the following person as my alternate surrogate, to carry out the provisions of this declaration should my surrogate be unwilling or unable to act on my behalf: Name: _____ Address: _____ _____ Zip Code: _____ Phone: _____
Add personal instructions (if any).	Additional instructions (optional): I understand the full import of this declaration, and I am emotionally and mentally competent to make this declaration.
Sign the document.	Signed:_____

Witnessing Procedure
 	
Two witnesses must sign and print their addresses.
	Witness 1:
	
	    Signed:_____
	
	    Address:_____
	
	Witness 2:
	
	    Signed:_____
	
	    Address:_____

© 1995 Choice in Dying, Inc.	

SAMPLE

Source: Choice in Dying. Reprinted by permission of Choice in Dying, 200 Varick St., New York, NY 10014; 800-989-WILL.

FLORIDA DESIGNATION OF HEALTH-CARE SURROGATE

Instructions	

Print your name.

Name: _____

(Last)   (First)   (Middle Initial)

In the event that I have been determined to be incapacitated to provide informed consent for medical treatment and surgical and diagnostic procedures, I wish to designate as my surrogate for health-care decisions:

Print the name, home address, and telephone number of your surrogate.

Name: _____
Address: _____
_____ Zip Code: _____
Phone: _____

If my surrogate is unwilling or unable to perform his/her duties, I wish to designate as my alternate surrogate:

Print the name, home address, and telephone number of your alternate surrogate.

Name: _____
Address: _____
_____ Zip Code: _____
Phone: _____

I fully understand that this designation will permit my designee to make health-care decisions and to provide, withhold, or withdraw consent on my behalf; to apply for public benefits to defray the cost of health care; and to authorize my admission to or transfer from a health-care facility.

© 1995
Choice in Dying, Inc.

(continued on page 160)

159

(continued from page 159)

Add personal
instructions
(if any).

Print the
names and
addresses of
those who you
want to keep
copies of this
document.

Sign and date the
document.

Witnessing
Procedure

Two witnesses
must sign and
print their
addresses.

© 1995
Choice in Dying, Inc.

Additional instructions (optional):

I further affirm that this designation is not being made as a condition or admission to a health-care facility. I will notify and send a copy of this document to the following persons other than my surrogate, so they may know who my surrogate is:

Name: _____

Address: _____

Name: _____

Address: _____

SAMPLE

Signed: _____

Date: _____

Witness 1:

    Signed:_____

    Address:_____

Witness 2:

    Signed:_____

    Address:_____

Source: Choice in Dying. Reprinted by permission of Choice in Dying, 200 Varick St., New York, NY 10014; 800-989-WILL.

care provider and acts on behalf of the person. The instructions an agent provides a practitioner, since they are expressed in person and considered in light of the practitioner's input, can hold greater weight than those wishes outlined in a living will. A living will, however, is a strong tool to outline wishes to an agent.

A woman must choose her agent carefully and only after family members have agreed to be supportive of the agent's authority and the individual's wishes. In many cases, those with durable power of attorney renege on their agreement to stand by the wishes outlined in the living will.

DO NOT RESUSCITATE ORDER

A "do not resuscitate order" (called a DNR order) means that cardiopulmonary resuscitative measures (CPR) will not be started or carried out should respiration or heartbeat fail. These orders also mean that the patient will not be placed on long-term mechanical life-support equipment.

It is important to talk with the attending physician about a DNR order before admission to a hospital, if possible. A person should discuss the matter with family members so they are aware of her wishes, and document a DNR order in a living will. The information should also be discussed with whoever holds the durable power of attorney. No matter how important a DNR order may seem under certain circumstances, it can be revoked if the woman changes her mind. In this case, the decision should be documented as well.

ASSISTED SUICIDE

The right-to-die issues have also given rise to the assisted-suicide controversy. Assisted suicide, which requires consent on the part of the dying person, should not be confused with refusing treatment or being allowed to die (euthanasia), which does not require the person's consent. Also called aid-in-dying, assisted suicide is the actual assistance in causing death, providing the means to stop the heart from beating, the lungs from breathing, and the entire brain from having any activity, perhaps through drugs.

Physicians are not legally able to assist in assisted suicide, such as with a lethal injection, because these suicides are criminal acts. The Hippocratic oath, under which most physicians swear to protect life, ethically prevents them from taking part and disallows them from intentionally causing death. (Some physicians today—some 20 percent of this generation of doctors—do not take the oath because they disagree with some of the concepts of it.) The Hemlock Society, a national organization that supports assisted suicide, is proposing a bill that would let physicians and nurses legally provide aid-in-dying measures to terminally ill patients. Thirteen states have also introduced aid-in-dying legislation that would allow legal options for those who are dying.

WILLS

While a living will outlines wishes about medical treatment, a will provides specific instructions about how to distribute or dispose of assets, property, and debts after death. It can also include information on how a spouse or child should be taken care of. There are three basic types of wills.

The **regular,** or **statutory, will** is a will that is written up and signed under the normal manner when the maker has had time to think out each term. It is written, not oral, and it is not written under an unusual circumstance or emergency.

THE DEATH WITH DIGNITY ACT

A group of organizations and individuals concerned about the right-to-die legislation in the state of Oregon has created and proposed the Oregon Death with Dignity Act, which would permit physician aid-in-dying for the terminally ill in that state. The act:

■ Permits a competent terminally ill adult the right to request and receive physician aid-in-dying under carefully defined circumstances.

■ Protects physicians from liability in carrying out a patient's request.

■ Combines the concepts of Natural Death Acts and Durable Power of Attorney for Health Care laws and makes them more usable.

■ Permits a patient to appoint an attorney to be reviewed by a hospital ethics or other committee before the decision is acted upon by the physician.

■ Allows a competent adult person to take advantage of the law by signing a Death with Dignity directive.

■ Requires hospitals and other health-care facilities to keep records and report to the Department of Health Services after the death of the patient, with the records remaining anonymous.

■ Permits a treating physician to order a psychiatric consultation, with the patient's consent, if there is any question about the patient's competence to make the request for aid-in-dying.

■ Forbids aid-in-dying to any patient solely because he or she is a burden to anyone, or because the patient is incompetent or terminal and has not made out an informed and proper Death with Dignity directive.

■ Forbids aiding, abetting, and encouraging a suicide, which remains a crime under the act.

■ Does not permit aid-in-dying to be administered by a loved one, family member, or stranger.

■ Forbids aid-in-dying for children, incompetents, or anyone who has not voluntarily and intentionally completed and signed the properly witnessed Death with Dignity directive.

■ Attempts to keep the decision-making process with the patient and health-care provider, and out of court.

■ Makes special protective provisions for patients with skilled-nursing facilities.

■ Permits physicians, nurses, and privately owned hospitals the right to decline a dying patient's request for aid-in-dying if they are morally or ethically opposed to such action.

For more information on right-to-die legislation, contact the Hemlock Society, an organization formed in 1980 to campaign for the right of a terminally ill patient to choose voluntary euthanasia. For a small fee, the organization can also supply you with forms for advance directives.

The **holographic, or olographic, will** is a will that is written and signed by the maker, in his or her own handwriting. It is commonly used by soldiers and sailors in active service. Only 25 states recognize holographic wills, and they must meet specific conditions.

The **nuncupative will** is an oral will that is made by an oral declaration, rather than writing. It must be made in front of witnesses, and it must be written down by a witness within a few days after it was made. This type of will is acceptable under certain special circumstances, such as when the maker is under imminent danger or extreme emergency and he or she dies as a direct result.

The first type of will is the most useful and desirable. It is an important part of estate planning, whether the maker is single or married, young or old. Without a will, wishes may not be carried out. A person will need a will to distribute property (even property that might have been forgotten), to designate a personal guardian for any children, and to appoint an "executor," who administers and represents the total estate.

COPING WITH DEATH

At death, there is a profound emptiness for those who experience the loss. This happens even when the death is expected. No matter what the circumstance, the loss of a loved one can come as quite a shock. The feelings of loneliness, loss, anger, or disbelief may be overwhelming.

You may feel that you are moving in slow motion, or you may find that you experience swings in mood and energy. You may be seized by erotic impulses or urges for high-risk activities. You may also experience physical symptoms related to stress, such as diarrhea, shortness of breath, and an upset stomach.

During this time, it is important that you take care of yourself to help you deal with the stress.

■ If a loved one dies in a hospital or at home, consider letting loved ones say their good-byes before having the body removed. In the hours that follow death, the body feels cold and the color pales, but the facial expressions soften with a peaceful look. This can help the process of grieving and recognizing love for the person.

■ Be sure to keep warm, as the shock of your loss may cause your body temperature to lower; you may be more susceptible to colds and flu.

■ Get plenty of rest. Sit or lie down as often as possible. Even if you don't fall asleep, closing your eyes will help calm your body for just a few minutes.

■ Keep up your nutrition and avoid alcohol and caffeine, as they will only add to your stress.

■ Practice some deep breathing. When we are under stress, we tend to hold our breath, which can make us tired and anxious. Close your eyes for a moment and breathe deeply; inhale through your nose and exhale through your mouth. Imagine inhaling new, cleansing air and exhaling old air.

■ Finally, let others help and care for you. Let friends and family make meals for you, draw warm baths, and give you neck massages. More important, let them listen to you talk about your deceased loved one and your feelings. Remember, friends and family need to show you their support; it is a gift they want to give you out of their love for you.

If a person dies without making a will (this is called dying intestate), all property would automatically be passed to relatives according to the court's formula. Without a will, the court appoints an executor and a guardian for children. It may be that the deceased would never personally consider the person appointed by the court (who may be an irresponsible child or an unfaithful spouse) for the responsibility.

A will can be drawn up using standard forms or customized with the help of an attorney. There is also a large selection of books and computer programs that can help to make a will that is legal and complete.

GRIEF

Grief following the loss of a parent, child, partner, or friend is a normal reaction to death and other irrevocable separations. American society tends to minimize the grief process; however, it is important to health and well-being to acknowledge losses. Rather than being something a person needs to "get over" in order to get on with life, grief is part of an ongoing healing process that colors a person's life for years or a lifetime. Grief may be a feeling of numbness, intense sadness, disbelief, or anger. As the fact of the loss becomes accepted, mourning

THE EMOTIONAL STAGES OF DEATH

Those who are terminally ill, as well as their loved ones, must come to terms emotionally with death and dying. Physician and psychiatrist Elisabeth Kubler-Ross, an expert on death, categorized the stages a terminally ill person goes through when faced with death. These stages do not always occur in order, and they often overlap. Moreover, a recent loss may revive various stages of grief related to previous losses. Other people dealing with the loss, or impending loss, of a loved one also go through similar emotions.

Stage 1: Denial and isolation. Faced with death, terminally ill people often deny that it is true and refuse to talk about the situation. Often they withdraw from friends and family. This is considered a natural defense to a painful situation.

Stage 2: Anger. A "why me?" attitude is displayed at this stage. Anger is often displaced—family members, nurses, and physicians are targets for harsh words and accusations.

Stage 3: Bargaining. In this stage, which is usually brief, the terminally ill person pleads for time, usually in exchange for good behavior. For example, a woman may pray that she will be "a better person" if only she could live to see her child's wedding.

Stage 4: Depression. When the reality and inevitability of death sets in, and the effects of the illness become apparent (such as hair loss from chemotherapy, loss of a job, or decreased function), depression sets in. During this stage, discussion of death is positive—a person should be encouraged to accept the situation.

Stage 5: Acceptance. At this stage, the person is neither angry nor depressed about death. While acceptance is not a happy stage, it provides rest and peace before death. It should not be considered "giving up hope."

recedes to a far less dominant role in life.

For some, the experience of grief is complicated by feelings of guilt, self-blame, or other overwhelming emotions. Physical illness or addiction to drugs or alcohol can complicate the grieving process. For those who have difficulty coming to terms with death or other loss, friends, members of the clergy, or bereavement counselors may be able to provide the support needed to work through grief.

A caregiver may experience what is called **anticipatory grief;** that is, grieving the loss of a loved one even though he or she has not yet died. Anticipatory grief can be elicited by the loss of the loved one's individual characteristics—his or her sense of humor, ability to manage affairs, or even simple physical skills. It can also be caused by the simple knowledge that a loved one is approaching death.

Anticipatory grief can be an emotionally difficult stage in caregiving. It comes at a time when the caregiver, and perhaps the loved one, know that death is near. It is part of the detachment process, the realization that this person will not be here for much longer. Although many people feel they should not allow themselves to grieve because their loved one is not yet gone, it is common and natural to do so. Some nursing homes and many hospices give anticipatory-grief counseling.

SEE aging; long-term care; medical rights.

For more information on grief, contact:

Living/Dying Project
75 Digital Dr.
Novato, CA 94949
415-884-2343

St. Francis Center
5135 MacArthur Blvd., N.W.
Washington, DC 20016
202-363-8500

For more information on death and dying issues, contact:

Choice in Dying, Inc.
200 Varick St.
New York, NY 10014
800-989-WILL
212-366-5540
http://www.choices.org

National Hemlock Society
P.O. Box 101810
Denver, CO 80250-1018
800-247-7421
http://www.hemlock.org/hemlock

National Hospice Organization
1901 N. Moore St., Suite 901
Arlington, VA 22209
703-243-5900
http://www.nho.org

DEPRESSION

Depression is a common condition that affects one in 20 Americans each year, and twice as many women as men. Depression, characterized by intense feelings of sadness, frustration, helplessness, and despair, is a clinical disorder requiring intervention and treatment. While most individuals experience symptoms of depression at times, clinical depression is not a passing blue mood. Without treatment, symptoms can last for weeks or years. However, appropriate treatment can help over 80 percent of those suffering from depression, according to the National Institute of Mental Health.

Some experts believe that women experience depression more often than men because of the psychosocial issues that they are likely to face. These factors include poverty, a bad marriage or relationship, absence of a partner, and being homebound with young children. Of the people living below the poverty line, 75 percent are women and children. Women also suffer a greater share of violence, ranging from childhood sexual abuse to rape and battering.

Premenstrual syndrome (PMS) may be an atypical form of depression in some women. Though it may cause temporary irritability and depression, it is not a source of ongoing clinical depression. Women with depression often have intensified flare-ups before their menstrual period begins each month.

Further, menopause has not been shown to be a source of depression in women, though the two were once thought to be linked because some menopausal symptoms, such as insomnia, fatigue, and irritability, are the same as some depressive symptoms. In fact, research suggests that many women find menopause, with its freedom from menstruation and contraception, liberating.

Depression is also common among older adults. One-third of people with Alzheimer's disease are clinically depressed. Depression is also attributed to difficulty adjusting to retirement, chronic ill health, financial hardship, and loss of purpose. Some medications, such as those used to lower blood pressure or relieve arthritis, may trigger depression.

CAUSES OF DEPRESSION

Depression can be triggered by life events, physiological changes within the body, or a combination of these two factors. When depression is linked to painful events, such as the breakup of a marriage or loss of a job, it is categorized as **psychological depression.** Symptoms are commonly psychological and emotional, though biological functioning also may be affected. People with low self-esteem, who are pessimistic and prone to stress, are at risk of developing psychological depression.

Biological depression is triggered by physiological events within the body rather than by painful experiences. It is accompanied by a variety of symptoms caused by chemical imbalances in the nervous and hormonal systems. Some conditions that can trigger biological depression are AIDS, heart disease, diabetes, allergies, chemical sensitivities, malnutrition, cancer, and influenza. Heredity is thought to play a role in biological depression (especially manic-depressive disorder), though it may occur in people who do not have a family history of depression.

TYPES OF DEPRESSION

Major depressive disorder is the most common form of clinical depression, characterized by symptoms of severe and lasting depression. **Melancholic depression** is a serious form of major depressive disorder, in which the individual has lost all interest and pleasure in all life activities. The most severe form of major depressive disorder is **psychotic depression,** marked by delusions (false beliefs in oneself or others), hallucinations, and a permanent sad mood. As many as 15 percent of people with major depressive disorders develop psychotic depression, which carries a major risk of suicide. These conditions are all classified as **unipolar depression.**

Manic-depressive disorder is categorized as a **bipolar** form of depression because it involves alternating episodes of serious mania and depression. More than 2 million Americans suffer from manic-depressive disorder each year. On average, the manic phase lasts one to three months, with the depressive phase lasting six to nine months. Symptoms of the manic phase include high energy, increased risk-taking, extreme euphoria, obnoxious behavior, and unrealistic beliefs in one's own abilities and powers.

DIAGNOSING DEPRESSION

The American Psychiatric Association uses the following criteria to diagnose depression, which is a collection of signs and symptoms. To be clinically depressed, a person must have at least five of the symptoms listed (including the first two) for the same two-week period. The symptoms cannot be a normal reaction to the death of a loved one.

1. Depressed mood (sometimes irritability in children and adolescents) most of the day, nearly every day

2. Markedly diminished interest or pleasure in all, or almost all, activities most of the day, nearly every day

3. Significant weight loss or gain when not dieting (more than 5 percent of body weight in a month) or decrease/increase in appetite nearly every day

4. Insomnia or hypersomnia (excessive sleep) nearly every day

5. Psychomotor agitation or psychomotor retardation, an abnormal speeding up or slowing down of one's physical activities or mental processes, nearly every day, as observed by others

6. Fatigue or loss of energy nearly every day

7. Feelings of worthlessness or excessive or inappropriate guilt (which may be delusional) nearly every day (not merely self-reproach or guilt about being sick)

8. Diminished ability to think or concentrate, or indecisiveness, nearly every day

9. Recurrent thoughts of death (not just fear of dying) or of suicide without a specific plan, or a suicide attempt, or a specific plan for committing suicide

167

POSTPARTUM DEPRESSION

Some 50 to 75 percent of new mothers experience "**baby blues**," a common, mild form of depression that comes on after giving birth. Marked by periods of crying and a feeling of disappointment, the baby blues usually last for a few days or a week.

But for some women, the problem is much deeper. One in 10 women will experience varying degrees of **postpartum depression (PPD)**. The onset of most cases of PPD occurs between six and 12 weeks after delivery, but it can occur up to a year later. For most women, the condition is characterized by a feeling of extreme disappointment following giving birth, coupled with fears about caring for the newborn baby.

Symptoms of postpartum depression include:

- Anxiety and panic attacks
- Uncontrollable crying
- Extreme mood swings
- Depression and feelings of inadequacy
- Feelings of anger toward the baby or partner
- Overconcern for the baby
- Lack of interest in the baby
- Fear of harming the baby
- Withdrawal from partner and friends
- Lack of interest in sex
- Insomnia or excessive fatigue and sleep

Some experts believe that postpartum depression may be caused by physical changes after delivery, such as the sudden drop in estrogen levels in the body, other hormonal changes, and the loss of blood. Discussing depression with a support group or other parents may prevent or alleviate postpartum depression. Because it may help a woman feel more confident in the care of her child, breast-feeding is also thought to help.

If postpartum depression does not disappear within two weeks, counseling should be sought. For some women, approximately one in 1,000, depression following delivery takes the form of a more severe temporary mental illness called **postpartum psychosis**. Symptoms include confusion, hallucinations, suicidal or destructive thoughts, and possibly severe psychotic episodes. A woman may become hyperactive or may have trouble caring for her child. Some studies indicate that this form of depression is a result of an endocrine imbalance that results in high levels of estrogen and low levels of progesterone. Treatments include medication, counseling, and even hospitalization.

For more information on postpartum depression or for names of support groups, contact:

Depression After Delivery
P.O. Box 1282
Morrisville, PA 19067
800-944-4773

National Association of Postpartum Care Services
P.O. Box 284
Glen Oaks, NY 11004
800-45-DOULA

Another form of depression is **seasonal affective disorder (SAD),** which begins in the fall and lifts in the spring. SAD has been linked to dark winter days, a poorly lit office environment, and unseasonable cloudy periods. People with SAD report their depression worsens the farther north they live and the more overcast the weather. SAD symptoms include those of depression, especially fatigue, decreased sexual appetite, and social withdrawal. In addition, SAD sufferers may crave carbohydrates. SAD affects 5 percent of Americans a year, though it has been estimated that 10 to 38 percent of those with recurring mood disorders actually have SAD. Women are three to four times more likely than men to suffer from it.

TREATMENT OF DEPRESSION

The major treatments for depression are antidepressant medication (pharmacotherapy), psychotherapy, and a combination of the two. Alternative therapies, including acupuncture, herbal and homeopathic medicines, massage, and yoga, are also used to treat depression.

ANTIDEPRESSANTS

Three groups of antidepressant medications have been used to treat depressive illnesses: serotonin-specific reuptake inhibitors, tricyclics, and monoamine oxidase inhibitors. Antidepressants work by increasing levels of neurotransmitters, chemicals in the brain that aid the transmission of the electrical signals that spark the neural interactions of the mind that shape behaviors and feelings.

The effectiveness of these drugs varies; different people respond differently to different medications. They require careful monitoring by a practitioner and should never be mixed with other medications without consulting a physician.

Serotonin-specific reuptake inhibitors, or **SSRIs** (Prozac, Zoloft, Paxil), "selectively" inhibit the reabsorption of the neurotransmitter serotonin. They are usually the first drugs prescribed when treating depression. SSRIs have fewer side effects than other antidepressants. These side effects include nausea, diarrhea, anxiety, headache, and rash. Lowered sex drive, difficulty achieving orgasm, and potential erectile dysfunction are also possible, but usually temporary, side effects. SSRIs, specifically Prozac, were once thought to be linked with aggressive or violent behavior; however, there is no evidence of this.

Tricyclics, or **TCAs** (Tofranil, Elavil), also work by affecting neurotransmitters. Side effects of TCAs include dry mouth, constipation, difficulty urinating, weight gain, drowsiness, and dizziness. They may not be effective in women also taking tamoxifen, a breast cancer drug. They should be avoided during breastfeeding and pregnancy. An overdose of TCAs may be fatal.

Monoamine oxidase inhibitors, or **MAOIs** (Marplan, Nardil, Parnate), increase the levels of neurotransmitters by inhibiting the production of monoamine oxidase, an enzyme that breaks them down. Side effects of MAOIs include those of tricyclics and also rapid heartbeat and decreased interest in sex. MAOIs can react with alcohol and some foods (including aged cheese, monosodium glutamate, and figs) to cause headache, nausea, seizure, stroke, and even coma. MAOIs are usually the last choice of treatment and are most often given to those who do not respond to tricyclics.

In addition, **lithium,** another antidepressant drug, is the treatment of choice for manic-depressive illness and some forms of recurring major depression. A side effect of lithium is possible kidney and liver damage, so patients on the drug need to be monitored very carefully by a practitioner. Other possible side effects are nausea, vomiting, muscle weakness, and increased thirst and urination.

There are several other antidepressant drugs available that do not fit into these categories. They include vanlafaxine (Effexor), which functions as an SSRI, and trazodone (Desyrel), which also inhibits serotonin reuptake but is chemically different from SSRIs. Bupropion (Wellbutrin) also inhibits reuptake of neurotransmitters, though no one knows exactly how it works.

PSYCHOTHERAPIES

The two major forms of psychotherapy are psychodynamic therapy and cognitive/behavioral therapy. Most therapists practice these forms of therapy. The most effective technique varies according to the individual's personality and disorder.

Psychodynamic therapy focuses on resolving the individual's internal psychological conflicts, often thought to be rooted in childhood. This type of therapy includes **psychoanalysis,** in which the patient is encouraged to express thoughts and emotions to the practitioner. Psychodynamic therapy also includes **interpersonal therapy,** short term (10 to 20

WHO CAN HELP?

Several types of professionals can treat depressive disorders:

A **psychiatrist** is an M.D. (a doctor of medicine) or a D.O. (doctor of osteopathy) who has completed four years of medical school and a residency and who holds a general medical license. Psychiatric training emphasizes the physical causes of mental illness. Psychiatrists are most familiar with the uses of antidepressant drugs.

Psychologists have completed four years in graduate school in psychology rather than in a medical school and usually hold a Ph.D. (doctor of philosophy) or a Psy.D. (doctor of psychology). Typically, a psychologist would have a subspecialty in clinical or counseling psychology and be licensed to practice psychology. While most psychologists cannot prescribe medication, they often work with medical doctors if drugs are needed.

Primary-care physicians (internists, family physicians, pediatricians, and specialists in adolescent medicine) may be qualified to medically diagnose and treat patients with depression; severe cases are often referred to psychiatrists.

Other practitioners who treat depression are **clinical social workers,** who usually complete a two-year graduate program to obtain a master's in social work (M.S.W.), and **family therapists,** who are licensed in marital and family therapy and have a degree in that type of counseling. A depressed person may also be treated by a **psychiatric nurse specialist,** a registered nurse who has specialized training in treating mental or psychiatric disorders.

HELPING YOURSELF

Depressive illness can make you feel exhausted, worthless, helpless, and hopeless. If you are prone to bouts of depression or are working to recover, it is important to realize that these negative views are part of depression and typically do not accurately reflect your situation. To fight depression and help negative thinking to fade:

■ Do not set difficult goals or take on a great deal of responsibility.

■ Break large tasks into small ones, set some priorities, and do what you can.

■ Do not expect too much from yourself. This may lead to increased feelings of failure.

■ Try to be with other people; it is usually better than being alone.

■ Participate in activities that may make you feel better. Try going to a movie or participating in religious or social activi-ties. Don't overdo it or get upset if your mood does not improve right away. Feeling better takes time.

■ Postpone any major life decisions, such as changing jobs or getting married or divorced, until your depression has lifted. If you must make a decision, consult others who know you well and have a more objective view of your situation.

■ Do not expect to "snap out" of your depression. People rarely do. Help yourself as much as you can and do not blame yourself for not being up to par.

■ Do not accept your negative thinking. It is part of depression and will disappear as your depression responds to treatment.

Source: "Depression: What You Need to Know," a pamphlet published by the National Institute of Mental Health.

weeks) therapy specifically for depression that focuses on personal conflicts.

Cognitive and **behavioral therapies** work to help the individual correct the behaviors and emotions that lead to depression. Cognitive therapy focuses on changing negative thinking, while behavioral therapy focuses on encouraging positive behavior.

These types of therapy may be used in several settings, including **individual therapy,** treatment that involves only the patient and the therapist; **family therapy,** in which partners, parents, or children are seen together by the therapist; and **group therapy,** in which people with similar problems gather together for support and discussion.

171

For more information on depression and where to find help, contact:

American Psychological Association
Office of Public Affairs
750 First St., N.E.
Washington, DC 20002
202-336-5700
pubinterest@apa.com

Depressives Anonymous: Recovery from Depression
329 E. 62nd St.
New York, NY 10021
212-689-2600

National Foundation for Depressive Illness
P.O. Box 2257
New York, NY 10116
800-248-4344

National Institute of Mental Health
Inquiries Branch
5600 Fishers Ln.
Rockville, MD 20857

Panic Disorder Information
800-64-PANIC

Depression/Awareness, Recognition, and Treatment Program (D/ART)
800-421-4211

National Mental Health Association
1021 Prince St.
Alexandria, VA 22314-2971
800-969-6642
703-684-7722
http://www.worldcorp.com/dc-online/nmha

DIABETES

Diabetes mellitus is a condition caused by the inability of the body to handle the breakdown of carbohydrates into sugar, the fuel the body needs to function. This inability is the result of low levels of insulin (a hormone produced in the pancreas that enables the cells to remove sugar from the blood for energy) or of the body's resistance to the actions of insulin. In those with diabetes, either the pancreas does not produce enough insulin or the insulin produced does not function properly. The disorder results in the accumulation of sugar in the blood and urine.

Uncontrolled diabetes can cause serious complications. When the cells are unable to receive the sugar to burn for fuel, they begin to use protein and body fat as a source of energy.

The breakdown of fats for fuel releases toxic acids called **ketones.** High levels of ketones poison the system. In extreme cases, they can cause unconsciousness and may lead to death.

Diabetes also has long-term effects. In premenopausal women, diabetes negates the natural protection from heart disease that estrogen provides. Diabetes also increases the risk of heart disease: a woman with diabetes is twice as likely to have a history of stroke and heart attack than is someone of the same age who does not have the condition. In addition, diabetes may cause damage to the eyes, the kidneys, and the nervous and circulatory systems. Unless carefully managed, it can also cause complications in pregnancy and childbirth.

SYMPTOMS

Diabetes often has no symptoms. When they do occur, symptoms include:
- Excessive urination
- Excessive thirst
- Excessive hunger
- Weight loss
- Genital and skin itching
- Blurry vision
- Numbness of extremities

DIAGNOSIS

Diabetes may be diagnosed using several blood tests that measure the amount of sugar present in the blood. If the level of sugar in the blood is higher than 200 mg/dl (milligrams per deciliter), two tests may be done to confirm diabetes. The first, the **fasting plasma glucose test,** simply measures blood sugar levels after a person hasn't eaten for eight to 12 hours. In an **oral glucose-tolerance test,** the blood sugar level is measured after the person has eaten a high-carbohydrate diet for three days. After that level is taken, the person is asked to drink a glucose solution, and the blood sugar levels are measured hourly for three to five hours to show how the body handles glucose. In both cases, if blood sugar levels are high, diabetes is present.

EFFECTS OF DIABETES

A cure for diabetes does not exist, but it can be controlled with medication, dosages of insulin, diet, or combinations of the three, depending on the type of diabetes and the specific case. Left unchecked, diabetes hastens the failure of several bodily functions. The most common organs and systems affected are:

- The circulatory system. According to the American Diabetes Association, diabetes leads to coronary heart disease, stroke, and circulation problems in the hands and feet. These conditions are two to four times more common in people with diabetes, and they account for most of their hospitalizations.

- The kidneys. The kidneys are stressed as they attempt to pump out the excessive sugar through the urine. Over a lifetime the exertion and vascular damage eventually brings on kidney failure. Diabetes is the leading cause of end-stage kidney disease.

- The eyes. Diabetic eye disease, or **diabetic retinopathy,** is the major cause of new vision loss in Americans 20 to 74 years old, according to the National Eye Institute.

- The nervous system. Nerve cells may be disturbed or damaged, causing severe pain or loss of feeling—a condition known as neuropathy.

TYPE-I DIABETES

Type-I diabetes is the most severe form of diabetes. It is also known as insulin-dependent diabetes because people with type-I diabetes generally depend on injections of insulin to regulate their sugar metabolism. In the past, this type of diabetes was often called juvenile diabetes because practitioners believed that it could only strike children and young adults. However, people of any age can develop type-I diabetes, although the majority of cases are discovered in people under 20 years of age. About 1 million Americans have type-I diabetes.

Type-I diabetes is an autoimmune disease: the body's own immune system attacks the pancreatic cells (beta cells) that produce insulin. Scientists are uncertain what causes the disease but have found a genetic link. At present, there are no preventive measures for type-I diabetes.

People with type-I diabetes are vulnerable to dangerous short-term complications of the disease. Two of these complications have to do with disruptive swings in blood sugar levels, such as **hyperglycemia** (too much blood sugar) and **hypoglycemia** (too little blood sugar). Those who have wide swings are said to have **brittle diabetes,** which is difficult to regulate. People with type-I diabetes are also at particular risk of **ketoacidosis,** or diabetic coma, in which poisons build up in the bloodstream.

TYPE-II DIABETES

Type-II diabetes is often called non-insulin-dependent diabetes. Formerly called adult-onset diabetes or maturity-onset diabetes, it seldom develops in people under the age of 40. Type-II diabetes in children and adolescents is sometimes called maturity-onset diabetes of the young and given the acronym MODY.

Type-II accounts for some 85 to 90 percent of all cases of diabetes. Four out of five of those with type-II are overweight. To an even greater extent than type-I, type-II runs in families. But it is generally thought that a combination of excess weight and age triggers the genetic predisposition.

People with type-II diabetes still produce the hormone insulin, but it does not function properly. The problem is linked to being overweight. Generally, someone who is chronically obese has a high carbohydrate intake, and that places strain on his or her body's glucose metabolism. At the same time, obesity causes insulin receptors on the cells' surfaces to resist insulin. Those cells (primarily muscle and fat cells) then cannot take glucose from the blood, and diabetes results. In response to the resulting

high blood sugar, beta cells in the pancreas struggle to produce more and more insulin. This eventually exhausts the beta cells, and the insulin secretion becomes inadequate.

GESTATIONAL DIABETES

Diabetes that arises during pregnancy is generally called gestational, or **type-III,** diabetes. It develops because of the distinctive hormonal environment and metabolic demands of pregnancy. Approximately 3 percent of pregnant women develop gestational diabetes, but it seems to be more common in women over 25.

While gestational diabetes symptoms are generally mild and not life-threatening to the woman, they can seriously jeopardize the health of the fetus. As a result, these pregnancies are often classified as high risk. For unknown reasons, women with diabetes tend to carry large fetuses with oversized organs. They are usually born prematurely and cause difficult labors because of their size. Respiratory problems, low blood calcium, jaundice, stillbirth, and infection are also common.

Many practitioners recommend routine diabetes screening for all pregnant women. But others cite the cost, duration, and inconvenience of the test as factors that make testing of all women impractical. Women who have diabetes prior to pregnancy need to maintain a strict treatment program to avoid any maternal or fetal complications. Oral contraceptives are often recommended for women with diabetes because they offer the most control when planning pregnancy.

In 95 percent of the cases, gestational diabetes disappears after childbirth. However, for about 5 percent of women, the diabetes remains. In addition, once a woman has had gestational diabetes, she is at risk for developing another form of diabetes (usually type-II) later in life, especially if she has a family history of diabetes, gains weight, and fails to exercise regularly.

TREATMENT

Treatment for type-I diabetes most often includes regular, daily injections of insulin in conjunction with a strict diet that helps keep blood sugar in a normal range. Exercise, which helps to lower blood sugar by making tissues more sensitive to insulin, should be part of a diabetic's self-care regimen as well. A woman with diabetes should work with her practitioner to develop a careful balance of insulin, diet, and exercise. In addition, a consistent and regular eating schedule should be followed. Some nutritional supplements may be of help.

Some people with type-II diabetes are able to control blood sugar levels with a regimen of diet and exercise. If that is not possible, drugs called oral hypoglycemic agents are prescribed to regulate blood sugar levels. These agents, which include acetohexamide, chlorpropamide, and glyburide, increase the secretion and effectiveness of insulin naturally produced in the body. Again, this treatment must be combined with a strict diet. Exercise, which helps people lose weight faster, reduces blood glucose levels, and makes insulin more effective, should be part of the self-care regimen as well. In some instances when all other treatments fail, a practitioner may prescribe insulin to a patient with type-II diabetes.

In some cases of gestational diabetes, diet alone can control the disease. Other women may need to take insulin. In these instances, the insulin doses and food required to control diabetes change as the pregnancy progresses—a woman may need close to three times more insulin by the time she is ready to deliver. The goal, as with all insulin therapy, is to keep blood sugar as close to normal ranges as possible. Women with diabetes who plan to become pregnant should first control their blood sugar levels. Well-managed diabetes reduces the risk of complications.

SEE endocrine system; pregnancy—prenatal concerns.

For more information on diabetes, contact:

American Association of Diabetes Educators
444 N. Michigan Ave., Suite 1240
Chicago, IL 60611
312-644-2233

American Diabetes Association
National Center
1660 Duke St.
Alexandria, VA 22314
800-232-3472
http://www.diabetes.org

American Dietetic Association
216 W. Jackson Blvd., Suite 800
Chicago, IL 60606-6995
312-899-0040
http://www.eatright.org

National Diabetes Information Clearinghouse
One Information Way
Bethesda, MD 20892-3560
301-654-3327
http://www.niddk.nih.gov

Diethylstilbestrol (DES)

Diethylstilbestrol (DES), a synthetic estrogen, was prescribed between the years 1941 and 1971 to an estimated 4.8 million pregnant women for the purpose of preventing miscarriages. While the drug proved ineffective at preventing miscarriages, it did have adverse effects on the reproductive systems, as well as the immune and cardiovascular systems, of the fetuses being carried in utero. There are an estimated 2.4 million women, and as many men, in the United States whose mothers used DES and who may be affected by it.

EFFECTS OF DES

The daughter of a woman who took DES may have changes to her vagina, cervix, and uterus. The most common conditions are:

■ Adenosis, the presence of glandular tissue in the vagina. This occurs in some DES daughters and often disappears after age 30. Simple adenosis does not have to be treated; a woman whose practitioner suggests this tissue be removed by freezing, burning, or surgery should get a second opinion.

■ An extra ridge of tissue in the cervix, called a collar or a hood. This condition may make it difficult to use a diaphragm.

■ A T-shaped uterus. Women with this condition may have complications during pregnancy.

The most serious consequence of DES exposure, **clear cell adenocarcinoma,** is rare. This cancer of the vagina and cervix develops in fewer than one in every 1,000 DES daughters, most often in women aged 15 to 22. However, the cancer has been known to develop in women as old as 41.

Up to half of all DES daughters will have difficulty with pregnancy, including infertility, ectopic pregnancy (in which a fertilized egg implants somewhere outside of the uterus), miscarriage, and premature delivery. If a DES daughter becomes pregnant, the pregnancy should be treated as high risk from the start to reduce the risk of complications. However, a DES daughter should not be discouraged from becoming pregnant. Some 80 percent of DES daughters who want children have successful pregnancies.

For men exposed to DES, effects may include testicular problems, such as undescended or underdeveloped testes and a higher risk of testicular cancer; sperm abnormalities; and reduced fertility.

UNKNOWN RISKS

Women's concerns about DES should not be minimized. DES-related health problems are still emerging. No one knows what possible cancer risks DES daughters face as they grow older, or if there will be an increased or decreased risk of cancer if they use birth control pills or hormone replacement therapy. (DES Action, a national consumer group representing the DES-exposed, suggests DES daughters and mothers avoid such drugs. However, there is no scientific data to support this view.) It is also known that DES mothers have an increased risk for breast cancer, making cancer screening important. There is no reason to believe that the effects of DES will be apparent in the children of DES daughters.

DIAGNOSING DES EXPOSURE

DES-related problems cannot be detected by a regular Pap test and pelvic exam. If you think you may have been exposed to DES, request a special "DES exam" from your gynecologist. It should include the following:

■ A Pap test including not only a smear of the cervix but four additional smears (called a four-quadrant smear) from the vaginal walls surrounding the cervix. These smears help to determine if a biopsy (tissue sample) needs to be taken to check for clear cell cancer.

■ Careful palpation (feeling) of the vaginal walls for any lumps or thickening

■ Use of an iodine stain to check the vagina and cervix for adenosis tissue, a glandular tissue not normally found in the vagina that can harbor clear cell cancer. (Regular tissue stains brown; adenosis tissue does not.)

Some practitioners also examine the cervix and vagina with a magnifying instrument called a **colposcope.** This viewing device helps them detect and biopsy areas of tissue abnormality.

DISCOVERING DES

Do you need to find out if you have been exposed to DES? Here are questions to ask your mother:

Did you take any drugs during the first five months of your pregnancy? (DES was given as pills, injections, and suppositories.)

If your mother says yes, ask her why she took the drugs and if she remembers the brand name. (DES Action has a list of the many brand names under which DES was marketed.) If she's uncertain, ask:

Did you have any problems during any pregnancy, such as bleeding, miscarriages, premature births, or diabetes?

If your mother did have any of these problems, there is more of a chance she took DES, even if she can't remember.

If your mother's physician is still practicing, DES Action suggests you ask in writing for

a copy of any records showing prenatal medication. (And send along a self-addressed, stamped envelope.) If the practitioner is retired, the practice may have been taken over by another who has the records. Your county medical society may know who has the records.

The information might also be on your mother's hospital records during the time of your birth. DES Action suggests you write to the medical records department of the hospital. Give the date of birth and mother's name and ask them to let you know what prenatal medicine is listed in the mother's record.

If your mother remembers the pharmacy she used, you can request copies of prescriptions filled for her during her pregnancy. Some pharmacies keep records going back many years.

"Blind," or unguided, biopsies are less accurate than those done with the aid of a colposcope. If an area of abnormal cells is small, a blind biopsy may miss it entirely.

On a Pap test, immature adenosis cells can be mistaken for **dysplasia** (abnormal cells) instead of what they really are, **metaplasia** (normal, fast-growing cells). To avoid misdiagnosis, a Pap test from a DES-exposed woman should be labeled as such before it is sent to the laboratory for analysis, with the request that it be examined by a pathologist familiar with DES cell changes.

Women who know they have been exposed to DES are advised to continue to have DES exams throughout their lives, perhaps more than once a year if their health-care practitioners think it necessary. If the exam shows no signs of abnormal cells, most practitioners agree that the woman can go back to annual Pap tests.

SEE cancer, vaginal; colposcopy; Pap test; medical records.

For more information on DES, contact:

DES Action East Coast Office
L.I.J. Medical Center
New Hyde Park, NY 11040
516-775-3450

DES Action West Coast Office
1615 Broadway, Suite 510
Oakland, CA 94612
510-465-4011
800-337-9288
http://www.desaction.org

DILATION AND CURETTAGE (D&C)

Dilation and curettage (D&C) is a procedure that involves widening, or dilating, the opening of the cervix, the narrow neck of the uterus, and removing all or part of the uterine lining (the endometrium) with a spoon-shaped instrument called a curette through the opened cervix. It may be done as a diagnostic procedure, after which the removed tissue is analyzed by a pathologist, or as a treatment.

A D&C may be done to:

■ Diagnose or rule out endometrial cancer.

■ Diagnose or remove suspected fibroids (also called leiomyomas, benign tumors, most commonly found in the smooth muscle cells of the uterus).

■ Diagnose and treat problems with heavy or abnormal bleeding. Analysis of a D&C sample may show overgrowth of the endometrial lining (hyperplasia). If the uterus is scraped thoroughly during the D&C, the overgrowth will be removed, alleviating some problems.

■ Diagnose problems with an intrauterine device (IUD) or aid in the removal of a "lost" IUD.

■ Follow up on an abnormal hysterosalpingogram (a diagnostic test in which dye is injected into the uterus and fallopian tubes to make the structures visible on x-ray) or abnormal endometrial cells on a Pap test.

■ Perform an abortion. Though abortion can be done through D&C, such procedures are very rare. They have been replaced with other methods.

■ Remove any placental remnants from the uterus after childbirth if there are signs that tissue remains in the uterus.

■ Remove any placental or embryonic remnants after miscarriage. However, studies show the procedure may not be necessary. Researchers found that 80 percent of women in their study who did not have a D&C following a miscarriage did not have any signs of remaining tissue in the uterus within three days. Some women may still choose to have a D&C to avoid the psychological effects that the lingering symptoms of a miscarriage may provoke.

PROCEDURE

The standard D&C may be done on an inpatient or outpatient basis by an obstetrician-gynecologist or by a general or family practitioner with special training. The woman is usually under general anesthesia; however, a paracervical block, supplemented with tranquilizers, sedatives, and other drugs, may be used.

With the help of a speculum inserted into the vagina to view the cervix, the practitioner begins to enlarge the cervix by inserting metal dilators (tapered rods) of increasing diameters. As an alternative, **laminarias** (dried seaweed stems) may be inserted several hours, often overnight, to dilate the cervix gradually and painlessly.

Once the cervical canal is wide enough, the practitioner inserts a **curette** (a spoon-shaped,

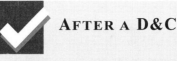

AFTER A D&C

A dilation and curettage procedure that scrapes too deeply could cause uterine scarring and possibly infertility. To avoid complications after a D&C, refrain from vaginal intercourse, douching, or the use of tampons, which may cause infection, for two weeks following the D&C. If you do have intercourse, use a condom.

It is normal after a D&C to have your next menstrual cycle come early or late, and it may be heavy for a few cycles. Other common side effects are mild cramps and mild backache. However, contact your practitioner if you have any of the following:
■ Fever
■ Foul-smelling discharge
■ Pain or severe cramps
■ Faintness
■ Profuse bleeding

sharp instrument) and scrapes the top and sides of the uterus. In a diagnostic D&C, the material removed by the curette is examined by a pathologist to determine if any disease is present. In addition, some conditions of the uterine lining can be treated by thorough scraping of the uterine cavity. The procedure usually lasts about 15 to 30 minutes.

RISKS AND COMPLICATIONS

Mild bleeding and cramps lasting for a couple of days are common following a D&C. More serious risks include heavier, prolonged bleeding; puncture of the uterine wall by the curette; and injury to the bladder and intestines. Forced dilation of the cervix may cause cervical incompetence (the inability for the cervix to remain appropriately closed) during subsequent pregnancies. The development of postoperative infection is also a possibility. As with any procedure using general anesthesia, death from reaction to the anesthetic drugs, error on the part of the anesthetist, or machine failure is a remote risk. In general, there are very few complications from a D&C.

ACCURACY
AND ALTERNATIVES

D&Cs are not foolproof diagnostic tools. Studies have shown that a D&C may be falsely negative, meaning that the test indicates no problems when problems actually exist. The chief problem with the procedure is that the practitioner cannot see the uterine lining to sample it. Since in a diagnostic procedure not all of the uterine surface is removed, some areas can be missed.

There are alternatives to this procedure that put less stress on the patient and may provide more accurate diagnoses. The alternatives are:

Hysteroscopy: A small fiberoptic telescope with an opening for a surgical instrument is inserted into the uterus through a minimally dilated (to about the diameter of a pencil) cervix during this procedure. Sometimes the cervix will open sufficiently from the application of prostaglandin gel, making a dilation unnecessary. Since the practitioner has a mag-

nified view of the tissue through the scope, suspicious areas can be sampled directly. Another advantage is that hysteroscopy can be done in a physician's office with a local anesthetic. However, the practitioner needs special additional training to peform and interpret hysteroscopy. A comparison of hysteroscopy and D&C has indicated that the D&C provided more information than the hysteroscopy in only 3.26 percent of the women studied.

Vacuum curettage (also known as endometrial aspiration): In this procedure, the uterine lining is removed with the help of suction from a small pump. In many women, the procedure can be used without general anesthesia, eliminating the small but real risk of anesthetic complications. In one study, the accuracy rate of diagnosis with vacuum curettage of the cervix was found to be twice as high as the traditional D&C.

Endometrial biopsy: A sample of tissue is taken with a cannula (a small plastic tube) during this procedure. The practitioner inserts a speculum in the vagina and holds the cervix open with a tenaculum (a grasping instrument) as the tissue sample is taken. The advantages of this procedure are that it does not stretch the cervix and is usually performed without anesthetics. Studies have shown it to be almost as effective as D&C in ruling out endometrial cancer.

Wait and watch: This course of treatment is usually most appropriate for women in their 20s or 30s who have abnormal bleeding but no other signs of disease.

SEE biopsy; hysteroscopy; medical testing (appendix B).

DISABILITIES

One in every six people in the United States has some sort of physical disability. Physical disabilities, which limit or destroy the body's ability to accomplish certain physical functions, result from birth defects, heredity, illness, and injuries.

Women with disabilities may have some special concerns. For example, disabled women are particularly vulnerable to sexual assault and abuse, especially by those who care for them. In addition, some health-care providers overlook the importance of reproductive health in women with disabilities, assuming them to be asexual, even though disabilities often have no effect upon menstruation, sexual desire, or the ability to have children.

The type of birth control used by a woman who is disabled should be chosen according to her needs and abilities. Oral contraceptives may have side effects, such as increased risk of blood clots in the veins, for those women who cannot be fully active. An IUD may cause heavy periods, which may be awkward to control, while the diaphragm and cervical cap may be difficult to insert for some women. A woman can usually find a suitable and effective method through a consultation with her practitioner.

The effects and types of disabilities vary from person to person. In order to master a particular disability, a woman should make an effort to learn about her disorder and its effects, and explore her own abilities. By becoming an expert on her own condition, a woman can gain more control over her health and her body and be sure she is getting appropriate medical care. With many disabilities, independence comes as a result of such knowl-

THE AMERICANS WITH DISABILITIES ACT

With the passage of the Americans with Disabilities Act (ADA) on July 26, 1990, disabled persons are entitled to have access to public buildings (use of ramps and other access areas specifically designated for those with disabilities) and to bathrooms and telephones; to use telecommunication devices (for hearing- and speech-impaired individuals); and to have the same number and quality of public services that a nondisabled person receives (transportation, state, and governmental services). Further, employers cannot discriminate against a qualified person with a disability.

The ADA stipulates that public accommodations (restaurants, hotels, theaters, practitioners' offices, pharmacies, stores, museums, parks, libraries, and so on) must be made accessible to persons with disabilities. If physical barriers exist in these public places, the barriers must be taken down, altered, or replaced with structures that provide the disabled with easy access. Elevators are required in buildings that have three or more stories or have more than 3,000 square feet of floor. Hotels that offer transportation for guests must provide this service to disabled persons as well.

The ADA further states that employers cannot discriminate against a qualified disabled person (in hiring or in promotion) and cannot screen out disabled applicants solely on the basis of their disabilities. Employers

(continued on page 182)

THE AMERICANS WITH DISABILITIES ACT—*CONTINUED*

who have more than 15 employees must also provide "reasonable accommodation" to disabled workers by modifying equipment or job restructuring.

Further, public transportation must be made accessible to disabled persons (Amtrak stations, for example, must be made accessible by July 26, 2010). Transit authorities must provide special transportation services to disabled persons who cannot use fixed-route bus services. Governments, both state and local, cannot discriminate against quali-

fied disabled persons, and their facilities, services, and communications must also be made accessible. Telephone companies must provide telecommunication devices and service for the hearing-impaired.

In legal matters, although individuals can bring private lawsuits to obtain court orders to stop discrimination, money damages cannot be awarded. Individuals can file complaints with the Attorney General's Office, which in turn can file discrimination lawsuits and obtain money.

edge. There are many support groups available to help women come to terms with their disabilities and work to overcome them.

Some physical disabilities can be overcome through operations, physical therapy, or the use

of specialized medical equipment, such as wheelchairs, artificial limbs, and hearing aids. The negative effects of some disabilities have been mitigated by construction of such public facilities as wheelchair ramps and elevators.

SEE birth defects; long-term care.

For more information on women and disabilities, contact:

American Paralysis Association
500 Morris Ave.
Springfield, NJ 07081
800-225-0292
800-526-3456 (New Jersey)
http://www.apa.uci.edu/paralysis

National Easter Seal Society
230 W. Monroe St., Suite 1800
Chicago, IL 60606-4802
800-221-6827
http://www.seals.com

National Multiple Sclerosis Society
733 Third Avenue
New York, NY 10017-3240
800-922-0484
212-986-3240 (New York)
http://www.nmss.org

National Rehabilitation Information Center
8455 Colesville Rd., Suite 935
Silver Spring, MD 20910-3319
800-346-2742
http://www.naric.com/naric

United Cerebral Palsy Association
1660 L St., N.W., Suite 700
Washington, DC 20036
800-USA-5UCP
202-776-0406
http://www.ucpa.org

DOMESTIC VIOLENCE

Each year, 4 million reported incidents of violence against women occur in the United States. Domestic violence is not limited by social or economic status. Women of any age or lifestyle may be affected. There is no typical profile of a battered woman because domestic violence occurs across religious, ethnic, racial, economic, and educational backgrounds.

According to the National Coalition Against Domestic Violence, half of all women will experience some form of violence from their spouses during marriage. In addition, 15 to 25 percent of pregnant women are battered. Though a man may be battered by a woman or another man, or a woman by a woman, 95 percent of all domestic violence cases involve a man assaulting a woman.

Domestic violence and battering is defined as a pattern of behavior used to establish control over another person using threats and fear. It is not limited to physical beatings, but also includes threats, sexual abuse, intimidation, isolation, and exploitation. Attacks usually begin with verbal threats, then progress to physical violence resulting in bruises, broken bones, choking, or even death.

The National Coalition Against Domestic Violence describes 12 characteristics likely in someone who commits domestic violence:

1. Grew up in a violent family.
2. Tends to use force or violence to "solve" problems.
3. Abuses drugs or alcohol.
4. Has poor self-esteem.
5. Has strong traditional ideas about gender roles.
6. Is jealous of relationships with other friends and family members.
7. Plays with guns, knives, or other weapons.
8. Expects partner to follow orders or advice.
9. Gets angry in a frightening way.
10. Experiences extreme mood changes.
11. Treats partner roughly.
12. Makes partner feel threatened.

Although the obvious answer for a woman in a violent relationship is for her to leave, this is not always possible. A woman may not have the financial means to leave home, especially if there are children whom she will need to support. Women also have real reason to fear retaliation—the violence becomes worse for 75 percent of women who attempt to leave. Some women believe that their partners can change or that the whole situation will simply disappear. Experts say a woman must admit that a problem exists before she can free herself from domestic violence. After that admission, she can take action to protect herself.

A woman can take several actions to make leaving a violent relationship easier. Money, car keys, and valuable documents (such as birth certificates and identification papers, which may be required to enter a shelter) should be kept in a safe, accessible place in case they are needed in a hurry. The phone number of the police should be kept on hand. A woman should also identify a place to go when she leaves, such as an emergency shelter, a social service agency, or the house of a trusted friend.

If an attack occurs, a woman should try to

protect herself, but she should call the police as soon as possible. The names and identification numbers of the police officers should be kept in case a record of the attack is needed. Most important, the woman should leave the house, with her children, if possible, and go to a safe place. Photographs of injuries should be taken and kept on record for possible use in a court case.

For help in dealing with domestic violence, contact the National Family Violence HelpLine at 800-222-2000, or 202-429-6695 in Washington, D.C., operated by the National Council on Child Abuse and Family Violence. The National Coalition Against Domestic Violence also operates a hotline at 800-799-SAFE.

LESBIANS AND DOMESTIC VIOLENCE

Experts speculate that women in lesbian relationships are just as likely to face domestic violence as women in heterosexual relationships. However, there are fewer resources and greater obstacles for victims of lesbian domestic violence.

Victims are often reluctant to report domestic violence because it means identifying themselves as lesbians, which may put friendships and careers in jeopardy. According to the National Coalition Against Domestic Violence, one of the biggest obstacles is homophobia. Because of such bias, they say, police are less likely to treat lesbian violence as a serious offense, and some judges dismiss charges.

Even when the violence is recognized, most communities do not have the counseling resources necessary to treat the victims. Some special circumstances apply to lesbians in violent relationships—for example, a "no male" rule at a local shelter may not keep a lesbian's partner from coming into the facility. However, these needs are beginning to be addressed.

Many shelters and hotlines now have information on same-sex battering. Local lesbian organizations may have services or resources for battered women. The National Coalition Against Domestic Violence operates a hotline at 800-799-SAFE and has resources for lesbians.

Most important, even if the resources are inadequate and the counselors are unable to respond appropriately, battered women should remember that their first priority is getting out of danger and that other problems may be addressed as they arise.

TO PROTECT YOURSELF AGAINST DOMESTIC VIOLENCE:

■ Do not tolerate abuse. By taking an early stand on abuse, you may be able to deter future incidents.

■ Keep up with friends and activities. An abuser may try to control you by cutting you off from friends and family and watching your every move. Keeping in touch also keeps self-esteem intact and can give you the confidence needed to leave a violent relationship.

■ Don't dismiss insults. Verbal abuse is an emotional form of domestic violence and may lead to physical assault.

■ Never excuse a slap, shove, push, or punch. Rarely does abuse occur just once. Violence during dating usually guarantees future incidents.

■ Tell a battering partner to seek counseling or you will leave the relationship. You do not deserve abuse. If your partner does not get help or change, it is not your fault.

SEE sexual assault.

For more information on domestic violence, contact:

National Clearinghouse for the Defense of Battered Women
125 S. Ninth St., Suite 302
Philadelphia, PA 19107
215-351-0010

National Coalition Against Domestic Violence
P.O. Box 18749
Denver, CO 80218
303-839-1852
NCADVI@IX.netcom.com

National Council on Child Abuse and Family Violence
1155 Connecticut Ave., N.W., Suite 400
Washington, DC 20036
202-429-6695

National Organization for Victim Assistance
1757 Park Rd., N.W.
Washington, DC 20010
800-879-6682 (for information and referrals)
202-232-6682 (for counseling and business)
http://www.access.digex.net/~nova

National Resource Center on Domestic Violence
6400 Flank Dr., Suite 1300
Harrisburg, PA 17112-2778
800-537-2238

For help or information on lesbian domestic violence, or for referrals to local groups with resources for lesbians, contact:

National Center for Lesbian Rights
870 Market St., Suite 570
San Francisco, CA 94102
415-392-6257
nclrss@aol.com

National Coalition Against Domestic Violence
Lesbian Task Force
P.O. Box 18749
Denver, CO 80218
303-839-1852
NCADVI@IX.netcom.com

EATING DISORDERS

Eating disorders, such as anorexia nervosa, bulimia, and binge-eating disorder, also known as compulsive overeating, are the result of many biological, psychological, and sociological factors. For most people with anorexia and bulimia, the disorder begins with a diet motivated by low self-esteem and poor body image that then develops into a pattern of compulsive behavior.

Eating disorders are mostly experienced by women; 90 percent of the victims of anorexia and bulimia are female. According to the American Anorexia/Bulimia Association, there are no firm figures on the number of people affected by eating disorders, though the count is thought to be in the millions. Anorexia and bulimia were rare until about 20 years ago, but now it is estimated that 5 to 20 percent of young women are affected by some degree of eating disorder.

The association reports that in the United States 1 percent of teenage women suffer from anorexia, and 10 percent of those may die as a result of the disorder. In addition, 5 percent of college-aged women have bulimia. Of people who are obese, 40 percent have binge-eating disorder.

The prevalence of young women with poor body images can become almost epidemic among college students. In a recent study of 643 college women, only 33 percent reported normal eating habits, while 3 percent were clinically bulimic. In the same study, 61 percent of the women exhibited some form of eating problem, such as chronic dieting, binge purging, or overeating.

ANOREXIA NERVOSA

Primarily affecting adolescent girls, anorexia nervosa is a disorder in which dieting leads to excessive weight loss that is a danger to health. Individuals with anorexia compulsively diet and generally do not eat, or eat only a small amount. Anorexia is treated as an illness in and of itself, although it is also a symptom of other psychological problems associated with family background, self-esteem, and social pressures.

Anorexia nervosa is characterized by:
- A relentless pursuit of thinness
- A refusal to eat
- A fear of becoming fat
- A distorted body image
- Excessive dieting leading to emaciation

The condition is commonly coupled with a high amount of physical activity and ritualistic eating habits. These rituals center on how food is prepared, arranged, and eaten, its type, and its amount.

Most symptoms of anorexia are reversible with weight gain but may be life-threatening if they remain untreated.

BULIMIA

As with anorexia, bulimia most often stems from feelings of poor self-esteem and the pressure to be thin. Bulimia is characterized by binging and purging. **Binge eating** involves taking in large amounts of food quickly. This is followed by **purging,** in which the person uses self-induced vomiting, laxatives, or fasting to

SYMPTOMS AND CONSEQUENCES OF ANOREXIA NERVOSA

■ Hunger, cravings, preoccupation with food, and, in many cases, binge eating

■ Dry, scaly skin. Skin may be yellow or gray.

■ Dull, brittle, thin hair

■ Loss of muscle as well as fat. Person may look like a skeleton covered only with skin.

■ Loss of menstrual periods and, sometimes, fertility in women

■ Loss of sexual desire

■ Icy hands and feet. Person is cold when others are warm.

■ Downy fuzz on face, limbs, and body

■ Shrunken, weakened heart

■ Anemia. Liver and kidney damage in some cases.

■ Loss of bone minerals. A young person may have the soft, brittle bones of an 80-year old.

■ Constipation, digestive discomfort, abdominal bloating

■ Dehydration

■ Muscle cramps, tremors

■ Dental problems

■ Death. Up to 20 percent of the people who have anorexia die.

Source: Reprinted with permission from *Eating and Exercise Disorders,* Anorexia Nervosa and Related Eating Disorders, Inc., P.O. Box 5102, Eugene, OR 97405.

control weight. Using these methods, bulimics can maintain their usually normal weight.

The binge purge cycle usually begins with a trigger, something that causes the woman to want to eat. Common triggers that lead to binges are anger, loneliness, rejection, resentment, helplessness, self-depreciation, depression, boredom, and even extreme happiness. However, after she eats, she usually experiences feelings of failure for having given in to the desire and compensates by giving in to the desire to purge.

BINGE-EATING DISORDER

Binge-eating disorder, or compulsive overeating, is a condition characterized by a pattern of overeating and/or a lack of exercise that begins in childhood. Food intake can be used as a way to deal with stress or to relieve anxiety. Other factors that may contribute to this eating disorder are genetic makeup, cultural background, and socioeconomic status.

Some compulsive overeaters tend to binge, while others eat continuously. Depression can occur. Other compulsive overeaters use their fat to hide or protect themselves from others, almost like a shell.

Treatment usually follows a plan that combines dieting with exercise and is geared toward maintaining body tone as weight is gradually reduced. Foods containing excess calories are eliminated while the balance of protein, carbohydrates, and fat required for growth is maintained. Exercise is encouraged because even a moderate increase in physical activity can lead to weight loss and appetite control. Self-help groups play an important role by providing moral support to help people overcome this disorder.

TREATMENT OF EATING DISORDERS

Emergency services for the treatment of eating disorders can be found at the nearest hospital emergency room or through a crisis hotline listed in the phone book. In a nonemergency situation, a health-care provider or friend can be asked to recommend a counselor. Students can often find low-cost services through the school counseling center.

PHYSICAL TREATMENTS

Initially, treatment for anorexia and bulimia involves medical assistance. A practitioner can monitor the woman's heart rhythms, nutritional status, and potential for bone loss. Occasionally, hospitalization is recommended. The woman is encouraged to eat more and, if necessary, is force-fed via a tube (called a nasogastric tube) inserted down the throat into the stomach. Hospitalization provides the structure needed to restore regular eating patterns.

If necessary, dental work will be done to help restore the damage caused by the effect of stomach acid on the teeth. Nutritional counseling will provide information about healthful eating. Vitamin and mineral supplements (particularly zinc sulfate) may also be used to help restore normal eating habits.

SYMPTOMS AND CONSEQUENCES OF BINGE EATING AND PURGING

■ Weight fluctuations because of alternating diets and binges
■ Swollen glands in neck under jaw
■ Loss of tooth enamel due to contact between stomach acid and teeth
■ Broken blood vessels in face; bags under eyes
■ Upset of the body's fluid/mineral balance leading to rapid or irregular heartbeat and possible heart attack
■ Dehydration, fainting spells, tremors, blurred vision
■ Laxative dependency, damage to bowels
■ Indigestion, cramps, abdominal discomfort, bloating, gas, constipation
■ Liver and kidney damage in some cases
■ Internal bleeding, infection
■ Death. Heart attack and suicidal depression are the major risks.

Source: Reprinted with permission from *Eating and Exercise Disorders*, Anorexia Nervosa and Related Eating Disorders, Inc., P.O. Box 5102, Eugene, OR 97405.

SYMPTOMS AND CONSEQUENCES OF COMPULSIVE OVEREATING

■ Weight gain, sometimes obesity
■ Increased risk of high blood pressure, clogged blood vessels, heart attack, and stroke
■ Increased risk of some cancers (breast, ovary, and endometrial cancers)
■ Increased risk of bone and joint problems
■ Increased risk of diabetes

Source: Reprinted with permission from *Eating and Exercise Disorders*, Anorexia Nervosa and Related Eating Disorders, Inc., P.O. Box 5102, Eugene, OR 97405.

New studies on eating disorders may lead to the development of improved treatments for sufferers. Research at the National Institute of Mental Health has indicated a link between anorexia and an abnormality within the brain. Women with anorexia and bulimia have abnormal amounts of certain brain chemicals; a similar condition occurs in depressive disorders. Women with anorexia are also thought to have excess levels of cortisol. Studies are also being done on the effect binging and purging have on the central nervous system.

PSYCHOLOGICAL TREATMENTS

The most successful long-term treatment for anorexia, bulimia, and binge-eating disorder is psychotherapy, a counseling technique used to change the behaviors that lead to the eating disorder. **Cognitive therapy** focuses on the attitudes of the woman, addressing issues such as self-esteem and body image. **Behavioral therapy** involves modifying eating habits, such as binge eating and purging, through conditioning and motivational techniques. **Family therapy** views the eating disorder as a symptom of problems with relationships. It views the condition as a symptom of dysfunction within the family.

PREVENTION OF EATING DISORDERS

To prevent eating disorders in young people, parents and role models should:

- Promote good nutrition and exercise.
- Make efforts to boost self-esteem and a positive self-image.
- Encourage the acceptance of natural body types despite media images.
- Avoid putting pressure on young people to attain unrealistic academic or social goals.
- Make communication a priority.
- Since dieting is a risk factor for developing an eating disorder, diets should be supervised by a professional.

Tranquilizers and antidepressants may be prescribed to relieve depression and anxiety.

There are many support groups to aid those with eating disorders, but they are more effective when combined with psychotherapy and medical care.

SEE depression; physical fitness; weight reduction.

For more information on eating disorders, or referrals to local support groups, contact:

American Anorexia/Bulimia Association
293 Central Park W., Suite 1R
New York, NY 10024
212-501-8351

Anorexia Nervosa and Related Eating Disorders, Inc.
P.O. Box 5102
Eugene, OR 97405
503-344-1144

Foundation for Education About Eating Disorders
One Country Creek Ct.
N. Potomac, MD 20878
301-424-6044

Take Off Pounds Sensibly (TOPS)
P.O. Box 07360
Milwaukee, WI 53207
800-932-8677

ENDOCRINE SYSTEM

The endocrine system is comprised of glands that produce hormones vital for the maintenance and regulation of the body's basic functions. The endocrine glands secrete directly into the bloodstream, rather than through ducts, as other types of glands (such as sweat glands) do. The endocrine system can be adversely affected by illness, stress, or age.

The endocrine system and the hormones it produces have a great effect upon the body of a woman. Female hormones are responsible for the shape the body develops during adolescence. They regulate the menstrual cycle. They improve cardiac function and provide natural protection against high cholesterol and osteoporosis. They promote healthy-looking skin, increase respiratory rate, and regulate body temperatures. When a problem with the endocrine system occurs, it can result in weight loss or gain, dry skin, fatigue, irregular periods, sweating, intolerance to cold, and a number of other symptoms.

COMPONENTS OF THE ENDOCRINE SYSTEM

The **hypothalamus** is located in the brain. It produces several types of hormones that interact with the pituitary gland and other glands of the endocrine system.

The hypothalamus is connected to the **pituitary gland** by a stem. The pituitary gland regulates many body processes, including growth, urine production, and skin darkening. It secretes prolactin, which is associated with the production of milk in the mammary glands.

Oxytocin, another of its secretions, triggers orgasm, the start of labor, and the release of milk from the breast. The pituitary gland also interacts with other endocrine glands by secreting trophic (stimulating) hormones.

Also located in the brain is the **pineal gland,** a small egg-shaped gland that produces melatonin, a hormone thought to suppress the development of sex glands before puberty. The hormone also affects the sleep/wake cycle.

The **thyroid gland** is located below the Adam's apple in the neck, making it the easiest gland to examine. It regulates the body's metabolism, bone growth, and body heat through the production of the hormones thyroxine, triiodothyronine, and calcitonin.

The **parathyroid glands** are two pairs of small oval glands adjacent to the thyroid gland in the neck. They secrete parathyroid hormone (PTH), which maintains the level of calcium in the blood. Overproduction of the hormone, a common disorder as women age, is called **hyperparathyroid.** It causes thinning of the bones (osteoporosis) and the formation of stones (calculi) in the urinary tract. Underproduction of PTH, which is exceedingly rare, is called **hypoparathyroidism.** It results in low levels of calcium and can lead to cramps, spasms, or seizures.

The **pancreas** produces and releases insulin, which helps to maintain blood sugar levels and to process carbohydrates. A malfunctioning pancreas may result in diabetes mellitus, a disorder in which the pancreas does not produce enough insulin, resulting in abnormal blood sugar levels. Symptoms of diabetes

DISORDERS OF THE THYROID

The thyroid gland, which regulates metabolism and other major body functions, can be the source of several different types of disease if it malfunctions. Women are five times more likely to have thyroid disease than men.

Hyperthyroidism, the most common thyroid disease, results when the thyroid produces too much thyroxine, the thyroid hormone. Early signs of hyperthyroidism include weight loss, increased appetite, intolerance to heat, and increased sweating. In more advanced cases, gland enlargement, muscle degeneration, anxiety, palpitations, shakiness, and mental hyperactivity are common symptoms.

The most common cause of hyperthyroidism is **Graves' disease,** an autoimmune disorder in which the body develops antibodies that stimulate the production of excessive amounts of thyroid hormones. A common symptom of the disease is bulging eyeballs, caused by the swelling of tissue behind the eyes. An overactive area of the gland, known as an **adenoma,** may also cause hyperthyroidism.

Hypothyroidism results from the underproduction of thyroxine. Common signs of this disorder are lethargy, muscle weakness, cramps, slow heart rate, dry and flaky skin, hair loss, a deep and husky voice, constipation, depression, weight gain, and high cholesterol. Hypothyroidism is usually caused by an autoimmune disease in which the body develops antibodies against its own thyroid gland. Its risk of occurrence increases with age.

Both hyperthyroidism and hypothyroidism may be confirmed with blood tests that measure the level of thyroid hormones in the blood. Hyperthyroidism may be treated with drugs that inhibit the production of thyroid hormones or with surgery to remove part of the thyroid gland. Hypothyroidism treatment consists of taking replacement hormones; in most cases, hormone replacement therapy continues for life.

include excessive hunger, thirst, and urination.

The **adrenal glands** are a small pair of glands located on top of the kidneys. The adrenal cortex, the outer region of the gland, produces steroid hormones, which include the sex hormones. The adrenal medulla, the inner portion of the gland, is closely related to the nervous system and secretes the hormones epinephrine and norepinephrine. These hormones speed up respiration and blood pressure in response to stimulants such as fear or anxiety.

Underproduction of steroid hormones in the adrenal cortex may result in a rare condition called **Addison's disease,** which is most often caused by an autoimmune disorder. Symptoms of Addison's disease include weakness, low blood pressure, and mottled skin.

Overproduction of these hormones results in **Cushing's syndrome.** People with Cushing's syndrome have a characteristic appearance: the face appears round and red, the trunk tends to become obese with a humped upper back, and the limbs begin to waste. Cushing's syndrome may also occur when people are given these steroid hormones (for example, prednisone) for an extended period of time as a treatment for diseases such as asthma or arthritis.

The **ovaries** are the female sex glands. They produce the hormones estrogen and progesterone, which are needed for menstruation, reproduction, feminine secondary sex characteristics, and skeletal development. Excessive production of these hormones is rare. Underproduction causes menstrual irregularities and, eventually, menopause. (Menopause typically occurs at age 50.) Menopause is considered premature when the ovaries stop functioning earlier than age 40. This

occurs in about 5 percent of all women and should be evaluated. The testes are the corresponding endocrine/sex glands in men.

The **placenta,** an organ that develops in the uterus during pregnancy to nourish the fetus, is also considered part of the endocrine system. During pregnancy, the placenta secretes estrogen and progesterone as well as human chorionic gonadotropin (HCG) and chorionic somatomammotropin, two hormones associated with fetal growth.

SEE androgens; estrogen; menstrual cycle and ovulation; reproductive system and sex organs of the woman.

ENDOMETRIOSIS

An estimated 5 million women in the United States suffer from endometriosis, which occurs most often in women between 25 and 40 years of age. There is no certain cause for endometriosis, but new evidence suggests that it may involve the immune system. Heredity also appears to be a factor. Women with immediate relatives who have endometriosis are seven times more likely to have the condition.

Endometriosis occurs when tissue from the lining of the uterus (called the **endometrium**) is present outside of the uterus. These "implants" are usually found in the pelvic cavity among other organs, usually the ovaries, bowel, or bladder. In these areas, the endometrial tissue grows and breaks down each month when the lining of the uterus breaks down into the menstrual flow. Since there is no outlet for the resulting blood and fluid, it remains in the pelvic cavity, where it

can cause severe pain and the formation of noncancerous cysts (sometimes known as chocolate cysts because of their dark color). As the tissue continues to grow, painful scar tissue also forms, which can block and damage abdominal organs, often causing infertility.

Endometriosis is often referred to as a career woman's disease because of the misconception that it is more common in affluent workingwomen in their 30s who have never had children. While endometriosis is most common in women between the ages of 25 and 40, it affects women of all ages regardless of social standing or the number of pregnancies they have had. Workingwomen may appear to be the majority simply because they have the means to seek diagnosis and treatment.

In 30 percent of infertile women, the infertility is related to endometriosis. The condition also puts women at higher risk for ectopic pregnancy (a potentially life-threatening condition in which the fertilized egg implants somewhere outside of the uterus) and miscarriage. Though mild cases of endometriosis may go unnoticed (one-third of women with endometriosis have no symptoms except infertility), symptoms of the condition can include:

■ Pelvic or abdominal pain that coincides with ovulation and menstrual periods

■ Heavy, lengthy, or irregular menstrual periods

■ Painful bowel movements and urination

■ Diarrhea or constipation

■ Pain during or after sexual intercourse

■ Nausea and vomiting

■ Lower back pain

■ Low-grade fever

■ Infertility

DIAGNOSIS

Endometriosis is difficult to diagnose because it can resemble other conditions, including pelvic inflammatory disease, bladder infection, ovarian cysts, and appendicitis. Definitive diagnosis can only be made through **laparoscopy,** an outpatient surgical procedure in which the internal organs are examined using a thin viewing scope that is inserted through a one-inch incision in the abdomen. A **laparotomy,** a more serious operation in which the surgeon opens the abdomen with a longer incision, may also be used.

Another diagnostic procedure, **MRI,** or **magnetic resonance imaging,** uses a strong magnetic field to create an image of the abdominal and pelvic area. MRI is claimed to be 96 percent accurate in detecting endometriosis, and some people think it may replace laparoscopy as the initial diagnostic procedure because it is noninvasive.

TREATMENT

There is no cure for endometriosis, though it may recede on its own after menopause or during pregnancy, when ovulation ceases. If the endometriosis is mild and is causing no symptoms, treatment may not be needed at all. Women diagnosed with endometriosis who wish to have children should consider becoming pregnant as soon as possible because the longer the condition is present, the more likely it is to interfere with fertility.

The goal of treatment with medications is to interrupt the menstrual cycle so the endometrial implants are not aggravated. Drugs that simulate the effects of pregnancy and menopause in the body are often used to treat endometriosis, but their ability to relieve symptoms is only temporary. **Oral contraceptives** containing estrogen and progestins, or progestins alone (Provera or Depo-Provera) can be used for mild cases to reduce growth. A stronger drug, **danazol** (Danocrine), inhibits the production of hormones by the pituitary gland, interrupting menstruation and suppressing ovulation. However, danazol has side effects that include weight gain, bloating, depression, cramps, and masculinizing effects, such as voice-deepening, which may be irreversible. **Gonadotropin-releasing hormone agonists (GnRH)** also stop menstruation and suppress ovulation. However, many women experience menopausal symptoms of hot flashes, insomnia, and emotional changes on this drug. In addition, prolonged treatment with GnRH can cause bone loss. Since endometriosis does recur once drug treatments end, medications are recommended only when there is a reason, such as to reduce symptoms long enough to allow a woman to conceive, or to reduce tissue growth before surgery.

New, experimental, immunological treatments for the condition include testing women for the presence of antibodies and giving them allergy-shot-like injections designed to encourage their immune cells to attack the patches of endometriosis.

The symptoms of endometriosis can also be treated through surgery. With the aid of laparoscopy or laparotomy, patches of endometriosis can be removed from organs by **dilation and curettage** (scraping), **cauterization** (burning), or **laser surgery** (vaporizing the tissue). Laser surgery can also be used to open cysts and repair the internal damage caused by scar tissue. Laser surgery results in the restoration of fertility in one-third to one-half of the cases.

Hysterectomy, the surgical removal of the uterus sometimes accompanied by removal of the ovaries **(oophorectomy),** is an option for women who have severe cases of endometriosis. Though 20 percent of hysterectomies are performed to alleviate endometriosis, experts say the surgery should be a last resort, since it may result in urinary tract, bowel, and back and joint problems as well as sexual dysfunction. In addition, hormone replacement therapy, prescribed after a hysterectomy and oophorectomy to relieve symptoms of early menopause, can reactivate endometriosis in 5 percent of women.

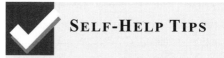

SELF-HELP TIPS

To relieve the symptoms of endometriosis:

■ Exercise regularly. Exercise can reduce the risk of severe endometriosis and some side effects of medications used to treat the condition, such as weight gain and depression.

■ Explore alternative therapies. Acupuncture, Chinese herbs, meditation, and homeopathy have been shown to be effective in reducing the pain and discomfort associated with endometriosis.

■ Cut back on fats in your diet. Saturated animal fat and hydrogenated vegetable oils can stimulate the production of prostaglandins, normal body chemicals produced during the menstrual cycle, which can prompt severe menstrual cramps.

■ Eat plenty of fruits and vegetables. Vitamins C, E, the B-complex vitamins, and the minerals selenium, calcium, and magnesium can help relieve endometriosis symptoms.

SEE biopsy; dilation and curettage (D&C); hysterectomy; laparoscopy; oophorectomy; second opinion.

For more information on endometriosis, contact:

Endometriosis Association
8585 N. 76th Place
Milwaukee, WI 53223
800-992-ENDO
800-426-2363 (Canada)

Endometriosis Treatment Program
St. Charles Medical Center
2500 N.E. Neff Rd.
Bend, OR 97701
800-446-2177 ext. 6904

ESTROGEN

strogen is the principal female sex hormone. First recognized around 1915, estrogen is responsible for the development of the secondary feminine sex characteristics, which include breasts, rounded hips, and pubic hair. The three principal forms of estrogen occurring naturally in a woman's body—along with 17 minor forms—are estradiol, estrone, and estriol. **Estradiol,** produced in the ovaries, is the dominant estrogen during the menstrual years. **Estriol,** produced in the placenta, reaches high levels during pregnancy. **Estrone,** manufactured by fat cells, becomes the dominant estrogen after menopause, when the ovarian production of estrogen decreases.

When a girl reaches puberty (usually around age 12), her pituitary gland signals the ovaries to begin to release estrogen.

The increased levels of estrogen cause the changes in the body commonly associated with puberty.

ESTROGEN AND MENSTRUATION

The pituitary gland, located in the brain, triggers the onset of the menstrual cycle when it releases a hormone, **follicle-stimulating hormone (FSH),** which causes the egg cells in one of the ovaries to ripen. FSH triggers the growth of the follicles of the ovaries, which begin to produce estrogen (in the form of estradiol). Estrogen also thickens the lining of the uterus, called the endometrium, in preparation for the implantation of a fertilized egg.

Two weeks into the menstrual cycle, when the levels of estrogen peak, the pituitary gland releases another hormone, **luteinizing hormone (LH).** LH stimulates the release of a ripened egg cell from the follicle of the ovary into a fallopian tube. This is called ovulation.

Under the influence of LH, the cells that line the egg follicle begin to produce **progesterone,** another hormone, in addition to estrogen. If the released egg is not fertilized and does not implant in the endometrium, estrogen and progesterone levels drop. As a result, the uterus sheds its thickened lining and expels the unfertilized egg in the form of menstrual bleeding. If fertilization occurs, progesterone (the pro-gestation hormone) is produced in large quantities to support the pregnancy.

Until menopause, the levels of estrogen increase and decline each month if the egg is not fertilized. If the egg does fertilize and implant, resulting in pregnancy, an organ known as the placenta forms to nourish the growing fetus. The placenta takes over the production of estrogen (in the form of estriol) and progesterone, and levels remain high until delivery.

ESTROGEN AND ORAL CONTRACEPTIVES

Oral contraceptives, commonly known as the Pill, contain estrogen (usually synthetic). Oral contraceptives prevent ovulation by halting the development of the egg in the ovary and by preventing implantation of a fertilized egg, should one be released.

Most oral contraceptives are "combination" pills, which contain synthetic estrogen

THE EFFECTS OF ESTROGEN

- Growth and development of breasts, uterus, fallopian tubes, and vagina during fetal development and puberty
- Decline and halt of the growth of the long bones: arms, legs, hands, and feet
- Promotion of feminine body shape (rounded hips and breasts) and increased thickness of fatty layers
- Variation of moods associated with the menstrual cycle (may be complicated by lifestyle)
- Promotion of healthy hair
- Thickening of vaginal lining and production of vaginal mucus
- Cyclic thickening of the endometrium (the lining of the uterus)
- Feedback to the brain needed for regulation and release of follicle-stimulating hormone (FSH) and luteinizing hormone (LH)—hormones produced by the pituitary gland that trigger ovulation and menstruation
- Increased fluid retention
- Production of abundant thin, stringy, cervical mucus during ovulation
- Protection against loss of bone density. Helps to build bones and maintain body's calcium balance.
- Protection against heart disease. Helps to increase amount of "good" high-density lipoproteins in the blood.
- Increased water content and thickness of skin. Promotes healthy, flexible, and moist skin.
- Decreased oil gland activity and oil secretion by skin
- Promotion of vaginal acidity
- Increased blood level of certain plasma proteins
- Increased protein metabolism rate

(usually 20 to 35 micrograms) and **progestins** (synthetic progesterone). By mimicking the effects of the body's own estrogen and progesterone, the combination pill suppresses the menstrual cycle. The combined effects of synthetic estrogen and progestins keep the pituitary gland from stimulating the ovarian follicle, and ovulation does not occur. Another form of the Pill, called the minipill, contains progestins only.

While high-dose Pills (50 micrograms) are associated with increased risk of blood clots, heart attacks, and strokes, the low-dose Pills (20 to 35 micrograms) that are common today are considered to be much safer for most women.

ESTROGEN AND MENOPAUSE

During menopause, the production of estrogen by the ovaries declines, and the levels of estrogen in the woman's body decrease. Estrone, the form of estrogen produced by the adrenal glands and the fatty tissue, becomes the dominant form of estrogen in the body. (This could explain why large women often have fewer menopausal symptoms linked to estrogen decrease than do small, thin women.)

Estrogen reduction after menopause can decrease bone mass, resulting in osteoporosis. The decline also changes lipid, or blood fat, levels, putting postmenopausal women at increased risk for heart disease. Even the slightest

RISKS OF ESTROGEN

Although estrogen has many benefits, women who take estrogen, either as an oral contraceptive or as a component of HRT, do face some risks. Estrogens in the bloodstream are deactivated by the liver and filtered by the kidneys into the urine. A woman with liver disease must consider this before taking estrogen, since her liver may not deactivate the estrogen properly, causing the levels to rise to a dangerously high level.

In addition, early studies of birth control pill users found that women who took the Pill had an increased risk of heart attack and stroke. The risk was even higher for women who smoked. Today, because the dose of estrogen contained in the Pill is much lower, most experts agree that oral contraceptives can be used by most women. However, the risk is still high for women over 35 who smoke and for those who tend to form blood clots.

Estrogen may stimulate the growth of uterine fibroid tumors. Similarly, endometriosis (the growth of endometrial tissue outside the uterus) may worsen when estrogen is used alone, but combining estrogen with progestins seems to minimize that risk. HRT has also been linked to an increase in gallstones and gallbladder pain. Studies show that women who take estrogen supplements are more likely to undergo procedures to have their gallbladder removed than those who do not.

In some studies, use of estrogens without progestins has also been shown to increase the risk of endometrial cancer and may possibly cause a slight increase in breast cancer in some women. Estrogen causes the endometrium to grow and thicken, which can lead to abnormal cell growth and subsequent cancer. To offset the endometrial cancer risk, progestins are prescribed. These progestins break down the uterine lining and allow it to shed as menstrual bleeding, which prevents cancer from forming. Studies have been inconclusive concerning breast cancer risks. While some experts say there is a substantial risk of breast cancer with the use of long-term HRT, others say the risk is small, and others have found no increased risk at all.

Although estrogen is approved by the Food and Drug Administration to alleviate some physical symptoms of menopause, its role in improving skin texture, curbing negative mood swings, and increasing sex drive is unclear to researchers.

Because of the conflicting information and the different risk factors of every woman, the decision to use estrogen requires knowledge and thought. Each woman, after reviewing the risks and benefits and discussing her situation with her practitioner, must decide for herself whether estrogen is the right choice for her.

decline in estrogen can disturb the hypothalamus (the body's regulating gland), which can lead to hot flashes and vaginal atrophy (thinning and dryness of the lining of the vagina)—both common conditions that often occur during menopause.

ESTROGEN AND HORMONE REPLACEMENT THERAPY

Hormone replacement therapy (HRT) is the use of hormones to offset the negative effects of menopause. Estrogen protects women from osteoporosis, hot flashes, and vaginal atrophy. In addition, it increases the levels of high-density lipoproteins, or HDLs, the "good" cholesterol that lowers the risk of heart disease.

The most commonly prescribed estrogen in HRT is Premarin, named for pregnant mares' urine, from which it is extracted. A conjugated equine estrogen, Premarin is a combination of estrogens, primarily estrone. Micronized estradiol or estrone alone may also be used.

Natural estrogens can be found in some plant foods, such as legumes and soy. Though no long-term data are available on natural estrogens, some experts believe these plant hormones may relieve mild hot flashes and lower the risk of osteoporosis and heart disease. The use of natural sources lessens the chance of an adverse reaction; however, there is no accurate way to measure dosage, since each plant may contain a different amount of estrogen.

SEE contraception; endocrine system; hormone replacement therapy; menstrual cycle and ovulation.

FEMALE GENITAL MUTILATION

Female genital mutilation (FGM), also called female circumcision, is a practice based on cultural and religious customs designed to control women's sexuality, prolong virginity, and enhance marriageability. This medically unnecessary surgery, used to alter the external sexual organs of a woman or girl, is most often performed in Africa, the Middle East, and Muslim areas of Indonesia and Malaysia.

FGM is a brutal practice, done without anesthesia and without the consent of the girl, that must be discouraged and eradicated. While it remains mostly an "underground" practice in the United States, more and more cases of FGM are being recognized. The 1995 women's conference in Beijing, China, declared FGM a violation of human rights.

American practitioners have begun to encounter immigrant women who have undergone the procedure, and some practitioners have also been asked by immigrant parents to perform the procedures on their young daughters. The American Medical Association (AMA) suggests that physicians strongly discourage the practice. The AMA and the American College of Obstetricians and Gynecologists support the movement to make the practice illegal in the United States, but caution health-care providers to treat women who have undergone the procedure with sensitivity and compassion.

TYPES OF GENITAL MUTILATION

According to the World Health Organization, there are four types of FGM:

■ Clitoridectomy. The clitoris and its hood are removed.

■ Excision. All or part of the labia minora is removed.

■ Infibulation. The clitoris, labia minora, and much of the labia majora are removed. The two sides of the vulva are sutured closed (sometimes with thorns), allowing only minimal passage of urine and menstrual flow.

■ The clitoris may be scratched, burned, or clipped. The labia minora may be enlarged, and the opening of the vagina may be cut and enlarged for childbirth.

The immediate risks of the surgery are death from hemorrhage, shock, and infection. The operations are usually performed by someone who is not medically trained, using unsterilized razors, scissors, or shards of glass. The procedure is done without anesthesia, and the death rate may be as high as 50 to 60 percent.

The long-term problems include chronic pelvic infection, abscesses on the vulva, thick scar tissue, damage to the urethra or anus, sterility, complications for the woman and the fetus at childbirth, incontinence, depression, anxiety, and sexual dysfunction.

Genital mutilation is usually performed on girls between eight and 12 years old, though it may be done as early as infancy and as late as 14 or 16 years. A woman may be reinfibulated—sewn closed a second time—after childbirth if her husband dies or leaves her or if he goes away for a long time.

Infibulation prevents sexual penetration, while clitoridectomy removes the source of a woman's sexual pleasure. Both procedures are done to decrease promiscuity and ensure a woman's fidelity. Young girls whose cultures encourage this practice face a difficult dilemma. They may not believe in FGM and be afraid of the procedures, but they may also recognize that their marriageability may depend on them. Women who have not consented to FGM may be considered to have a questionable sexual history and may have a great deal of difficulty marrying within their culture.

FIGHTING GENITAL MUTILATION

The World Health Organization, United Nations, and several other political forces are joining together to pass legislation to stop the practice of FGM. To date, in Sweden, Great Britain, France, and several other countries, those who perform FGM may be imprisoned. In the United States, efforts are being made to outlaw FGM, though attempts are hampered by its underground nature. On a grassroots level, groups are working to form anti-FGM support groups and educational programs for schools and health clinics.

For more information on FGM, contact:

Research Action Information for the Bodily Integrity of Women (RAINB♀)
915 Broadway, Suite 1109
New York, NY 10010
212-477-3318
http://www.rainbo.org

FIBROIDS

ibroids, also called leiomyomas or myomas, are benign, muscular growths on the inside, outside, or even within the wall of the uterus. Fibroids are common and seldom life threatening—in fact, many women have no symptoms at all. Twenty percent of all women, and 50 percent of all women aged 50 or older, have these growths. Though fibroids are considered tumors, there is only one chance in 1,000 that they will become cancerous.

Firm, round, and gray-white in appearance, fibroids range in size from one-sixteenth of an inch to more than six inches. They are usually discovered during a routine pelvic exam. Fibroids, which usually occur in clusters, can grow either slowly or rapidly, and their rate of growth is thought to be affected by estrogen. Fibroids are likely to grow during pregnancy, when hormone levels are high, and shrink after menopause, when levels drop. Because they are located in the wall of the uterus, fibroids can also interfere with pregnancy and fertility. African-American women, women who have never been pregnant, and those with a family history of fibroids are most likely to have them.

SYMPTOMS AND DIAGNOSIS

Though there may be no symptoms at all, fibroids can cause heavy bleeding during periods, cramping, frequent urination, and pelvic pain and pressure. If the fibroids cause no symptoms, treatment is not necessary; they often shrink and disappear on their own after menopause.

To confirm the presence of fibroids, a practitioner may need to do diagnostic procedures such as an **ultrasound** (an "x-ray" of the body using sound waves rather than radiation), **laparoscopy** (insertion of a viewing scope into an incision in the abdomen), or **hysteroscopy** (insertion of a scope into the uterus).

TREATMENT

Fibroids may be relieved with **gonadotropin-releasing hormone agonists (GnRH),** estrogen-blocking drugs that can cause the tumors to shrink temporarily. GnRH should be used for a specific reason (such as infertility) because the growths do recur after treatment ends. However, GnRH creates a time frame during the first few months after treatment ends, during which tumors are reduced, and this may allow for conception. Because GnRH drugs will create a false menopause, triggering hot flashes and bone loss, there is a six-month limit on their use. Hormone replacement therapy can be used to counteract the effects of GnRH.

If the fibroids are small enough and located on the inner lining of the uterus, they can also be removed by **dilation and curettage,** the scraping of the uterine lining, or during **hysteroscopy,** a diagnostic procedure.

Myomectomy is a procedure in which the fibroids are cut from the uterus, but the uterus is preserved. A myomectomy is often requested by younger women who still wish to bear children. If the growths are extensive or difficult to reach, a myomectomy can be complicated and risky and may involve extensive blood loss and the formation of painful scar tissue. About 15 to 20 percent of the time, additional surgery is required because fibroids have continued to grow. Because of the uterine scarring involved in the procedure, a repeat myomectomy may be difficult or impossible.

Another option is **endometrial ablation,** a procedure in which the uterine lining and the fibroids are burned off using an electric current. While ablation stops heavy menstrual flow, it leaves the woman infertile.

A **hysterectomy,** removal of the uterus, is often recommended for fibroids; in fact, 30 percent of all hysterectomies are done to remove fibroids. In many cases, however, a hysterectomy is not necessary. Indications that a hysterectomy is needed include chronic pelvic pain, excessive bleeding, or fibroids that cause severe symptoms and that cannot be treated with myomectomy.

Traditionally, fibroids have been the number one reason for hysterectomy, accounting for almost one-third. At one time, gynecologists followed the standard that called for a hysterectomy if and when fibroids grew to the point where the uterus is the size of a 12-week pregnancy (about 3 $^1/_2$ inches in diameter), even if symptoms were not severe.

However, conservative gynecologists now believe treatment should depend on fibroid symptoms, not size. If the symptoms are not causing serious problems, a practitioner may

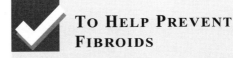

TO HELP PREVENT FIBROIDS

■ Stay physically fit. Exercise can remove estrogen and fat from the body and may help prevent fibroids from growing.

■ Take care of your liver. The liver removes excess estrogen from the blood. Cut back on alcohol and caffeine and eat more foods rich in vitamin B$_6$ (such as beets and garlic), to help your liver function better.

■ Consider alternatives to hormone replacement therapy. The estrogen in the treatment may fuel the growth of fibroids, even after menopause.

■ Add more fiber to your diet. It aids in removing excess estrogens from the body.

track the growth and effects of a fibroid before recommending treatment or surgery.

Alternative therapies, such as acupuncture, herbal and homeopathic remedies, massage, and yoga, may be effective in treating some of the symptoms of fibroids.

SEE dilation and curettage (D&C); hysterectomy; hysteroscopy; laparoscopy.

For more information on fibroids, contact:

HERS Foundation (Hysterectomy Educational Resources and Services)
422 Bryn Mawr Ave.
Bala Cynwyd, PA 19004
610-667-7757
tzht72a@prodigy.com

FIBROMYALGIA

Fibromyalgia, also called fibrositis, is a common condition characterized by chronic, generalized muscle pain and fatigue. Fibromyalgia has no known cause. Women are 10 times more likely than men to contract fibromyalgia, which affects 5 million Americans each year. The condition is difficult to diagnose because of its unexplained nature and wide variety of symptoms.

While some researchers believe fibromyalgia is related to arthritis, others believe it is caused by infection, thyroid disease, or stress. Another theory maintains that neurochemical abnormalities lead to sleep disorders, which cause the symptoms. There has also been speculation that fibromyalgia is tied to chronic fatigue syndrome and Lyme disease, an acute inflammatory disease believed to be transmitted by a tick-borne organism.

Unlike arthritis, fibromyalgia does not involve inflammation and does not lead to permanent damage to connective tissues and organs. Aside from unexplained pain, symptoms include disrupted sleep, chest pain, headaches, menstrual cramps, and dizziness. A woman with fibromyalgia has what practitioners call tender points, muscular nodules that hurt when pressed.

There is no laboratory or blood test to diagnose fibromyalgia, and x-rays reveal nothing.

Treatments focus on alleviating pain rather than curing the fibromyalgia. Exercise, heat, and muscle stretching can help ease symptoms, and analgesics and anti-inflammatory drugs are often used. Tricyclic antidepressants are prescribed to promote deeper sleep. Some alternative therapies, including acupuncture and massage, are also used to treat fibromyalgia.

SEE arthritis; chronic fatigue syndrome.

For more information on fibromyalgia, contact:

American Massage Therapy Association
820 Davis St., Suite 100
Evanston, IL 60201-4444
708-864-0123

Arthritis Foundation Information Line
30 W. Peachtree St.
Atlanta, GA 30309
800-283-7800
404-872-7100
http://www.arthritis.org

Chronic Fatigue and Immune Dysfunction Syndrome (CFIDS) Association
P.O. Box 220398
Charlotte, NC 28222
800-442-3437
704-362-CFID
http://cfids.org/cfids

Fibromyalgia Network
P.O. Box 31750
Tucson, AZ 85751
520-290-5508

GYNECOLOGIC EXAMINATION

Annual gynecologic examinations by a practitioner are an important part of maintaining good health and help to ensure fertility and uncomplicated pregnancy and childbirth. They may also detect sexually transmitted infections before symptoms are apparent. In addition, many life-threatening conditions, such as breast cancer and cervical cancer, are first detected at a woman's annual exam.

Many women feel uncomfortable or anxious before a gynecologic exam, especially if they have never had one before. These women should let their practitioners know that it is their first gynecologic exam and ask any questions they may have. To reduce anxiety, the procedure should be explained and the instruments to be used should be shown to the woman beforehand. Many practitioners will give first-time patients more time and will try to be sensitive to any special needs.

RECOMMENDATIONS FOR GYNECOLOGIC EXAMS

Women over 18 years old and women who are sexually active should have gynecologic exams at least once a year. The exam is done each year so that symptoms of any problems, such as sexually transmitted infections or precancerous conditions, can be found early, when treatment is most successful. Usually, gynecologic examinations include a pelvic exam with a Pap test, a breast exam, and sometimes blood and urine tests.

Gynecologic examinations should be scheduled between menstrual periods because the menstrual fluid may affect some of the laboratory tests. Douching or using vaginal preparations should be avoided for 24 hours before an exam because they can mask symptoms of some conditions. Women may also want to prepare a list of questions and concerns in preparation for the exam.

BEFORE THE EXAMINATION

The practitioner will need a medical history in order to diagnose any possible problems and may ask a series of questions or ask you to fill out a questionnaire. The questions may address the following issues:

■ Family history of breast cancer or cancer of the reproductive organs

■ The date of your last menstrual period; the number of days in your cycle; the number of days your period lasts; the amount of flow (light, moderate, or heavy); symptoms that might indicate a problem: pain, swelling, fever, discharge, or bleeding

■ Whether or not you are planning to become pregnant

■ The number of children you have and their ages; any miscarriages, abortions, or stillbirths; any suspicion of infertility

■ Type of birth control you are using, if any, and whether or not you are aware of emergency contraception

■ Whether you have been practicing safer sex as protection against sexually transmitted infections (STIs)

■ Whether you have had new sex partners, multiple sex partners, or sex partners with STIs or risk factors for STIs since your last exam

■ Whether any STIs have been diagnosed in the past

■ Your general health and mental health (if there is any stress, anxiety, or worry, or if tranquilizers or any other drugs are being used)

■ Whether there is any pain or bleeding during or after sex

■ Sexual practices, satisfaction, and abuse

It is important to answer all of the questions honestly; the information is needed in order to provide the best possible care.

A urine sample may also be requested before the exam begins. The practitioner checks the color, clarity, acidity, and concentration of the urine. The sample may be tested for diabetes, pregnancy, and signs of bladder or kidney infection. Urinating before a pelvic exam also makes the examination more comfortable for the patient.

THE PELVIC EXAMINATION

There are several parts to a pelvic examination: the external genital exam, the speculum exam, the bimanual exam, and the rectovaginal exam.

A drape sheet is supplied for the pelvic exam. You may use it to cover yourself during the procedure to feel less exposed and more comfortable. If the practitioner is a man, usually another woman—a nurse or support person—will be present during the exam, to answer questions and provide support. You may request that any practitioner, man or woman, have another woman present during the exam.

The exam table has metal footrests, and you

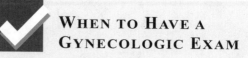

WHEN TO HAVE A GYNECOLOGIC EXAM

Annual gynecologic exams are a necessary part of good health. However, you should also consider scheduling a gynecologic exam:

■ If you are 16 years old and haven't begun menstruating

■ If your mother took diethylstilbestrol (DES) while she was pregnant with you. This drug is now banned but was widely used between 1941 and 1971 to prevent miscarriage.

■ If you have been suffering from severe menstrual cramps

■ If your menstrual flow is very heavy or lasts more than 10 days

■ If you experience any bleeding between periods

■ If you experience any burning, itching, or unusual discharge

■ If you experience burning when you urinate

■ If you have been experiencing painful intercourse, especially if you also have chills or a fever

■ If you are sexually active and have missed one period

■ If you have not been sexually active and have missed three or more periods

■ If you are planning to become pregnant

will be asked to lie down and place your feet on them, spreading your knees apart. This position, known as the lithotomy position, gives the practitioner the best view of the visible internal reproductive structures, which include the vagina and the cervix.

THE EXTERNAL GENITAL EXAM

The practitioner begins by visually inspecting the external genitals—the vulva, the labia, and the opening of the vagina—for irritation, herpes sores, genital warts, discharge, or anything else that appears unusual.

THE SPECULUM EXAM

After the external exam, a speculum (a duck-bill-shaped device made of metal or plastic) is inserted into the vagina and is opened to spread apart the walls of the vagina and view the cervix, the opening of the uterus. There may be a feeling of pressure or slight discomfort when the speculum is opened. It may be warmed first to take away the chill.

The speculum permits the practitioner to examine the cervix and to insert other instruments as needed. The practitioner looks at the vagina and the cervix for signs of redness, discharge, and rough spots, which could be precancerous cell changes.

While the speculum is open, the practitioner will also take samples for analysis. Cervical mucus may be collected on a cotton swab to test for gonorrhea, human papilloma virus, chlamydia, or other sexually transmitted infections. A woman who has risk factors for STIs should ask her practitioner to take a sample for testing if he or she does not normally do so.

At this time, a **Pap test** will also be done. This procedure is used primarily to detect cancerous and precancerous cells on the cervix. The Pap test involves taking a sample of cells from the cervix with a wooden spatula that looks like a popsicle stick and a small brush, known as a cytobrush. The sample is later tested in a lab for the presence of abnormal cells.

The Pap test is the most accurate way of testing for abnormal cervical cells, cells that indicate an infection is present, or cells that may become cancerous. The Pap test is done each year, in part, because 15 to 30 percent of those who are tested are said to have normal readings when in fact there are abnormal cells present. While improvements are being made in the accuracy of Pap tests, the best strategy for a woman is to have a Pap test done each year.

THE BIMANUAL EXAM

After the speculum is removed, the practitioner inserts two gloved, lubricated fingers into the vagina until they are against the cervix. The other hand is placed on the abdomen and pressure is applied, enabling the practitioner to feel the size and shape of the uterus and check for masses that might be on the ovaries or fallopian tubes. The practitioner will also check for tenderness or pain (which may indicate infection) and the position of the uterus.

THE RECTOVAGINAL EXAM

Many practitioners end the exam by inserting a gloved finger into the rectum and one into the vagina to determine the tone and alignment of the pelvic organs, the ovaries, the fallopian tubes, and the ligaments of the uterus. The practitioner looks for rectal lesions and tests the tone of the rectal sphincter muscles. Women over 35 are also checked for masses or blood in the rectum that may be an early sign of colon cancer.

BREAST EXAMINATION

At least once a year, you should have your breasts examined for lumps by a health professional. Usually, this test is done at the same time as the pelvic exam. You rest on your back and stretch your arm above your head as the

✓ MAKING THE EXAM MORE COMFORTABLE

There are several things you can do to make your annual gynecologic exam more comfortable:

■ Find a sensitive health-care provider. A sensitive practitioner is gentle, takes things slowly, and explains everything that is being done. Some practitioners warm the speculum before inserting it into the vagina. A smaller speculum may be available for women with smaller vaginas, and some practitioners will only use one finger instead of two to perform the internal portion of the exam. Some practitioners put covers over the metal stirrups so that your feet stay warm. All of these measures may seem simple, but they can make the exam much more comfortable.

■ Consider taking someone with you. You may feel much more comfortable if you have your mother, partner, or a close friend along during the exam to offer moral support. Some health centers discourage bringing a friend into the exam, since this may compromise the woman's ability to speak freely about experiences such as abuse or sexual satisfaction.

■ Consider whether you will be more comfortable with a woman or a man for a health-care provider. Whether your practitioner is a man or a woman, don't hesitate to request the presence of a woman nurse if that will make you more comfortable. This is your right and may make you feel much more relaxed.

■ Ask questions. If you don't know why something is being done, or if you have other questions about your reproductive health, your practitioner can provide the answers. The exam will be a much more positive experience if you leave it with all of your questions answered. Open communication with your practitioner can also make you feel more comfortable during the exam.

■ Try to relax. Some women experience pressure in the bladder or rectum when the speculum is in place. Relaxing your muscles can relieve this pressure and can also make the rectal exam less uncomfortable. Before your annual exam, you can practice relaxing your muscles while doing a self-exam with a speculum or while inserting a tampon. You'll feel less tense if you:

—Breathe slowly and deeply with your mouth open.

—Try to relax your muscles. Let your stomach muscles go soft. Relax your shoulders and relax the muscles between your legs.

—Ask your practitioner to let you know what is being done as it is happening.

■ Remember that you're in charge. Though you may feel you are in a vulnerable position during a pelvic exam, you are the one who has the final say. Let the practitioner know if anything is too uncomfortable or painful and ask as many questions as you like. You can remove the drape sheet, if you wish, in order to see what the practitioner is doing. Some offices and clinics can set up a mirror so you can see the examination, if it is requested in advance. Most important, remember that you can stop the examination if you feel it is necessary.

practitioner checks the breast and armpit for lumps. The practitioner will also ask if you perform monthly self-exams and should instruct you on the proper technique.

ADDITIONAL PROCEDURES

Several other tests may be done before or after the pelvic exam in order to help the practitioner make the most accurate diagnosis possible. These tests may also be done if the gynecologic exam is part of a **general medical examination.**

The practitioner may check height and weight, blood pressure, and pulse. There may also be an examination of the fingernails, skin, and head as well as the eyes, nose, and throat. Swollen glands, a sore throat, and rashes on the palms of the hands may be symptoms of syphilis, for example. The practitioner may also listen to the lungs and the heart using a stethoscope.

There may also be an abdominal examination. For this exam, the practitioner gently presses down on the abdomen, feeling for signs of liver or spleen enlargement. The practitioner may also check your back for any pain or tenderness in the area of the kidneys.

If necessary, blood may be taken for analysis; it can be used to detect anemia and some sexually transmitted infections, including syphilis.

AFTER THE EXAMINATION

When the examination is finished, the practitioner should take a few minutes to discuss the results of the exam and any questions or concerns. This is the time to discuss birth control, menopause, the breast self-exam, or any other questions that have gone unanswered.

If the lab tests indicate anything unusual, the practitioner will contact the patient with the results. Pregnancy test results are usually available during the office visit; Pap test and blood test results may take three to 10 days.

SEE breast self-examination; Pap test; practitioners, how to choose.

For more information on a gynecologic exam, contact:

Planned Parenthood Federation of America, Inc.
810 Seventh Avenue
New York, NY 10019
For the Planned Parenthood nearest you, call:
    800-230-PLAN
http://www.ppfa.org/ppfa

HEART DISEASE

Coronary heart disease (CHD) is the narrowing of the blood vessels that nourish the heart, most often caused by the buildup of fatty deposits called **plaque** on the artery walls. This degeneration, known as **atherosclerosis** or hardening of the arteries, obstructs the flow of oxygen- and nutrient-rich blood to the heart, causing damage to the heart muscle. One may experience chest pain, heart attack, or sudden death.

Coronary heart disease is the leading cause of death among American women, taking the lives of 250,000 a year. This accounts for 28 percent of fatalities among women annually. One in every nine women between the ages of 45 and 64 and one in every three women over the age of 64 have some form of heart disease.

CHD is only one form of cardiovascular disease (diseases of the heart and blood vessels). Other conditions aree **high blood pressure**—also called **hypertension**—and **stroke,** which occurs when the blood supply to the brain is interrupted. The heart may also be affected by **arrhythmias,** irregularities in the heart's rhythm, and **valvular heart disease,** which occurs when the valves that regulate the flow of blood through the heart are not functioning properly.

RISK

According to the American Heart Association, the following factors contribute to coronary heart disease:

■ Heredity. Children of parents with cardiovascular disease are more likely to develop it themselves, especially if the parent suffered a heart attack at an early age (less than 55 for men and 65 for women).

■ Gender. Men have a greater risk of heart disease earlier in life. After menopause, the women's death rate from heart disease eventually increases to equal men's.

■ Increasing age. Four out of five people who die from heart attack are 65 years of age or older.

■ Smoking. Smokers' risk of heart attack is more than twice that of nonsmokers.

■ High cholesterol levels. The risk of heart disease increases as cholesterol levels increase. Levels of 200 mg/dl (milligrams per deciliter) in adults is associated with a low risk of heart disease, while levels of 240 mg/dl and over double the risk. For women, a low HDL, or good cholesterol, level (below 50 mg/dl) is a more important indicator of risk than total cholesterol. High levels of triglycerides are also important risk factors for women.

■ High blood pressure. High blood pressure increases the workload of the heart, resulting over time in an enlarged, weakened heart.

■ Physical inactivity. Lack of exercise can lead to obesity, high blood cholesterol levels, hypertension, and diabetes.

■ Diabetes. More than 80 percent of people with diabetes die of some form of heart disease because diabetes affects many systems of the body that can contribute to heart disease. The risk of heart disease is increased 150 percent for women with diabetes. Often those with diabetes have high cholesterol and atherosclerosis.

■ Obesity. Excess weight increases the strain on the heart. People more than 30 percent over their ideal weight are more likely to develop heart disease.

■ Stress. Researchers have noted a relationship between the levels of stress in a woman's life and the risk of heart disease. While stress is common in today's lifestyles, it appears to be the stresses that women have little or no control over that are dangerous to their health.

SYMPTOMS

Symptoms of heart disease in women may be more subtle than those for men. Symptoms may include:

■ Subtle yet constant pressure or heaviness in the chest

■ Pain in the shoulders, neck, or jaw that runs down the arms or back

■ Dizziness, fainting, sweating, nausea, unusual shortness of breath, or weakness with chest discomfort during minimal exertion (such as climbing stairs)

■ Chest pain during exertion or stress that subsides during a period of rest

■ Indigestion that cannot be relieved with antacids

■ Difficulty breathing

When the heart does not get enough oxygenated blood, chest pains known as **angina pectoris** occur. An angina attack usually lasts for no more than 15 minutes; if it does not subside, the woman should be taken via ambulance to the hospital emergency room to diagnose possible heart attack through blood tests and electrocardiogram (EKG).

A **heart attack,** medically known as a **myocardial infarction,** most often occurs when a clot blocks the coronary artery, the major artery to the heart. This results in **ischemia,** a diminished blood flow to a portion of the heart muscle. The blockage is usually the result of the buildup of plaque within the arteries and spasm of the blocked artery. Heart attacks are also caused by other factors, such as shock, overexertion, congestive heart failure, and other conditions that force the heart to require more blood.

CHOLESTEROL AND HEART DISEASE

Cholesterol, a fatty substance found in the body as well as in certain foods, has long been associated with CHD. While cholesterol is necessary to the body, high levels of a type of "bad" cholesterol known as **low-density lipoproteins,** or **LDLs,** contribute to the buildup of plaque within the arteries. **High-density lipoproteins,** or **HDLs,** are known as good cholesterol because they help to clear excess bad cholesterol from the bloodstream. In addition, high total cholesterol can be the result of an inherited genetic trait. Medications may be used to lower high cholesterol levels. Changes in diet can also help regulate the level of cholesterol in the body.

ESTROGEN AND HEART DISEASE

The relationship between coronary heart disease and estrogen, a hormone produced mainly in the ovaries, is a controversial subject. In premenopausal women, naturally occurring estrogen can help to protect against CHD because it raises HDL cholesterol levels and lowers the levels of the clogging LDL cholesterol. For this reason, the risk of heart disease for women

NATIONAL CHOLESTEROL EDUCATION PROGRAM CHOLESTEROL CLASSIFICATION GUIDELINES FOR ADULTS

**Cholesterol Level (mg/dl)
Classification**

Total Cholesterol
Less than 200	Desirable
200-239	Borderline
240 or higher	High

HDL Cholesterol
50-75 or higher	Desirable
35-49	Borderline low
Less than 35	Low

LDL Cholesterol
Less than 130	Desirable
130-159	Borderline high
160 or higher	High

Triglycerides
200 or less	Safe
200-400	Borderline
400-1,000	High
1,000 or above	Very high

increases after menopause, when ovarian production of estrogen ceases.

Oral contraceptives, which contain estrogen, were once thought to increase the risk of CHD by three times by contributing to high blood pressure and blood clots. Blood clots are dangerous because they may clog arteries and possibly lead to heart attack or stroke. This has some truth for women who are over age 35 who smoke and take oral contraceptives. However, recent studies show no increase of heart attack associated with the Pill, possibly because the amount of estrogen contained in oral contraceptives has decreased as they have been refined.

Hormone replacement therapy (HRT) is often prescribed to replenish the level of estrogen in the blood. The American College of Physicians' 1992 Clinical Guideline for preventive hormone therapy reports that estrogen prescribed alone reduces the risk of heart disease by 35 percent. Some experts believe that when estrogen is taken in conjunction with another hormone, such as progestin, some of its protection against heart disease disappears. Conflicting evidence shows that estrogen in combination with progestin actually improves the protection against heart disease.

However, if estrogen is prescribed without progestin, it may increase the risk of endometrial cancer because estrogen promotes the growth of the uterine lining. HRT has also been linked to breast cancer and may fuel the growth of endometriosis and fibroids. In addition, estrogen may decrease the anticlotting factors of the blood and may cause blood clots in women with a history of them.

A woman considering oral contraceptives, HRT, or estrogen in another form should discuss her specific risk factors with her practitioner, then weigh the risks and benefits before making a decision.

DIAGNOSIS

If any of the symptoms of heart disease are present, a woman should immediately seek medical help. If a problem is suspected, the practitioner may recommend an **electrocardiogram (EKG),** a test in which electrical leads placed on the body measure the electrical currents of the heart. The currents are transcribed

CUTTING BACK ON CHOLESTEROL

Reducing dietary cholesterol may help to lower the levels of cholesterol in your blood. To help reduce cholesterol:

■ Cut your intake of saturated fats. This should lower your cholesterol and your weight, reducing your risk of heart disease.

■ Try soy proteins, found in tofu and soy milk. It has recently been found to lower cholesterol levels in those who eat 30 to 40 grams a day.

■ Eat foods rich in fiber, such as carrots, celery, and breads and cereals made with whole grains.

■ Eat more fruits and vegetables. Replace animal fats—especially those that are solid at room temperature—with vegetable oils, such as corn, safflower, soybean,

olive, and sesame. A vegetarian diet may be protective.

■ Keep track of what you eat. Get yourself a chart of foods and their dietary cholesterol content and place a ceiling of 300 mg a day on your meals.

■ Cut down on coffee. Caffeine can elevate heart rate and cause arrhythmias that may be dangerous to those with heart disease.

■ If it is necessary for you to severely limit your dietary cholesterol, talk with your practitioner or a dietician about a strict diet. The Pritikin diet, for example, eliminates fatty meats, sugar, salt, eggs, oils, and nuts from the diet, and relies on fruits, vegetables, and whole grains.

into a pattern along a continuous strip of graph paper, then read for any abnormalities. EKGs are often inaccurate, showing abnormalities in women and men who do not have heart disease.

A **stress test** calls for the patient to have EKG readings before, during, and after exercise, usually done on a treadmill. Stress tests are designed to diagnose symptoms of heart disease that occur with exertion. However, it may be difficult for some women to raise their heart rate enough to make the test accurate. This test may also show abnormalities where none exist.

In addition, a standard **x-ray** may be done to examine heart structures. **Angiography,** used to examine blood flow and heart function, may be done by injecting dye or another contrast material into the blood vessels to make them visible, then taking an x-ray. Another test is an

echocardiogram, in which ultrasonic waves are used to create an image of the heart.

Cardiac catheterization, a form of angiography, is an invasive test in which a plastic tube is inserted through a blood vessel in the groin into the heart of a patient. Then, dye is injected and an x-ray is used to obtain detailed images of the heart's blood vessels. It is also possible to monitor the pressure in the heart chambers, and take blood samples. Some people have chest pain and abnormal stress tests but normal coronary arteries. This may mean the pain is due to problems in the smaller blood vessels within the heart. However, cardiac catheterization is still the most definitive test available.

In addition, new variations of **CAT scans** (computerized axial tomography scans, which create three-dimensional x-rays) and **MRI,** or **magnetic resonance imaging** (which uses a

DIAGNOSING HEART DISEASE

To ensure a reliable diagnosis:

■ Seek a complete cardiac workup with a practitioner who uses an echocardiogram.

■ Find a practitioner who begins the examination from scratch and does not rely on information from other practitioners. A practitioner should also ask about your medical history and habits, such as whether or not you smoke and exercise.

■ Get a second opinion if there is any doubt about the diagnosis. Heart disease is a serious issue and should not be taken lightly.

magnetic field to create an image), offer noninvasive ways of diagnosing problems with the heart's blood supply. These tests are expensive and not yet widely available.

TREATMENT

There are several drug treatments for coronary heart disease. **Calcium channel blockers** block calcium, the primary factor in coronary spasm, and are used to treat angina. **Vasodilators,** which include nitroglycerin and other drugs, such as Isordil and Cardilate, work by dilating the blood vessels to allow the blood to flow more easily. In addition, **diuretics,** which promote urination and speed the elimination of sodium and water from the body, are used to lower blood pressure. While these drugs may prevent attacks of angina, they do not change the underlying physical problems of heart disease.

If a heart attacks occurs, **beta blockers** (such as Inderal) may be used to slow blood pressure and keep heart attack damage to a minimum. **Clot-busting drugs** (such as streptokinase, tPA, and Eminase) are enzymes that disintegrate the blood clot blocking the artery. While these drugs are as effective in women as in men, women are at higher risk of internal bleeding, a complication of the drugs.

Surgery may be necessary for individuals with severe symptoms of heart disease and those with narrowing of the left main coronary artery, no matter what the symptoms, because it can lead to sudden death. The most common surgery is **coronary bypass,** in which a vein is removed from the leg and is used to create a detour around the blocked portion of the coronary artery.

Laser coronary angioplasty is a procedure in which a thin catheter is inserted into a blocked vessel and a laser is used to disintegrate the blockages. **Balloon angioplasty** is the insertion of a balloon, which when inflated pushes the blockage out of the way and stretches the artery. When the ballon is removed, the artery should be more open to blood flow.

HEART DISEASE AND GENDER BIAS

Coronary heart disease has long been considered a "man's disease" by many practitioners. However, women who have heart attacks are twice as likely as men to die from them, and there are many theories as to why this is true.

Studies have shown that women are on average 10 years older than men when they first suffer symptoms of heart disease and 20 years older when they first suffer heart attack. Some experts speculate that this advanced age may

LIFESTYLE AND HEART DISEASE

Lifestyle changes are an important part of the treatment for heart disease. There are many steps you can take to reduce your risk of heart disease or increase your chances of recovery:

■ Quit smoking. Nearly three times as many smokers die from CHD than from lung cancer.

■ Reduce your levels of cholesterol. (See previous discussion.)

■ Eat oily varieties of fish at least twice a week. Omega-3 fatty acids, found in fish such as salmon, flounder, and cod, may help to prevent blood clots from forming.

■ Drink alcohol in moderation. While a small amount of alcohol (one to two drinks per day) may increase the levels of HDL cholesterol, more may cause high blood pressure, and alcohol is more toxic in women than in men—in lower amounts and in shorter periods of time. Women who have a history or potential for alcoholism should not drink at all.

■ Ask your practitioner about the benefits of aspirin. Aspirin helps to thin the blood and prevent clots from forming. However, aspirin is not safe for everyone and in some may increase the risk for stroke.

■ Exercise regularly. Exercise is an important preventive of heart disease, since heart disease is twice as likely to develop in inactive people than in those who are active.

■ Reduce stress. Relaxation techniques, such as meditation and yoga, can help relieve tension.

■ Monitor diabetes carefully. If you have diabetes, you probably have less natural resistance to heart disease. By controlling diabetes with insulin or other medications, the risk of CHD is lowered.

■ Lower high blood pressure. High blood pressure puts a strain on the heart. Alcohol, caffeine, cigarettes, and stress can all increase blood pressure.

■ Control weight gain. A 1995 study from Harvard Medical School found that a weight gain of as little as 10 pounds after age 18 could result in an increased risk of CHD for middle-aged women.

lead to more complications and therefore the higher mortality rate. In addition, some feel that older women are treated less aggressively because they are "past their prime." Men, for example, are more likely to undergo the standard cardiac catheterization test than women and are much more likely to undergo surgery as a treatment for CHD.

It has also recently been acknowledged that the symptoms of heart disease manifest themselves differently in women than in men. As a result, some experts say, symptoms in women are not recognized and instead are downplayed as psychological symptoms of depression and anxiety. Women may receive inadequate or delayed treatment as a result.

In addition, the majority of the medical studies done on heart disease and research on treatments have used men as their subjects. However, many treatments and diagnostic tests that are effective for men may not be as effective for women. Women-centered studies are needed, some experts say, to determine how to best diagnose and treat heart disease in women. The Women's Health Initiative current heart disease study involving 140,000 women, sponsored by the National Institutes of Health, may provide some answers.

SEE blood pressure; cholesterol; hormone replacement therapy; stroke.

For more information on heart disease, contact:

American College of Advancement in Medicine
P.O. Box 3427
Laguna Hills, CA 92654
714-583-7666

American Heart Association
7272 Greenville Ave.
Dallas, TX 75231-4596
800-AHA-USA1
214-373-6300
http://www.amhrt.org

Coronary Club, Inc.
9500 Euclid Ave., EE37
Cleveland, OH 44195
800-478-4255
216-444-3690

High Blood Pressure Information Center
National Heart, Lung, and Blood Institute
P.O. Box 30105
Bethesda, MD 20824-0105
301-251-1222
http://www.nhlbi.nih.gov/nhlbi/nhlbi.html

Mended Hearts
7272 Greenville Ave.
Dallas, TX 75231
214-706-1442

Women's Heart Research Fund
P.O. Box 7827
West Trenton, NJ 08628
609-771-9600

HERBAL MEDICINE

Herbal medicine is a healing art that uses plants to prevent and cure illnesses. A person skilled in the art of herbal medicine who can compound herbal mixtures made from the various plants is an herbalist.

Herbology, the use of plants as medicine, is probably as old as humankind. People have practiced herbal medicine throughout the world and throughout history. According to historians, many ancient peoples, including the Chinese, Egyptians, Babylonians, and Aztecs, practiced herbal medicine. African Americans and Native Americans were also herbalists and educated the early European Americans on the use of herbs as coital and postcoital methods of birth control.

Humans probably learned how to use herbs to treat illnesses by watching animals and noting what plants they ate when they were sick. Herbalists claim that their remedies do not have the harmful side effects that are so common with modern medicines. However, if taken improperly, the herbs themselves can be dangerous to a person's health.

Herbs can be used as astringents, tonics,

laxatives, and mild diuretics. Nervines are herbs that can either relax or excite the nervous system. Herbs are taken in many different forms depending on their type and use. They may be taken naturally, as capsules, powders, tinctures, or oils. Often they are steeped in boiling water to create herbal infusions.

Anxiety, premenstrual syndrome, and symptoms of menopause can be treated with herbal medicine. Phytoestrogens, plant-derived estrogens, are used to relieve hot flashes, night sweats, and mood swings. Foods that contain phytoestrogens include soy products and leafy greens.

A consultation with an herbalist is recommended when choosing herbs and doses for treatment. Certain herbal preparations should never be taken during pregnancy because they can cause premature labor. An herbalist should be informed of all medical conditions including pregnancy or potential pregnancy, and a practitioner should be consulted before using herbs. One's traditional practitioner should also be informed of all herbs that are being used. Some herbs can cause harmful side effects or are toxic in certain amounts. Some are especially dangerous when taken with prescription medications.

Since herbal remedies do not need to be evaluated by the Food and Drug Administration, their

HERBAL REMEDIES AND THEIR USES

The following list gives just a few of the many remedies available along with the symptoms that they treat:

Chamomile—diarrhea; migraine headaches; gastritis; colitis; overindulgence in food or drink; insomnia; nightmares

Evening Primrose Oils—rheumatoid arthritis; premenstrual syndrome; heart disease; obesity

Garlic—high blood pressure; reduced resistance to infection

Ginseng—stress; lack of energy; tiredness

Peppermint—indigestion; colic; anxiety

Rosemary—nervous tension; headaches

Sage—insomnia; depression; increased perspiration; bad breath

Valerian—insomnia; anxiety; tension

manufacturers may make unsubstantiated claims about their products. As with medications, the key to using herbs is to carefully research the claims for each one. Libraries and health food stores usually have books on herbal medicine.

SEE Chinese medicine.

For more information on herbal medicine, contact:

American Botanical Council
P.O. Box 201660
Austin, TX 78720
512-331-8868
http://www.herbalgram.org

American Herbalists Guild
P.O. Box 746555
Arvada, CO 80006
303-423-8800

Association of Natural Medicine Pharmacists
8369 Champs de Elysses
Forestville, CA 95436
707-887-1351

HOMEOPATHIC MEDICINE

Homeopathic medicine treats illnesses by using natural substances that stimulate a person's own healing powers while avoiding harmful side effects. Most practitioners skilled in homeopathy today are allopathic physicians (doctors of medicine, or M.D.'s) or osteopathic physicians (doctors of osteopathy, or D.O.'s) who have additional training in homeopathic principles. Homeopathy is used to treat many conditions women experience, including menstrual disorders, infertility, stress, endometriosis, and urinary tract infections.

Homeopathy dates back to Hippocrates, though its scientific foundations were set down in 1810 by Samuel Hahnemann, a German physician. It follows the philosophy that "like cures like" and that minute amounts of substances that cause symptoms of diseases in healthy people will bring about cures in sick people. Another basic tenet of homeopathy is that the whole person must be treated and not just the disease.

Homeopathic medicine requires the use of a single remedy. Homeopaths administer only one medicine at a time. If the condition persists, a second medication is used, but they are never combined. Homeopathic medicine uses the smallest dose possible in order to allow the body to absorb the medication and to prevent rejection or reactions due to strong doses.

OVER-THE-COUNTER REMEDIES

Homeopathic medications are extracted from naturally occurring substances such as plants, animal material, and natural chemicals. The substances are soaked in water and alcohol for more than a month, then filtered several times and shaken vigorously for several seconds. The preparations are taken by mouth, tend to be tasteless, can be stored for periods of time, and do not produce toxic side effects.

A basic belief of homeopathy is that no matter how many times a solution has been diluted from the original material, it will remain effective. In fact, the remedy is thought to become more powerful through dilution. The labels of the remedies usually indicate how many times they have been diluted.

Homeopathic remedies can be found in health food stores and drugstores. The remedies should be taken in the correct doses. Allergic reactions to remedies are uncommon, but any reaction should be reported to a regular practitioner. A regular practitioner should also be made aware of any homeopathic medications being taken. If a condition persists despite homeopathic remedies, a doctor or homeopathic physician should be contacted.

For more information on homeopathy or a listing of local homeopathic physicians, contact:

International Foundation for Homeopathy
P.O. Box 7
Edmonds, WA 98020
206-776-4147

National Center for Homeopathy
801 N. Fairfax St., Suite 306
Alexandria, VA 22314
703-548-7790
http://www.healthy.net/nch

HORMONE REPLACEMENT THERAPY

Hormone replacement therapy (HRT) is a regimen used to treat and prevent osteoporosis, prevent heart disease, and relieve many symptoms of menopause. During menopause, the ovaries' production of estrogen declines. This causes an increased loss of bone density and has a detrimental effect on cholesterol levels and blood vessel tones. It also upsets the body's thermostat, which can lead to hot flashes and vaginal atrophy (dryness and thinness of the vaginal lining). Women on HRT take natural or synthetic hormones to supplement these diminishing levels of estrogen and restore the balance of hormones in the body.

ADVANTAGES OF HRT

More than 11 million women choose HRT to relieve menopausal symptoms. The benefits of HRT include:

■ Relief from hot flashes, which usually subside after about two weeks of HRT

■ Relief from vaginal atrophy

■ Protection from osteoporosis. HRT works by slowing down the loss of bone mass due to estrogen withdrawal during menopause.

■ Prevention of heart disease. HRT, particularly estrogen, is believed to help prevent heart disease, the number one killer of postmenopausal women, by directly affecting the blood vessels and by raising blood levels of high-density lipoproteins (HDLs), the beneficial cholesterol that lowers one's risk for heart disease.

No one is sure whether HRT helps prevent skin aging, mood swings, depression, or insomnia. A National Institutes of Health Conference found no evidence that estrogen relieves depression and prevents skin aging, but some practitioners still prescribe it for emotional stability or to preserve youthful appearance.

DISADVANTAGES OF HRT

On the surface, HRT may seem like an ideal way to relieve bothersome menopausal symptoms, but it is not without risks and disadvantages. Medical research findings on HRT are contradictory and confusing, and its possible long-term effects are unknown.

■ When taken alone as HRT, estrogen causes the uterine lining to grow and thicken, which can lead to abnormal cell growth and eventual cancer of the endometrium (uterine lining). However, if progestin is prescribed to balance the estrogen, there is no increase in risk. Progestin causes the thickened lining of the uterus to shed as monthly bleeding (similar to a menstrual period), even in women beyond menopause.

■ HRT has also been linked to breast cancer, although there is no solid evidence for such a connection. A few studies show increased risk of breast cancer for women using long-term (seven years or more) HRT; most others show no increase in risk.

■ HRT may also increase gallstones and gallbladder pain. Women who take estrogen as a part of HRT are more likely to have their gall-bladder removed than women who don't.

■ In premenopausal women, HRT can fuel estrogen-dependent fibroid tumors or endometriosis, and it can cause painful, lumpy breasts. HRT may be taken by premenopausal women in the few months or year before menopause occurs to help control the irregular bleeding and hot flashes.

■ Reported short-term side effects of HRT are rare. They include bleeding between monthly "periods," water retention, bloating, breast tenderness, nausea, increased cervical mucus, cramps, weight gain, headaches, hair loss, itching, and corneal changes that prevent the use of contact lenses. Side effects may be minimized by adjusting dosage.

COMPONENTS OF HRT

ESTROGEN

The primary hormone of HRT is estrogen, the hormone produced in the ovaries that thickens the uterine lining, regulates menstruation, and is responsible for the development of breasts, rounded hips, and pubic hair during puberty. The most commonly prescribed estrogen of HRT is Premarin, named for pregnant mares' urine, from which it is extracted. Premarin is a combination of estrone (a type of estrogen naturally produced in the fat cells of women) and other estrogens. Other types of estrogen, such as estrone and micronized estradiol, are also prescribed. Estrogen is available in many forms, including pills, injections, patches, and vaginal creams.

PROGESTIN

Progestin, synthetic progesterone, or natural progesterone is the second component of HRT,

often added to estrogen to offset the risk of endometrial cancer. Progestin breaks down the uterine lining and allows it to shed as menstrual bleeding, which prevents cancer from developing.

A new study, called the Postmenopausal Estrogen and Progestin Interventions (PEPI) Trial, found that a mixture of estrogen and progestin is better than estrogen alone for protecting women against the risk of both endometrial cancer and heart attacks. Some experts, however, believe that progestin reduces the cardiovascular benefits of estrogen and do not prescribe progestin for women who have had a hysterectomy. In these cases, estrogen alone is considered safe because there is no need to worry about endometrial cancer.

ANDROGENS

Androgens, male hormones that include testosterone, may also be used in HRT. They are prescribed when estrogen and progestin therapy does not completely relieve symptoms and are especially useful in treating hair loss and diminished sex drive. They are thought to provide an increased sense of well-being, a higher level of sexual desire, relief from headaches and depression, and increased bone mass. Side effects include excessive hair growth (hirsutism) and oily skin. Generally only small amounts of androgens, combined with estrogen, are used.

WEIGHING THE PROS AND CONS

Because of the conflicting evidence on HRT, it is difficult for health professionals to reach a consensus on whether to recommend it. Whether to take HRT is an individual decision each woman must make. Before deciding, she must consider her risk factors and the severity of her symptoms. She should also consider her lifestyle, such as whether or not she smokes, because smoking interferes with estrogen protection against heart disease and osteoporosis.

The benefits of HRT may outweigh the risks. For example, at age 50, one out of every 50 women develops breast cancer. By 60, the rate increases to one out of every 24. However, if it is detected and treated early, there is a five-year survival rate of 94 percent. On the other hand, after 50, women's risk of heart disease increases threefold. Therefore, a woman may consider taking HRT, since it significantly reduces the risk of heart disease, while the statistical chances of developing breast cancer are small. Even if breast cancer does develop, it is highly treatable if detected early.

Most practitioners recommend HRT if a woman's HDLs (high-density lipoproteins) are low and:

■ Heart disease runs in her family.

■ Osteoporosis runs in her family, or a bone density test shows that her hip or backbone is very thin.

■ Her ovaries were surgically removed before age 45.

HRT is not recommended if a woman has a history of any of the following:

■ Breast or endometrial cancer, or if the cancers run in her family

■ A tendency to form blood clots

■ Unexplained vaginal bleeding

A health-care provider should carefully monitor the health of women who use HRT and have a history of:

■ Migraines

■ Endometriosis

■ Fibroid tumors

■ Diabetes

■ Gallbladder disease

FORMS OF HRT

HRT comes in many forms. A woman, with the help of her practitioner, should find out about them all and decide which is best suited to her needs.

Pills: For women at high risk of heart disease, oral therapy is the best form of HRT because it travels through the liver first and has the most positive effect on increasing HDL cholesterol, the good cholesterol which is made in the liver.

Vaginal creams: Estrogen-containing cream applied directly to the vagina reduces vaginal atrophy, itching, and irritation. The creams are used continually, not on an "as needed" basis. Because the estrogen is absorbed directly into the bloodstream, this form has fewer side effects than other methods. However, it does not travel to the liver and so does not have cardiovascular benefits.

Estrogen-releasing patches: These patches release estrogen continuously through the skin into the bloodstream. The steady flow of estrogen means there are no fluctuating levels (meaning fewer side effects), and practitioners can be sure the proper dosage is being taken. However, patches have not yet been shown to provide protection from cardiovascular disease. They are best for women who suffer short-term side effects from estrogen and who are at low risk of heart disease. The patches need to be changed once or twice a week.

Implants: Pellets containing estrogen or progestin can be implanted under the skin by a practitioner. The pellet slowly releases the medication into the body for three to four months. They have few side effects. However, they do not provide protection from heart disease and may be difficult to remove if side effects do occur. It is also difficult to tell when a pellet has been used up.

219

ALTERNATIVES TO HRT

HRT is not the ideal solution to menopausal relief, nor is it the only one. There are many other ways to offset the effects of diminishing estrogen levels.

Though heart disease may be prevented using HRT, it may be treated and prevented in many other ways. Drugs are available to lower blood pressure and cholesterol, and lifestyle factors can be adjusted to lower your risk. A program of proper diet and regular exercise will lower risks significantly.

Osteoporosis, too, can be slowed through programs other than HRT. Medications, such as the drug calcitonin, can be prescribed to halt bone loss. Weight-bearing exercise, a good diet, and plenty of calcium in the premenopausal years can also help prevent brittle bones.

The drug **Fosamax,** which does not contain hormones and was recently approved by the FDA, increases bone strength and reduces fractures in older women. An advisory committee reported that Fosamax seems to pose fewer risks than estrogen; so far, the only identified side effect is mild stomach discomfort. Another drug, **slow-release sodium fluoride**, is awaiting FDA approval (at time of publication). Studies have shown the drug may help to actually reverse bone loss.

Hot flashes and vaginal atrophy can be treated through other means as well. The hormone progestin can be taken to stop hot flashes, and over-the-counter lubricants (such as Replens) may be used for vaginal atrophy.

Another possible way to replenish lost estrogen and prevent menopausal symptoms is to eat plant foods containing natural estrogens, such as legumes, papaya, and soy. These plant estrogens may relieve mild hot flashes and lower the risk of osteoporosis, breast cancer, and heart disease. Yams are also a good source of progestins; however, they need to be eaten raw and in large amounts. While phytoestrogens are all-natural, they are still a form of estrogen replacement therapy—and the dose of estrogen you are eating cannot be determined. Be sure to discuss plant estrogens with your practitioner, especially if you have a history of estrogen-dependent cancer or if there is a reason you cannot take hormone replacement therapy.

Alternative therapies for menopause include homeopathy and Chinese medicine. Biofeedback, in which the woman learns techniques that allow her to control her heartbeat and monitor brain waves, may also be effective.

Some herbal remedies have proven effective for some of the symptoms linked to menopause. Panax ginseng, fennel, licorice, anise, dong quai, motherwort, and chamomile are among the herbs available. These herbs ease hot flashes and promote relaxation, but they may have drawbacks, such as increased blood pressure (licorice is such an herb). Herbs are all-natural, but many can be toxic in large doses. Herbal creams containing natural alternatives, such as yams, dong quai, black cohosh, and panax ginseng, are also available. Contact an herbalist for correct dosage and possible side effects.

Injections: Intramuscular injections of estrogen can provide effects for up to four weeks. However, they offer varying levels of estrogen in the blood, are difficult to monitor, and do not provide protection against heart disease.

LONG-TERM HRT

Experts are unsure of how long it takes for women on HRT to receive the benefits of protection against osteoporosis and heart disease. While only a few years of treatment may be necessary for menopausal symptoms, some experts are now saying it may take at least seven years to derive the best heart benefits, and possibly 10 years for osteoporosis benefits. Some practitioners feel HRT should be perpetual.

Still, no one is quite sure about the long-term effects of HRT either. Because of the lack of comprehensive research over the years, and the number of conflicting studies, it will be some time before all the questions are answered. One major study by the National Institutes of Health will be completed in 2005 and is expected to provide some definitive results. Until more information is available, however, women should weigh the pros and the cons, talk with their practitioners, and make individual decisions on the use of HRT.

SEE androgens; cancer, breast; estrogen; heart disease; menopause; osteoporosis.

For more information on HRT, contact:

National Institute on Aging Information Center
P.O. Box 8057
Gaithersburg, MD 20898-8057
800-222-2225
niainfo@access.digex.net

National Women's Health Network
514 10th St., N.W., Suite 400
Washington, DC 20004
202-347-1140

National Women's Health Resource Center
2425 L St., N.W., 3rd floor
Washington, DC 20037
202-293-6045

North American Menopause Society
c/o University Hospitals of Cleveland
Department of OBGYN
11100 Euclid Ave.
Cleveland, OH 44106
216-844-3334
http://www.menopause.org

Office of Alternative Medicine
National Institutes of Health
9000 Rockville Pike
Bldg. 31, Room 5B-38
Bethesda, MD 20892
301- 402-2466

HYSTERECTOMY

Hysterectomy is the surgical removal of the uterus, a procedure that is often accompanied by removal of the ovaries and fallopian tubes. According to the National Center for Health Statistics, hysterectomy remains one of the most commonly performed major surgeries in the United States, with 562,000 performed in 1993. The National Center for Health Statistics reports that one third of the women in the United States have a hysterectomy by the age of 60.

Radical hysterectomies—removal of the uterus, the upper one-third of the vagina, and the lymph nodes—are done to stop the spread of cancer of the uterus, vagina, fallopian tubes, and ovaries. An emergency hysterectomy may be warranted for severe, uncontrollable bleeding and for some rare complications of pregnancy, such as uterine rupture or abnormal placentas.

In non-life-threatening circumstances, there is much controversy about when a hysterectomy is appropriate. Many hysterectomies are performed for abnormal bleeding. Statistics show that 40 percent of hysterectomies are performed for fibroid tumors, 20 percent for uterine prolapse, and 20 percent for endometriosis; however, all three conditions can sometimes be relieved with less invasive alternatives. Only 10 percent of hysterectomies are performed because of cancer.

TYPES OF SURGERIES

Several different types of hysterectomies and related surgeries can be performed.

A **total hysterectomy** removes the entire uterus with the cervix. It does not always involve removal of the ovaries or the fallopian tubes. Ovulation may continue while menstruation stops—the egg is released into the pelvic cavity and absorbed by the body.

Removal of the ovaries and fallopian tubes often accompanies hysterectomy. Removal of one ovary is an **oophorectomy;** removal of both is a **bilateral oophorectomy.** Removal of the fallopian tubes is called a **salpingectomy.** If ovaries and fallopian tubes are removed along with the uterus, it is called a **total hysterectomy with bilateral salpingo-oophorectomy.**

A **subtotal,** or **supracervical, hysterectomy** involves amputation of the uterus above the cervix. The cervix remains in place, which some practitioners believe helps to augment sexual response. The procedure is not recommended in cases where cancer is a concern because the cervix can still be affected. Less tissue is cut during this surgery than with a total hysterectomy, so bladder, bowel, and sexual functions may be less affected.

A **radical hysterectomy,** reserved for invasive cancer, involves removal of the uterus, removal of the upper one-third of the vagina, and extensive removal of lymph nodes. It does not *necessarily* include removal of the ovaries or fallopian tubes. Complications are more common than with a total or subtotal hysterectomy.

Hysterectomies can be performed in two ways. An **abdominal hysterectomy** removes the uterus through an incision in the lower abdomen, which may be horizontal or vertical. An abdominal hysterectomy is recommended when there is widespread cancer; when fibroids are too large to remove through the vagina; or when there is abdominal scarring due to previous operations. While an abdominal hysterectomy allows the surgeon access to the entire abdominal cavity, it may mean a longer recovery period and more postoperative pain for the woman.

A **vaginal hysterectomy** removes the uterus through an incision in the vagina near the cervix. The main advantages of this technique are a hidden incision and faster healing. It is also more commonly recommended than the abdominal hysterectomy for uterine prolapse. However, when abdominal scarring or adhesions are present, as a result of previous surgery or infection, it may be more difficult to perform a vaginal hysterectomy. In this case a laparoscope, a flexible viewing device, may be inserted into the abdomen and may be used in conjunction with a vaginal hysterectomy. It may also be used to assess and treat scarring prior to surgery so that vaginal hysterectomy is easier to perform.

BENEFITS AND SIDE EFFECTS OF HYSTERECTOMY

Hysterectomies for nonmalignant conditions are intended to improve a woman's health and quality of life. In some women, removal of the uterus can bring relief from pelvic pain, fatigue, depression, and sexual or urinary tract dysfunction caused by an underlying disorder.

However, other women report depression, fatigue, urinary disorders, and pain after the surgery. If the ovaries are removed as well, instant menopause will occur, increasing the risk of osteoporosis and heart disease unless hormone replacement therapy is begun. A small percentage of women report a decreased sex

THE SAVING-THE-OVARIES QUESTION

In 40 percent of hysterectomies, the ovaries are also removed. Some experts contend the ovaries could become cancerous and that ovarian cancer is a deadly and hard-to-diagnose disease. Others maintain that while that is true, ovarian cancer is also less common than other cancers, affecting less than 1 percent of all women. Researchers have calculated that one in 700 women whose ovaries are removed would have developed ovarian cancer.

Some practitioners feel that, if a woman is approaching menopause, the ovaries are no longer needed and that hormone replacement therapy will restore her blood hormone levels. But researchers now know that the ovaries continue to produce an array of hormones well past menopause and that hormone replacement therapy is far from perfect and has side effects and risks.

Even when the surgeon leaves the ovaries intact, there is a chance they will decrease production of hormones after hysterectomy, at least temporarily, or even shut down, most likely because the surgery disrupts their blood supply.

drive or lack of orgasm after hysterectomy. Women may also feel "incomplete" or less "womanly" after a hysterectomy.

A hysterectomy is a procedure that should be carefully considered:

■ It is major surgery with death or serious injury to other organs occurring in one to two per 1,000 operations performed.

UNNECESSARY HYSTERECTOMIES

Close to 90 percent of all hysterectomies are performed for nonmalignant conditions that, in some cases, might have been treated by other means. A 1993 study by the Health Maintenance Organization Quality of Care Consortium found that 25 percent of hysterectomies were performed for questionable reasons, while 16 percent were performed for inappropriate reasons.

No one knows for sure why unnecessary hysterectomies are performed. One reason may be training: physicians were once taught to recommend hysterectomies if fibroids reached the size of a 12-week pregnancy, whether symptoms were severe or not. Some physicians still follow this rule of thumb. Economic incentives may also play a part in some practitioners' recommendations. Hysterectomies are more lucrative than medical management of a chronic gynecological problem. In some cases, medical therapies may not be tried long enough before resorting to hysterectomy, or they are not chosen correctly to treat the condition.

■ Up to 10 percent of women have complications of fever or hemorrhage following the operation.

■ All surgery carries a risk of postoperative depression. Hysterectomy may be more likely to be associated with depression and other hormone-related psychological problems, especially in women who have the surgery for other than life-threatening conditions. If there is any question about the necessity of the surgery, a second opinion should be sought.

THE IMPORTANCE OF A SECOND OPINION

With one out of every three women in the United States facing a hysterectomy by the age of 60, a second opinion should be sought by all women to whom the procedure is recommended. All information and alternatives should be thoroughly explored before a woman makes the decision on whether or not a hysterectomy is going to improve her health and quality of life.

A practitioner may say that a hysterectomy is "indicated," or standard medical practice, but that doesn't mean it is the best choice for every woman. Alternatives to hysterectomy include **myomectomy** (removal of fibroids), **dilation and curettage,** and **hysteroscopy** for removal of fibroids; **laparoscopy, laparotomy,** and drugs for endometriosis; and the insertion of a pessary or surgical positioning for uterine prolapse.

A woman should ask the practitioner to be specific and state why the surgery is necessary, which organs should be removed, which organs will not be removed, and which organs might be removed. The practitioner can be asked to put the information in writing or can add it to a surgical consent form.

SEE endometriosis; fibroids; hysteroscopy; laparoscopy; oophorectomy; second opinion; uterine prolapse.

For more information on hysterectomy, contact:

American College of Obstetricians and Gynecologists
409 12th St., S.W.
Washington, DC 20024
202-863-2518
http://www.acog.com

Endometriosis Association
8585 N. 76th Place
Milwaukee, WI 53223
800-992-ENDO
800-992-2363 (Canada)

HERS Foundation (Hysterectomy Educational Resources and Services)
422 Bryn Mawr Ave.
Bala Cynwyd, PA 19004
610-667-7757
tzht72@prodigy.com

National Women's Health Network
514 10th St., N.W., Suite 400
Washington, DC 20004
202-347-1140

HYSTEROSCOPY

A hysteroscopy, a procedure in which a viewing instrument is inserted into the uterus, allows the practitioner to examine the cervical canal and the inside of the uterus for fibroids or other abnormal tissue. If necessary, instruments can be inserted through the hysteroscope to perform surgery, such as removal or cauterization of abnormal tissue. In this way, hysteroscopy can be used for both diagnostic and therapeutic procedures.

REASONS FOR HYSTEROSCOPY

A hysteroscopy is done for the following reasons:

■ To find and remove minor adhesions

■ To locate and remove sore tissues, uterine polyps, uterine cancer, and fibroids that are inside the uterine cavity

■ To find a missing intrauterine device (IUD)

■ To find the cause of infertility and repeated miscarriages

■ To relieve menorrhagia, heavy bleeding caused by fibroids in the uterus. This condition requires hysteroscopic resection, a new technique in which uterine fibroids are shaved away.

PROCEDURE

A hysteroscopy is usually performed by a gynecologist. As in a pelvic exam, a speculum is inserted into the vagina to separate the vaginal walls. Then a hollow, thin, slender, telescope-like instrument called a hysteroscope is inserted through the vagina and cervix. This instrument allows the practitioner to view the inside of the uterus and view IUD position, growths, scars, or other disorders. A sample of tissue for microscopic examination may also be taken with an instrument inserted through the hysteroscope in a procedure called a **biopsy.**

Any growths, such as fibroids, that are found may be removed either by burning them away with a laser that attaches to the hysteroscope or by shaving them off with an electric current that is provided by an instrument called a resectoscope.

If laser ablation therapy is being performed, the practitioner uses a laser that is attached to the hysteroscope to dissolve the uterine lining. This is done to relieve excessive bleeding caused by fibroids in the uterus, though it results in infertility.

RISKS AND SIDE EFFECTS

The procedure is performed on an outpatient basis and has very few major complications. After the procedure, women may experience mild cramps for a few days, but most women are able to resume regular activities in less than a week. Perforation of the uterus and infection are possible complications. Following a myomectomy (a procedure done to remove fibroids in the uterus), some women experience hyponatremia, a condition of the kidneys that occurs when the body's sodium levels are below normal.

There is also the possibility that the fibroids can grow back. If this occurs, another hysteroscopy or a hysterectomy may be necessary.

SEE biopsy.

INCONTINENCE, URINARY

Urinary incontinence, the involuntary loss of urine, is a condition of the urinary system that affects some 10 million individuals in the United States, according to the National Institutes of Health. Of those, 85 percent are women. Women are more susceptible to bladder control problems as a result of childbirth, surgery, and postmenopausal changes.

Urinary incontinence can be uncomfortable and embarrassing. However, 90 percent of those who have it can be treated successfully. In addition, it is gaining recognition as a common problem, and much of the shameful stigma associated with incontinence is disappearing as people are able to discuss the disorder more openly.

THE URINARY SYSTEM

The urinary system consists of the kidneys, ureters, bladder, and urethra. The kidneys (a pair of bean-shaped, reddish brown organs the size of mangoes) filter the blood and remove waste products that are sent then to the bladder (a balloon-shaped reservoir) via the ureters (tubes connecting the kidneys with the bladder) and stored there until excreted from the body. About two quarts of this fluid, called urine, are produced daily.

As urine collects in the bladder, the bladder gradually expands until it becomes full. Muscles in the bladder neck help hold the urine until enough has been collected for urination, the process by which urine is eliminated from the body. At the bottom of the bladder, the urinary sphincter muscle contracts to hold urine in the bladder. When it is relaxed, urine is then allowed to pass into the urethra (the tube that carries the urine from the bladder and out of the body). If either the sphincter or the bladder does not work properly, a person may have a urinary incontinence problem.

TYPES OF INCONTINENCE

There are three common types of incontinence. **Urge incontinence** is the inability to retain urine long enough to reach an appropriate place to urinate. It is not triggered by pressure or strain to the bladder. With urge incontinence, the muscle in the bladder called the detrusor unexpectedly pushes the urine out as soon as the urge to urinate is felt. This type of incontinence is associated with neurological disorders (which may occur after a stroke), allergies, or a bladder infection or injury.

Stress incontinence is the involuntary leakage of urine during activities that put pressure on the bladder. These activities include coughing, laughing, sneezing, and exercising. Stress incontinence may be caused by weak pelvic floor muscles (the muscles which support the uterus and bladder) or weak sphincter muscles (the muscles that hold urine in the bladder). This condition often occurs in women over the age of 50 and may be caused by damage to the muscles during childbirth, multiple childbirth, or the weakening of muscles due to hormone deficiency.

Overflow incontinence is involuntary leakage from a bladder that does not completely empty. When a person with overflow incontinence urinates, the bladder does not completely empty, leaving the person with the feeling of having to urinate. Incontinence may occur at any time, even when the bladder feels empty. Often this problem is caused by nerve damage, drug side effects, a stretched bladder, or a blockage in the urinary tract.

Urinary leakage that is associated with the inability to use a toilet because of mental or physical impairments is known as **functional incontinence.**

DIAGNOSIS

The treatment of urinary incontinence depends greatly on the correct diagnosis of its cause. Before diagnosis, the person should record the volume of fluids taken in, the frequency of urination, and the events surrounding each episode of incontinence for one week. Then a complete medical history and physical examination should be done by a practitioner experienced in incontinence problems. Incontinence may sometimes be traced to medications (including diuretics, over-the-counter sleep aids, Valium, and some decongestants), allergies, neurological disorders, constipation, or other treatable disorders.

A complete examination for incontinence includes a pelvic exam, which includes a rectovaginal exam and a speculum exam. This enables the doctor to determine if a physical problem such as a **cystocele** (sagging of the urinary bladder into the vaginal wall) is contributing to the incontinence. The practitioner may also order a urinalysis and urine culture to rule out infection.

If the simpler tests are inconclusive, **urodynamic studies** may be done to finalize a diagnosis. This series of tests includes uroflowmetry, cystometry, and endoscopic procedures.

Uroflowmetry is a noninvasive procedure that records the volume of urine voided and the length of each urination. The practitioner will also note the effort needed to start the urine stream, continue the stream, and the presence of any dribbling after urination.

Cystometry is an invasive procedure that involves threading a catheter (a thin, flexible tube) through the urethra and into the bladder. Gradually, the bladder is filled with sterile water or carbon dioxide gas until it is full. Pressure monitors in the catheter take a series of readings indicating how well the bladder is functioning as it fills. Once the bladder is full, the person is directed to urinate, and the force of the stream is measured. After urination, a measurement is also made of the retained urine left in the bladder.

Endoscopic procedures, which involve the use of thin viewing scopes, look inside the urethra and bladder for physical causes of incontinence such as a genitourinary fistula (an abnormal passage) or a urethra diverticuliae (a weakness in the urethral wall that causes a pocket to develop). Some women develop urinary tract fistulas, which lead to incontinence, as a result of a difficult childbirth.

Other tests may include the **post-void residual test,** which measures the amount of urine left in the bladder after emptying; **electromyography,** which checks bladder and urinary sphincter coordination and muscle tone; and **profilometry,** which measures urethral resistance and length.

CAUSES OF INCONTINENCE

Although advanced age does tend to present more opportunities for urinary incontinence, bladder control problems are not an inevitable part of growing older. Only 30 percent of

STRENGTHENING THE PELVIC FLOOR

Kegel exercises are done by tightening and relaxing the muscles used to stop urination. Strengthening the muscles can prevent and improve urinary incontinence, improve sexual sensations, and aid recovery from childbirth. Because they are undetectable, Kegel exercises can be done anywhere, anytime. Do at least five in a row several times daily:

■ Tighten muscles a little and hold for five seconds.

■ Tighten a little more. Hold five seconds more.

■ Tighten as much as possible. Hold for five seconds.

■ Relax in reverse steps, holding five seconds at each step.

Another method for strengthening the pelvic floor muscles is the use of vaginal cones. The vaginal cones are all the same size but differ in weight, with each one progressively heavier. A normal exercise routine is to insert a cone in the vagina twice a day and retain it for 15 minutes. The muscles of the pelvic floor are gently squeezed to keep the cone in place. As the muscles of the pelvic floor become stronger, the next heavier cone is used and so on until the entire set has been used. In three studies of 103 women using the vaginal cones, 68 to 79 percent reported improvement within four to six weeks.

women over 65 are reported to have incontinence problems. Urinary incontinence has many different sources. They include:

■ Menopause. After menopause, the reduction in the level of estrogen frequently causes the tissues of the vagina and the urinary tract to thin and become less flexible, possibly causing incontinence.

■ Weak muscles, possibly due to childbirth, age, or lack of exercise and hormones

■ Chronic bladder infections

■ Restricted mobility

■ Excessive urine production

■ Blockages of the urinary tract. Obstructions of the urinary tract in females usually involves an organ protruding into the vagina, the case with a very large cystocele or uterine prolapse.

■ A deficiency of vitamin B_{12} leading to pernicious anemia

■ Spinal cord injuries. These also affect the way the sphincters contract and therefore result in a loss of urinary retention.

■ Multiple sclerosis

■ Postviral nerve damage

Incontinence may often be treated by treating the condition that is contributing to the bladder control problem.

TREATMENT

Behavioral treatments are a common type of treatment for incontinence. They include bladder training, habit training that involves sched-

 SELF-CARE FOR INCONTINENCE

■ Regulate the amount of fluid you take in. Your incontinence may be linked to drinking too little throughout the day rather than too much. Talk to your practitioner about finding the right amount.

■ Avoid coffee, tea, pepper, and alcohol. These are diuretics—they promote urination.

■ Quit smoking. Nicotine irritates the bladder, and a smokers' cough can trigger stress incontinence.

■ Eat a proper diet. A diet high in whole grains, fruits, and vegetables with some fish and low in white flour, sugar, fats, and meat can help to prevent constipation and urinary tract infections which can lead to urinary incontinence.

■ Cross your legs before sneezing. Researchers have found that women with urinary incontinence who cross their legs before sneezing, laughing, or coughing lose nearly one-tenth less urine than when they do not cross their legs.

■ Don't rely exclusively on pads, padded undergarments, or catheters to handle urinary problems. While these products can provide a sense of confidence to an incontinent person in public, they should not take the place of treatment. Delaying medical treatment may make the problem worse. Dependence on pads should be a last resort.

■ Concentrate on other things when you feel the urge to urinate. Instead of thinking about your bladder, concentrate on the work in front of you, the voice on the radio, or the view out the window.

■ Develop a urination schedule. Urinate more often—perhaps every two or three hours. Work with your practitioner and experiment with timing to see how it works for you.

uled urination, and pelvic muscle exercises. These techniques help strengthen and control the muscles surrounding the bladder. A woman should work with her practitioner to determine what program and schedule would work best for her problem.

Medications may also be used to treat incontinence. However, some have severe side effects, and most are only effective when used with mild cases of incontinence. For stress incontinence, a class of medications known as alpha-adrenergic agonist (pseudoephedrine, ephedrine, phenylpropanolamine) works primarily by increasing the strength of the bladder sphincter. Urge incontinence may be treated with a class of medications called anticholinergic and antispasmodic (propantheline, imipramine, oxybutynin), designed to reduce the spasms within the bladder.

In addition, postmenopausal women can often be relieved of stress incontinence through hormone replacement therapy (HRT), which helps to thicken the vaginal lining and the walls of the urinary tract. However, if improperly used, HRT may increase the risk of uterine cancer, so the risks and benefits of the hormones should be weighed before treatment begins. Once on an HRT regimen, a woman must visit her practitioner regularly and report any abnormal bleeding.

Surgery is also an option for some women with incontinence. Collagen implants may be effective in the treatment of stress incontinence. In a relatively noninvasive procedure, the tissue surrounding the urethra, at the base of the bladder, may be injected with collagen, causing it to firm up, which prevents urine from leaking during normal activities. This procedure can be done under local anesthesia in less than an hour. One to three sessions may be needed, leading to a total of three to six injections.

Collagen implants reportedly relieved symptoms of incontinence in 60 to 80 percent of the female patients who underwent the procedure, depending on the number of injections they receive. Unfortunately, 4 percent of the women who had the procedure reported an allergic reaction to the bovine collagen gel. A simple skin test performed before any implant can determine whether or not a woman would be allergic to the collagen.

Several types of surgery may also be done to repair a cystocele that is interfering with the flow of urine through the bladder. Other procedures treat incontinence by tightening weakened pelvic muscles to provide the bladder with more support.

SEE hormone replacement therapy.

For more information on urinary incontinence, contact:

Help for Incontinent People (HIP)
P.O. Box 9
Minneapolis, MN 55440
800-328-3881

Simon Foundation for Continence
P.O. Box 835
Wilmette, IL 60091
800-237-4666
708-864-3913 (Illinois)

INFERTILITY,
DIAGNOSIS OF

Infertility affects more than 4.9 million couples in the United States. Defined as the inability to conceive after a year of unprotected intercourse, or the inability to carry a child to term, infertility is a growing problem among women and men. Experts say this is because more women are waiting until they are older to have children, which increases the chances that their fertility has been affected, possibly by a previous sexually transmitted infection, pelvic inflammatory disease, scarring from earlier surgery, or the aging process itself.

While 86 percent of couples do conceive a child within two years without assistance, one in seven has difficulty. The cause of infertility may lie within the body of the woman or the man, or it may be a combination of factors from both partners. It is estimated that 40 percent of infertility problems can be attributed to causes within the man, and 40 percent to the woman, while 20 percent are caused by problems within both the man and the woman or are unexplained. An estimated 25 percent of infertile couples have more than one factor causing infertility.

If conception is not successful after more than a year of unprotected intercourse (six months if the woman is aged 35 or older), it may be time to seek help. A gynecologist or a specialist known as a reproductive endocrinologist can recommend simple self-help measures to improve the chances of conception. A woman can chart ovulation using fertility awareness methods (FAMs). Intercourse prior to or at ovulation is critical for pregnancies to occur. It is also important to be sure that the semen is placed high in the vagina, at the level of the cervix.

In addition, some practitioners recommend alternative therapies, such as acupuncture, herbal medicine, and homeopathic remedies, for treatment of infertility.

INFERTILITY IN MEN

In men, infertility results from low **sperm count** (the percentage of sperm per milliliter of semen), a decrease in sperm **motility** (the percent of sperm moving rapidly), or poor sperm **morphology** (the shape of the sperm which allows it to penetrate the egg). An enlargement of the veins surrounding the spermatic cord, called a **varicocele,** may be present, causing a drop in sperm count. Sperm ducts may become blocked, or sexual dysfunction may prevent ejaculation. Trauma or injury to the scrotum and testes, sexually transmitted infections, excessive drug and alcohol use, and hormone imbalances can also affect fertility.

Before any testing for the woman begins, experts recommend a semen analysis, a simple, noninvasive procedure to check sperm number, shape, and viability. If the problem is found to be an infection or sexual dysfunction, infertility may be solved by curing that condition. Low sperm count and motility can be remedied with hormone injections, and variceles and blockages can sometimes be surgically repaired. A man may also opt to avoid surgery and choose donor insemination to achieve conception. A urologist generally treats fertility problems in men.

INFERTILITY IN WOMEN

There are many causes for infertility in women. The **fallopian tubes** may be blocked, preventing the egg from being fertilized and delivered to the uterus. **Endometriosis,** sexually transmitted infections, or scarring from previous surgery can cause such damage. **Ovulation** can be affected by hormonal imbalances, thyroid disorders, or chronic diseases, such as diabetes. The **uterus** may be shaped incorrectly for implantation or may contain tissue that interferes with implantation. In some women, antibodies that block sperm from the uterus may be present in the **cervical mucus.**

There are many diagnostic tests that can be used to determine the cause of infertility in women. An **endometrial biopsy** can be done to examine the lining of the uterus and check whether ovulation has occurred. **Urine** and **blood** tests are used to measure hormone levels. A **postcoital pelvic examination** may be done a few hours after intercourse to examine the progress of the sperm and check for antibodies in the cervical mucus.

More invasive tests include a **hysterosalpingogram,** in which dye is slowly injected into the uterus as x-rays are taken. The dye allows the clinician to see the shape of the uterus and fallopian tubes, along with any abnormalities and blockages. A **laparoscopy** is a minor but technically difficult procedure done under general anesthesia, in which a viewing scope is inserted into a small incision in the abdomen to search for endometriosis or scar tissue and to look at the functioning of the fallopian tubes. A

hysteroscopy is the insertion of a viewing instrument through the vagina into the uterus to look for a cause of infertility.

Infertility problems linked to endometriosis, fibroids, or a specific infection may be solved by treating the condition itself. If the problem is determined to be hormonal, a fertility drug, such as clomiphene citrate (Clomid), can be used to stimulate the pituitary gland. The pituitary gland releases follicle-stimulating hormones (FSH) and luteinizing hormones (LH), which increase the ripening and number of eggs being released. Human menopausal gonadotropin (Pergonal) contains FSH and LH and therefore acts directly on the ovary in the same way. Multiple embryos can result from the use of fertility drugs, since several eggs may be released at once. A injection of HCG (human chorionic gonadotropin) is then given to prompt release of the eggs in a predictable way. A side effect of fertility drugs is **hyperstimulation syndrome,** which results in swollen, painful ovaries.

Some recent studies indicate that clomiphene may double the risk of ovarian cancer (which has a lifetime risk of 2 percent) when used for a long period of time, though this risk is not confirmed. The risk of ovarian cancer is related to the number of ovulations. The number is increased with the use of fertility drugs and decreased with the use of contraceptive drugs, such as oral contraceptives, that suppress ovulation.

Fallopian tubes can be reconstructed or repaired surgically (but never completely) if the damage is not severe. **Balloon tuboplasty,** a variation on a technique developed to treat heart conditions, is sometimes used to clear fallopian tubes, though success varies. In the procedure, a tube with a small balloon is inserted into the fallopian tube; when the balloon is

THE WOMAN'S INFERTILITY SPECIALIST

The reproductive endocrinologist is a physician specializing in the treatment of hormonal and infertility problems in women. This is a subspecialty of obstetrics and gynecology. While the first steps of diagnosing infertility can be taken by a physician or gynecologist, this specialist may be recommended for more invasive tests, procedures, and surgeries. If treatment of infertility is not successful, it is the reproductive endocrinologist who usually performs assisted fertility procedures such as donor insemination and in vitro fertilization.

To find a fertility specialist, ask your friends or gynecologist for a recommendation. Your library may have a copy of the *American Medical Directory: Physicians in the United States,* which contains information on every doctor who is a member of the American Medical Association. Another source is the *Official ABMS Directory of Board Certified Medical Specialists,* published by Marquis Who's Who.

As with any physician, a reproductive endocrinologist should be chosen carefully. Some questions to ask:

■ Are you a board-certified reproductive endocrinologist?

■ What is your training? Where and when were you trained?

■ What is your success rate for my type of fertility problem? How many of the related procedures have you done?

■ What definition of success is being used? Is it based on fertilizations? Pregnancies? Live births?

■ Do you have any restrictions on treatment? Is there an age limitation or limit to number of treatments?

■ What will this cost? Many insurance companies do not cover infertility testing, procedures, and surgery.

To verify the credentials of a reproductive endocrinologist or a urologist, call the American Board of Medical Specialties at 800-776-CERT.

Lists of physicians, and information on infertility and treatment, are available from:

RESOLVE
1310 Broadway
Somerville, MA 02144
617-623-1156
http://www.resolve.org

American Society for Reproductive Medicine
[formerly the American Fertility Society]
1209 Montgomery Hwy.
Birmingham, AL 35216-2809
205-978-5000
http://www.asrm.com

expanded, the tube is stretched and the blockage pushed aside. Scar tissue and adhesions can also be removed surgically in some cases. A specialist is recommended for such procedures because the organs are very delicate and can be easily damaged further.

SEE endometriosis; fibroids; gynecologic examination; hysteroscopy; infertility, procedures for; laparoscopy; menstrual cycle and ovulation.

INFERTILITY, PROCEDURES FOR

It is estimated that as many as 42 percent of infertile women seek advanced methods of achieving pregnancy, such as donor insemination (also known as artificial insemination), in vitro insemination, and embryo transfer when conventional medical treatments are not successful. The high-tech procedures can be expensive as well as emotionally taxing. Couples and individuals face complicated tests, trials, and procedures as well as the pressure of possible failure. Still, many people view these procedures as their last chance to have a biological child. Assisted fertility procedures are also an option for single women, lesbians, or gay men who wish to have children.

DONOR INSEMINATION (DI)

Usually considered the easiest and least expensive of the advanced treatments, donor insemination involves the placement of sperm in or near the cervix at the most fertile times of a woman's menstrual cycle. It is performed when sperm is not available or present in the semen and when low sperm counts make conception unlikely. According to the American Society for Reproductive Medicine, donor insemination has an average pregnancy success rate of 10 percent per cycle. Most women who get pregnant do so in the first three to five cycles.

Sperm can be donated by a woman's partner or by an anonymous donor. The sperm is usually collected through masturbation, though it can also be collected in specially designed condoms worn during sexual intercourse. The semen with the sperm may be placed in a small cup under the cervix and left in place for six to 12 hours to allow the sperm to swim up the cervix and enter the uterus. Or the semen may be washed to remove chemicals called prostaglandins, which can cause cramping in the uterus, and to concentrate the most motile sperm. The sample may then be inserted through the cervix into the uterus using a small tubing and a syringe (this is called **intrauterine insemination**). If the sperm has been donated, it may be frozen for storage before insemination occurs. Studies say that using frozen sperm, which is less viable, decreases the chances of pregnancy by about 50 percent.

All donors must be screened for sexually transmitted infections, including HIV. Voluntary guidelines for screening from the Centers for Disease Control and Prevention have been in place since 1986 (the guidelines are mandatory in New York and Indiana), and individuals should be certain that they undergo insemination only at centers that follow these guidelines. Donor sperm also raises psychological and moral questions. Some religious groups feel DI is adultery; some men have trouble dealing with the idea of a child who is not biologically his and his partner's.

IN VITRO FERTILIZATION (IVF)

Meaning "fertilization in glass," in vitro fertilization is used to conceive what are commonly known in the media as test-tube babies. It is most often used in women with blocked fallopian tubes but functioning ovaries, but may also be used to treat infertility caused by endometriosis or a low sperm count. With this technology, the ovaries are stimulated using fertility drugs to prompt the ripening of several eggs for ovulation rather than just one. Common fertility drugs include clomiphene citrate (Clomid) and human menopausal gonadotropin (Pergonal). A side effect of fertility drugs is **hyperstimulation syndrome,** in which the ovaries become swollen and painful. In addition, some studies have shown clomiphene to double the risk of ovarian cancer (which has a lifetime risk of 2 percent) in women who take it for a long period.

A few days before ovulation, the ripened eggs are collected from the follicles of the ovaries using a needle that is guided by **transvaginal ultrasound aspiration,** a minor surgical procedure in which an ultrasound probe is inserted through the vagina to create an image of the pelvic organs. Then a hollow needle is guided through the vagina into the follicles, and the eggs are removed through the needle by a suction device. **Laparoscopy,** a surgical procedure in which a long viewing scope is inserted through a small incision in the abdomen to guide surgical instruments, is less frequently used for egg retrieval in IVF.

At the time the eggs are collected, some women opt to have extra eggs removed. If surplus eggs are available, they are collected, fertilized, and frozen for use in future trials with a procedure known as **cryopreservation.** While this cuts costs if more IVF attempts are necessary, the process creates legal and ethical questions, including custody of the frozen embryos and the method of disposal of unused embryos.

Once the eggs are retrieved, they are fertilized in a glass dish using prepared sperm collected from a partner or donor. **Microinsemination,** a process that concentrates sperm near the eggs in the dish, may be done to increase chances of fertilization. Another procedure, **micromanipulation,** involves the insertion of a single sperm directly into the egg to facilitate fertilization. A few days after fertilization, the practitioner inserts up to five fertilized eggs (or embryos) into the uterus using a long, thin tube inserted through the cervix. The more eggs transferred, the greater the chance of pregnancy; however, multiple eggs could also mean multiple pregnancies, which are considered high risk.

According to the American Society for Reproductive Medicine, the rate of pregnancies resulting in live birth for women undergoing IVF in the United States was approximately 18.3 percent in 1993. For women undergoing three trials of IVF, the rate rose to 50 percent in the best of hands.

The process of **"natural" in vitro fertilization** is similar to IVF except that it abandons the use of fertility drugs. Instead, a single egg is collected through aspiration or laparoscopy after it ripens naturally before ovulation. While the odds of pregnancy are better with stimulated IVF because more eggs are produced, natural IVF is preferred by women who cannot take fertility drugs or who fear side effects. Natural IVF is also less expensive than stimulation on a per-cycle basis; however, its success rate is much lower, making the average cost of a successful pregnancy higher.

GIFT AND ZIFT

A variation of IVF is **gamete intrafallopian transfer (GIFT)**. As with IVF, the ovaries are stimulated with fertility drugs. However, with GIFT, the eggs are collected through **laparoscopy** rather than transvaginally, then mixed with sperm and transferred to the fallopian tubes during the same procedure. Within the fallopian tubes, it is hoped, fertilization can take place in its natural environment rather than in a laboratory.

For this procedure, a woman must have at least one unblocked fallopian tube and one functioning ovary. GIFT is used to treat male fertility problems, mild endometriosis, cervical mucus problems, and unexplained infertility. The American Society for Reproductive Medicine reports that pregnancy rates are 23 to 28 percent for GIFT—5 to 10 percent higher than for IVF.

RATING A FERTILITY CLINIC

The success of a fertility clinic cannot be determined by its rate of pregnancy alone. Many clinics have age limits for their clients or a limit to the number of attempts that can be made—restrictions that increase their statistical success rate. Some clinics include the total number of conceptions in their rates, even if the pregnancies ended in miscarriage, or compile rates over months rather than years.

A good indicator of success is the clinic's "take-home baby" rate, the number of clients whose pregnancies end in live births. Experts say a reasonable success rate is somewhere between 10 and 15 percent.

The American Society for Reproductive Medicine recommends asking the following questions to fully understand the success of an IVF clinic:

■ When did this program perform its first IVF procedure? First GIFT procedure?

■ How many babies have been born from this program's IVF efforts? GIFT efforts?

■ In the past two years, how many stimulation cycles have been initiated for IVF? For GIFT?

■ In the past two years, how many embryo transfer procedures have been done in the IVF program? GIFT program?

■ In the past two years, how many pregnancies have resulted from IVF? GIFT?

■ In the past two years, how many miscarriages have occurred from pregnancies initiated by IVF? By GIFT?

■ In the past two years, how many live births have occurred in your program from IVF? From GIFT?

■ How many ongoing pregnancies are there from IVF? From GIFT?

■ How many deliveries were twins or other multiple births?

For more information on clinic success rates or infertility procedures, contact:

American Society for Reproductive Medicine
[formerly the American Fertility Society]
1209 Montgomery Hwy.
Birmingham, AL 35216-2809
205-978-5000
http://www.asrm.com

ADDITIONAL OPTIONS FOR INFERTILE WOMEN AND MEN

For men and women who continue to have trouble conceiving a child, there are options beyond the medical procedures that can be performed. Embryo transfer and surrogacy, two of the primary choices, involve bringing in a third individual, a woman who will donate her own egg or carry the child to term. While these options involve aspects of donor insemination and in vitro fertilization, they are not technically infertility treatments.

Embryo transfer is similar to IVF, except that the egg is provided by a surrogate, a woman who is a volunteer donor. In the procedure, the egg is fertilized within the surrogate by donor insemination, then washed out of the uterus and transferred to the recipient. There are risks for the donor, such as ectopic pregnancy and the chance that she will remain pregnant because the embryo is not washed out. This option is appropriate for women who cannot conceive but can carry a child to term.

The opposite of embryo transfer is **surrogacy,** in that it is used for women who can conceive but not carry a child to term. With surrogacy, an egg fertilized through IVF is transferred into the uterus of a woman who did not produce the egg. The surrogate then carries and delivers the child. Because of the myriad legal and moral issues surrounding this practice, many states have outlawed surrogacy.

Zygote intrafallopian transfer (ZIFT), also called **pronuclear stage transfer (PROST),** is a variation of GIFT. With this procedure, the egg is collected transvaginally, then fertilized outside of the body, which is helpful if the infertility is due to a male factor. Then the **zygote** (a fertilized egg that has not yet divided) is surgically placed by laparoscopy into the fallopian tube about 18 hours later. In some cases, the egg is allowed to divide several times before it is transferred to the fallopian tube in a slightly different procedure known as **tubal embryo transfer (TET).**

The advantage of ZIFT or TET over GIFT is that fertilization is assured; they are recommended for women whose egg quality is deemed poor, or if the ability of the sperm to penetrate and fertilize the egg is questionable.

SEE adoption; infertility, diagnosis of; laparoscopy.

INSOMNIA

Insomnia, the most common sleep disorder, is the inability to fall asleep or stay asleep. An adult with insomnia cannot get the proper amount of rest (seven to nine hours a night, on average) needed to function on a daily basis. The disorder may occur only occasionally, or it may become chronic and last for months or even years. At least 40 million Americans suffer from chronic sleep disorders, and 20 to 30 million more suffer from intermittent insomnia. Women tend to suffer insomnia during pregnancy and menopause.

Sleeplessness is associated with a number of physical and emotional conditions. It may be caused by a medical condition, such as heart disease, diabetes, or anemia, by prescription and over-the-counter medications that contain ingredients that deter sleep, or by chemicals (such as monosodium glutamate, MSG) or allergies. Physical pain and discomfort can also result in insomnia. Before prescribing medications to induce sleep, a practitioner should rule out medical causes for insomnia and review all prescription medications being taken to ensure that they are not the source of the insomnia.

Depression, stress, and anxiety may also lead to insomnia. Jet lag (when a change in time zone throws off the body's natural sleep patterns) and advanced age also contribute to

MAINTAINING GOOD SLEEP HYGIENE

Some 60 to 70 percent of individuals with sleep disorders can learn to sleep better without treatment by learning better sleep habits.

Sleep, specifically the sleep/wake cycle, is regulated by an internal body clock called a **circadian rhythm.** Without the circadian rhythm functioning properly, a person may not be able to fall asleep or awaken at desired normal times. Proper sleep habits can help to keep this internal clock on schedule and alleviate circumstances that lead to sleeplessness.

To get a better night's sleep:

■ Keep a regular sleep schedule and limit daytime naps.

■ Avoid caffeine and nicotine especially late in the day. They contain stimulants that may disrupt the normal sleep cycle.

■ Don't drink too much alcohol. Though at first alcohol appears to induce sleep, gradual withdrawal over the course of the night (which happens with even a few drinks) may interrupt sleep.

■ Avoid illegal drugs. Such drugs (such as heroin) promote insomnia.

■ Exercise outdoors during the day on a regular basis.

■ Don't exercise too close to bedtime. Physical exertion stimulates the release of adrenaline, which energizes the body's systems. Ideally, a workout five to six hours before sleep can lower the body's core temperature and help induce sleep.

✓ HELP YOURSELF TO BETTER SLEEP

To combat the occasional night of sleeplessness, the following self-help techniques may be used:

■ Create a comfortable sleeping environment just for the purpose of sleep. By keeping work, arguments, and television out of the bedroom, you may keep stress and stimulation from interfering with sleep.

■ Snack on complex carbohydrates (English muffins, cereal, or crackers) one to two hours before bed to promote deeper sleep. However, avoid foods with sugar and protein, which stimulate the body.

■ Take a warm bath before bed.

■ Try a glass of warm milk. Experts say that in some individuals, the amino acid L-tryptophan contained in milk acts as a sedative. However, the amino acid tyrosine, also present in milk, energizes others. So if it helps you sleep, drink it.

■ Drink mild herb tea. Herbal remedies known for their sedative effect include teas brewed from valerian root, chamomile leaves and flowers, and catnip. (Consult your practitioner before taking herbal remedies. They may have side effects or react with prescribed medication. Some remedies should not be taken during pregnancy or in the case of diabetes or heart disease.)

■ Try sex. Sexual stimulation releases endorphins, hormones that make you mellow and relaxed.

■ Listen to repetitive white sounds. Small machines are available for this purpose, though a fan or humidifier may also help.

■ If wakefulness persists, go to another room to read, write a letter, or do some other task. Productive activity can reduce the stress caused by trying to get to sleep.

---

insomnia. An older individual tends to sleep less and experiences natural periods of insomnia, the result of a slowing metabolism.

WOMEN AND INSOMNIA

Pregnancy and menopause are causes of sleeplessness unique to women. Women in the last months of pregnancy may suffer from sleeplessness because of excitement, nervousness, heartburn, fetal kicking, or their inability to find a comfortable sleeping position. The night sweats and hot flashes (hormone imbalances that cause a woman to wake up soaked in sweat) of menopause may also cause sleeplessness.

TREATMENT

A complete medical and psychological examination should be done to pinpoint the cause of insomnia before treatment begins. A sleep disorder center can be sought to help make the diagnosis. If a medical condition is causing sleeplessness, that condition may be treated in order to relieve the insomnia. **Hormone replacement therapy** may be prescribed for insomnia related to menopause because estrogen is thought to alleviate night sweats and improve the quality of sleep.

Over-the-counter (OTC) sleep aids, which usually contain antihistamines, are not recommended for insomnia because they further disrupt the sleep cycle. OTC medications may perpetuate insomnia and cause psychological dependence. Pregnant women should not take any medications for sleep loss because of potential harm to the fetus. Instead, they should try to take short naps, if possible, during the day to make up for sleep loss.

Prescription sleep medications work by suppressing nerve-cell activity within the brain. They include two major classes of drugs: benzodiazepines and antidepressants.

Benzodiazepines, prescribed to relieve anxiety and promote sleep, are effective for short periods of time—about two weeks—and are used to treat short-term insomnia caused by emotional stress or travel. Side effects include sweating, nausea, rapid pulse, depression, and nausea, and they can be addictive. Common benzodiazepines are diazepam (Valium) and triazolam (Halcion).

Tricyclic antidepressants are prescribed for insomnia related to fibromyalgia, other chronic pain, or nonrestorative sleep. Because tricyclic antidepressants are effective in very small doses, their side effects are generally mild. They include dry mouth, constipation, urinary problems, and tremors. Because these drugs can have side effects, they should not be taken without the supervision of a physician. Common tricyclic antidepressants are Elavil and Tofranil.

When the reason for insomnia is psychological, psychotherapy may be used, possibly in conjunction with drugs, to treat the disorder that is causing sleeplessness.

Some alternative therapies have also been shown to be effective in treating insomnia, including yoga, herbal medicines, massage, self-hypnosis, and relaxation techniques. An experienced practitioner should be consulted for details. Herbs useful in treating insomnia include valerian and passionflower. Lately, melatonin has also been used.

For more information on insomnia, contact:

American Sleep Disorders Association
1610 14th St., N.W., Suite 300
Rochester, MN 55901-2200
507-287-6006
http://www.wisc.edu/asda

Better Sleep Council
P.O. Box 13
Washington, DC 20044
703-683-8371

INSURANCE

Traditional types of indemnity insurance include **hospital insurance, medical/surgical insurance,** and **major medical insurance.** These plans work on a fee-for-service basis, which means the providers of medical care are paid according to the services they render. The fees are based on "usual, customary, and reasonable (UCR) rates." It is generally recognized that the UCR method of paying for medical services contains incentives that can lead to inefficient cost management.

Managed-care programs, which include **health maintenance organizations,** provide health care through a system of practitioners and hospitals. These are reimbursed on a preset fee schedule. Other major insurance programs are **Medicare,** a federally funded plan for people 65 years and older, and **Medicaid,** which provides coverage for individuals whose incomes are below the poverty line.

The services covered and the fees paid for medical care vary according to the type of insurance plan. One may pay for cosmetic surgery, while another will not. There may be dollar limits on some services, such as infertility treatments. Additional coverage is often available, based on what the insurance company offers and what an individual, union, employer, or government is willing to purchase. Nonmandated benefits may be removed from coverage due to state laws or religious reasons. For example, some states restrict Medicaid coverage of abortion.

A review of the insurance policy's "schedule of benefits" will explain benefit coverage, exclusions, and limitations. Specific questions concerning coverage should be directed to an insurance agent or claims manager who knows the details of the policy. Medicare beneficiaries may direct their questions to the Social Security Administration at 800-772-1213, while a caseworker at the welfare department can help with Medicaid concerns.

HOSPITAL INSURANCE

Hospital insurance provides coverage for inpatient and outpatient facility services. The policy usually specifies the number of days of hospitalization and the percentage of costs that will be covered in a certain time period, or sets a dollar limit on the total benefits payable. The policy will also state what is excluded from coverage—for example, substance abuse or rehabilitation. After an initial **deductible**—an amount that must be paid by the policyholder before the insurance company will pay costs—or percentage, the plan generally pays for all covered expenses. Blue Cross plans and commercial carriers (Travelers, Prudential, etc.) are common providers of hospital insurance.

MEDICAL/SURGICAL INSURANCE

Medical/surgical insurance is divided into two parts. The medical portion pays for practitioner's visits to the hospital while the individual is in the hospital and may cover office visits that lead to inpatient or surgical care. It also pays for some drugs, x-rays, anesthesia, and laboratory tests performed outside of the hospital. The surgical portion covers fees for the surgeon, assistant surgeon, and anesthesiologist, whether surgery was performed in the hospital or an ambulatory surgical center. It may also cover procedures performed in a practitioner's office. There may be a dollar limit on benefits payable. Medical/surgical insurance (e.g., Blue Shield) is often sold in conjunction with hospital insurance.

MAJOR MEDICAL INSURANCE

Major medical insurance covers most medical and surgical expenses associated with all levels of illness. While it provides extended coverage for hospital and medical services, it does not cover preventive care. This plan usually requires that the consumer contribute an initial amount, called a deductible, toward the covered expenses. A deductible typically ranges from $100 to $500 per covered individual (although some plans may impose a $1,000 deductible). Once the deductible is paid, major medical pays up to a certain percentage of covered expenses, while the consumer pays the remaining percentage, called a **coinsurance.** For example, if insurance would cover 80 percent, the consumer would pay 20 percent. If the provider does not participate with the insurance plan, the consumer may have to pay the difference between the provider's charge and the insurance plan's reimbursement. This is called **balance billing.** It is wise to find out before being treated if the insurance company's benefits will be accepted as payment in full. If they are not, some practitioners may be willing to negotiate the fee of the service to lower the cost to the patient.

Once out-of-pocket expenses reach a certain amount, some policies have a "stop-loss" provision which protects the consumer from further outlays of cash (with the exception of balance billing). For example, a policy with a stop-loss limit of $5,000 and a 20 percent coinsurance requires the consumer to pay $1,000 (plus deductible), while the insurance company covers the remaining $4,000. Once the stop-loss limit is reached, the policy covers 100 percent of all additional expenses up to the maximum limit. **Catastrophic coverage** refers to major medical with a deductible greater than $1,000.

COMPREHENSIVE INSURANCE

Comprehensive insurance is a term applied to a plan that combines hospital, medical/surgical, and major medical coverage in one policy. It usually requires a single deductible and a coinsurance up to a stop-loss limit, like major medical insurance. A comprehensive policy may have a lifetime benefit of $1 to $5 million.

Comprehensive plans, known as fee-for-service plans, generally do not have conditions on the cost or quality of services or how they are used. (Exceptions may include psychological care or prescription medication.) An individual can visit any practitioner and may be charged whatever fee the practitioner feels is appropriate. In an effort to contain costs, many plans require "precertification"—contacting the insurance company before certain services, such as hospitalization or emergency room admittance, are approved. Failure to do so could result in large out-of-pocket expenses.

MANAGED CARE

Managed care, a rapidly expanding, relatively new form of health-care delivery, regulates the cost of services it provides and measures the quality of the practitioners who provide them. The goal of the system is to give people access to high-quality, cost-effective health care. In managed care, the provider is contractually bound to accept the reimbursement offered by the insurance company as payment in full, so patients do not have to deal with balance billing.

Health maintenance organizations (HMOs), a form of managed care, are prepaid health-care plans that provide members with medical care in return for a fixed monthly premium. All care is provided through a system of HMO-approved physicians, hospitals, and medical professionals. Members are required to choose a primary-care physician—known as a gatekeeper—from the HMO's approved list, and then visit that practitioner for medical care or a referral to another practitioner. Primary-care physicians receive a fixed monthly payment per member—known as capitation—or are reimbursed for services according to a set fee schedule.

HMOs usually cover physician's fees and services, hospital and surgical fees, home health care, outpatient surgery, some nursing home services, and preventive care such as routine checkups and immunizations. Most people join an HMO through their employer.

In an HMO, all but a small portion of medical care is prepaid. However, members are usually responsible for a small **copayment,** a set amount charged regardless of the cost of the services, on each visit—usually $5 to $10. Some consider the limited choice of physicians the HMOs biggest drawback. Services provided by physicians who are not approved by the HMO are not covered, or only partially covered, unless the HMO offers a point-of-service option, described below.

Preferred provider organizations (PPOs) operate much like HMOs, offering a closed panel of physicians. However, participants in a PPO are not required to visit a primary-care physician for services or for referral to another practitioner. Instead, members are only required to stay within the designated groups of physicians. If a provider outside of the panel is used, additional fees or higher copayments are charged. In addition, members must pay any difference between the covered fee of the PPO and the actual charges of the out-of-network provider.

Point-of-service (POS) plans are an option for HMO and PPO members that allows visits to participating or nonparticipating providers, but with different levels of coverage. POS plans simply cover less of the cost of medical care to the consumer if a preferred provider is not used. Many PPOs can be considered point-of-service plans, which offer the option of care from a practitioner or hospital outside the plan, but with an additional copayment. At any time, a member can opt out of the network and seek care without the approval of the primary-care physician. If this is done, the member is subject to additional fees and copays. Self-referral to a specialist, even within the network, may in some cases be considered an out-of-network service.

EMPLOYER PLANS

Employer self-insured plans are health-care programs that are designed and paid for by employers. Each employer is free to decide what type of coverage is provided and the extent of that coverage without regard for any legal mandates. Employers who provide self-insured plans are exempt from the federal Employee Retirement Income Security Act (ERISA), which mandates certain benefits (maternity, pediatric wellness) when provided by traditional insurance plans.

TRENDS IN HEALTH CARE

In the United States today, there is a strong movement toward managed health care, driven by the twin forces of employers seeking to purchase cost-effective care for employees, and several large insurance companies (including Prudential, Aetna, Metropolitan Life, Travelers, and Cigna) competing for a share of the marketplace. While at one time these insurance corporations offered mostly traditional, fee-for-service indemnity plans, they are now working to establish their own networks of primary-care providers, specialists, and hospitals. The practitioners and hospitals in these networks agree to provide all necessary medical services as well as referrals to those members of the plan for a set monthly fee.

This development puts the insurance companies in the dual role of not only determining the cost and reimbursement of medical services but also controlling the services delivered. This runs counter to the traditional indemnity insurance market where patients and practitioners usually determined how services were rendered, with the insurance companies paying on a fee-for-service basis.

Some say the trend will lead to an oligarchy, where the largest managed-care companies and their practitioners will dominate the market. Practitioners in private practice who are not part of a managed-care network are already finding that their patients are disappearing, obligated to go to a practitioner in a managed-care network. Small insurance carriers, once able to compete in the insurance market, are finding themselves overwhelmed by the dominance of the larger managed-care networks. To protect themselves from being wiped out by the big companies, many small groups are joining together to create larger networks of providers to allow them to compete in the market. Those looking on hope the competition will lead to lower overall health-care costs and more efficient service.

These plans are funded by the employer up to a certain dollar amount per employee, which may be subject to change from year to year. For example, an employer may cover all medical expenses up to $2,000, after which all services are covered by insurance. Self-insured plans may be administered by the employer, or an outside firm, such as an insurance company, may be contracted to handle all claims. Employers protect themselves from unlimited liability by carrying what amounts to a major medical policy to cover all expenses over a certain dollar amount.

Two other aspects of insurance to consider are **ERISA,** the Employee Retirement Income Security Act of 1974, and **COBRA,** the Consolidated Omnibus Budget Reconciliation Act of 1986. ERISA is a set of laws governing how employers are to administer health insurance benefits. The legislation requires an employer to provide employees with all information and documents about health benefits and to pay all claims made by beneficiaries. If a claim is denied, a written explanation must be provided, and an appeal process must be in place.

COBRA requires employers to offer to employees, their spouses, and dependents an opportunity to maintain their medical coverage in the event that they are fired. COBRA also applies to such situations as termination of employment, reduction of hours, death, divorce or legal separation, eligibility for Medicare, and loss of independent status by a child. The employee is responsible for making premium payments under the COBRA plan, which is offered for a period of 36 months for widows, divorced spouses, spouses of Medicare-eligible employees, and dependent children, and 18 months for employees with reduced hours or who have been terminated.

MEDICAID

Medicaid, the joint federal and state health insurance plan for low-income individuals, was created in 1965. Aside from California, which calls its program MediCal, the program is known in most states as Medicaid or medical assistance. Medicaid provides coverage for low-income individuals, including the aged, blind, disabled, pregnant women, adults with dependent children, and children under age six. States also have the option to cover other groups, such as the residents of long-term-care facilities (nursing homes) or single adults.

The Medicaid law, and subsequent federal regulations, mandate a basic list of services that must be included in any state Medicaid program. These services are:

■ Inpatient hospital services
■ Outpatient hospital services
■ Physician services
■ Medical and surgical services of dentists
■ Laboratory and x-ray services
■ Nursing facility services for individuals 21 and over
■ Home health care for persons eligible for nursing facility services
■ Family planning services and supplies
■ Rural health clinic services
■ Federally qualified health center services
■ Nurse-midwife services
■ Services of certified pediatric or family nurse-practitioners
■ Early and periodic screening, diagnostic, and treatment services for children under 21 and treatment for conditions identified in screening
■ Assurance of the availability of necessary transportation

In addition to these mandated services, states have the option of offering up to 32 more categories of care, such as podiatric and chiropractic services, private-duty nursing, and physical therapy. Definitions and limitations on eligibility for services are available from local welfare offices.

To determine eligibility for Medicaid, an individual must submit an application to the local office of the state welfare department—the official state agency of Medicaid. Only the state can determine if a person meets the criteria for any of the specific Medicaid programs.

About 38 states are currently putting into place **Medicaid managed-care** programs to enroll some of those insured through Medicaid in a health maintenance organization. Under the arrangement, the state pays the monthly fee to the private HMO, which then enrolls the Medicaid individual as a member. The HMO is required to provide all of the services offered by the traditional HMO plan in that state, and some offer more than is required. The plan is designed to give those with Medicaid an option in health care and to allow easier access to service. It is also hoped that the arrangement will stabilize state spending for health care. Those who enroll in a Medicaid managed-care program are limited to approved providers only.

MEDICARE

Medicare is the federal insurance plan that covers individuals 65 years of age and older, those who are permanently and totally disabled, and those who have end-stage renal disease. Social Security Administration offices across the country take applications for Medicare and provide information about the program. Part A of Medicare, which is free, deals with hospital insurance and helps to pay for hospital stays and care in a skilled nursing home or a home health agency. Part B, which had a premium of about $46 per month in 1994, deals with doctor insurance, covering doctor bills, outpatient hospital services, and some medical supplies and services. Supplemental medical insurance, called Medigap policies, is available to beneficiaries to help them cover the deductibles and copayments found in the Medicare program.

Everyone who is eligible for Medicare, in any of the coverage groups, has to be a citizen of the United States, by either birth or naturalization, or an alien admitted for permanent residence who has resided in the United States for at least five years. In addition, to be eligible, individuals must be entitled to payments under the Social Security Act or the Railroad Retirement Act. This means, in general, that they must have worked for at least 10 years (or, alternatively, six quarters out of the last 13 quarters) in jobs that were covered under the Social Security Act, or be covered based on the earnings record of someone who is covered.

A person who has not fulfilled the work requirement may be eligible based on the earnings record of someone who is covered. For example, widows and widowers are covered if they were married to their spouses at least one year before the death of the spouse. Divorced persons are eligible if they were married to the covered person for at least 10 years. In addition:

■ Wives who have reached age 65 are eligible if their husbands are covered.

■ Divorced wives are eligible if they were married to the person on whose earnings record they are covered, have attained age 65, and have not remarried.

■ Widows and widowers are eligible if they are over 65.

■ Mothers of covered children are eligible if they have attained the age of 65.

■ Parents of children eligible for Social Security who were receiving at least one-half of their support from their child at the time of the child's death or disability are eligible when they reach age 65.

Being 65 or older does not mean automatic enrollment in Medicare. The woman may have to take action when she turns 65. People who are in doubt about their status should apply; the worst that can happen is that they will find out the enrollment is already taken care of. The present situation is as follows:

■ Individuals who are 65 or older and have been receiving Social Security or Railroad Retirement benefits will automatically be enrolled for participation in Parts A and B (the hospital and doctor insurance portions of Medicare). They will receive a notice and their card about three to four months before their 65th birthday. The card will *not* be valid until they turn 65. Individuals are covered for Medicare even if they do not have their card; the hospital can bill under the Social Security number even if the card is not available. A Temporary Notice of Medicare Eligibility can be obtained from the Social Security office.

■ If people are 65 or older when they apply for Social Security benefits, they will automatically be enrolled in Medicare as part of the application process for Social Security. The card will be sent in the mail automatically. If they have been found eligible for Social Security, individuals are covered for Medicare even if they do not have their card.

■ End-stage renal (kidney) disease patients are automatically enrolled if they are receiving Social Security disability benefits; otherwise, they must apply.

Those who have not applied for Social Security or Railroad Retirement benefits before age 65 must file an application to enroll in Medicare. Formerly, persons were notified by mail when they were eligible to enroll. This service has been dropped as a cost-cutting measure. Individuals can apply for Part B Medicare coverage to begin on their 65th birthday anytime between three months before the month of their 65th birthday and three months after. The Social Security Administration calls these

seven months the personal enrollment period. If the application is submitted later than three months after one's 65th birthday, the Part A (hospital insurance) coverage will begin on the date of application, not on the 65th birthday.

If there is any doubt about Medicare eligibility and requirements, individuals can contact a Social Security representative to clarify their status. Medicare standards can vary with certain circumstances.

Medicare HMOs were made available in 1985 by the Health Care Financing Administration as an option for Medicare beneficiaries and retiring employees who already belonged to HMOs. HMO Medicare coverage is a supplement to, not a substitute for, Medicare coverage. The Medicare HMO plan provides all basic

FINDING A COMPATIBLE PRACTITIONER

Just as some insurance plans have restrictions on which practitioners their members can visit, many practitioners do not accept all forms of insurance from their patients. Ask what your practitioner accepts and what is not accepted. Many hospitals and clinics also have policies on insurance coverage.

Large insurance carriers, such as Blue Cross/Blue Shield, are widely accepted and can provide lists of participating physicians for their customers. Insurance from smaller companies, however, is less likely to be accepted by practitioners. Contact a representative of the company for a list of practitioners in your area who do accept coverage.

A practitioner who accepts Medicare can be found through the local Social Security office. In the case of Medicaid, caseworkers at the state welfare office can provide lists of participating practitioners. Health mainte-

nance organizations, by nature, provide a list of practitioners for members to choose from.

If your practitioner does accept your insurance, make sure your carrier's benefits will be accepted *as payment in full.* Even if a practitioner does accept your plan, the amount paid by the insurance carrier may not completely cover the bill for the service. In that case, the difference must be paid by you. Find out the cost of a service up front to avoid any surprise expenses.

If there will be a cost to you even with your insurance coverage, you can try negotiating the price of the procedure with the practitioner. For example, if your practitioner charges $800 for a service, and the insurance company will only reimburse $600, you will owe $200. If your health-care provider is willing to adjust the price of the procedure, you may only need to pay $100.

Medicare services and some additional services, usually including a deductible for hospital and skilled-nursing services, a deductible and copayment for physician services in hospital and office settings, diagnostic and rehabilitation services, prescription drugs, hearing aids, and eyeglasses.

Medicare beneficiaries may be required to pay the HMO a monthly premium for coverage of hospital and medical expenses over and above basic Medicare coverage. Some company retirement plans contribute to the HMO monthly premiums.

SEE medical records; practitioners, how to choose; second opinion.

For more information on insurance, contact:

Health Insurance Association of America
555 13th St., N.W., Suite 600
Washington, DC 20004-1660
202-824-1600

LAPAROSCOPY

Laparoscopy is a procedure used to examine the pelvic organs, including the fallopian tubes, the ovaries, the exterior of the uterus, and the pelvic cavity. Because the viewing instrument, called a laparoscope, is inserted through an incision near the navel, the procedure is often called belly button surgery, or Band-Aid surgery. It may be used for diagnostic or therapeutic reasons.

REASONS FOR LAPAROSCOPY

Laparoscopy is most commonly used to diagnose:

- Ovarian cysts
- Ectopic pregnancy
- Endometriosis
- Unknown causes of abdominal pain
- Infertility caused by blocked fallopian tubes
- Pelvic inflammatory disease

Laparoscopy is frequently used to determine if a hysterectomy is necessary and can be used during some vaginal hysterectomies. A number of other surgical techniques can also be done via laparoscopy as well, including:

- Treatment of endometriosis
- Removal of benign growths or scar tissue
- Removal of an intrauterine device (IUD) that has perforated the uterus
- Removal of an ovarian cyst or tumor
- Removal of fibroids
- Removal of all or part of the uterus
- Removal of eggs for in vitro fertilization
- Certain sterilization procedures such as tubal sterilization

PROCEDURE

The procedure is usually performed in a hospital operating room or in an outpatient surgical center. A gynecologist or surgeon performs the procedure, which requires local or general anesthesia. First, the surgeon makes a half-inch incision at the navel. Then a hollow needle is inserted through the incision, and carbon dioxide is pumped into the abdomen, inflating it like a balloon. This is done to lift the skin, muscle tissue, and intestines away from the pelvic organs so that the practitioner has a better view of them.

The surgeon then inserts an instrument called a **laparoscope** through the same incision. The laparoscope is a long, slender metal tube with a lens and a light source at one end and a telescopic eyepiece at the other. The practitioner uses this viewing instrument to look for any scar tissue, endometrial tissue, cysts, tumors, or other growths. During the procedure the surgeon may insert other instruments through the laparoscope to take samples of tissue for biopsy (microscopic analysis) or to remove minor endometrial implants or scar tissue. A second or third tiny incision may be made to more easily introduce other special instruments for more complicated procedures.

After the surgery, the carbon dioxide is released from the abdomen via the hole through which the instruments were inserted, and the incision is closed with a single absorbable stitch.

RISKS AND SIDE EFFECTS

Most women are able to leave the hospital the same day, but practitioners recommend they restrict their activity for three to seven days following the laparoscopy. During the procedure, women who are put under local anesthesia may feel an uncomfortable pressure or fullness. For the first two to three days after the procedure, women often feel some pain under their ribs or in their shoulders, an effect of the medications given during surgery and of the abdominal distension from the carbon dioxide.

Most complications are minor. As with any procedure that involves anesthesia, rare complications that may occur include cardiac irregularity, cardiac arrest, infection, internal bleeding, and perforation of a major blood vessel.

Other possible complications include internal organ or skin burns (if cauterization is involved), perforation of the uterus, puncturing tissues or organs such as the intestines, and carbon dioxide embolism (which occurs when the carbon dioxide blocks a blood vessel or organ and may cause immediate death). Complications resulting in death occur in less than one in 3,000 cases.

SEE biopsy; contraception—sterilization.

For more information on laparoscopy, contact:

American Association of Gynecological Laparoscopists
13021 E. Florence Ave.
Santa Fe Springs, CA 90670
310-946-8774
http://pages.prodigy.com/CA/jmp/jmp.html

LONG-TERM CARE

According to the National Health Information Center, the number of Americans over age 85 is expected to triple to 8.5 million in the next 40 years, increasing the proportion of the population at high risk for chronic health problems. Women must deal with long-term-care issues on two levels; they not only require long-term care more often than men, they are also traditionally in the role of caregiver when a family member or friend requires care. According to the National Family Caregiver Association, 75 percent of all family caregivers are women.

Even relatively healthy older people may need some regular assistance with personal care or household chores. For younger chronically ill or disabled Americans, their needs are similar to the elderly. Depending on an individual's needs, preferences, and resources, long-term care can range from at-home care from a family member to institutional care with continuous professional supervision.

HOME HEALTH CARE: FAMILY CAREGIVERS

A caregiver is anyone who is caring for someone who is ill or disabled at home. He or she does this over a long period of time, and it is a major part of daily life. A caregiver is usually a spouse, brother, sister, son, daughter, daughter-in-law, or son-in-law.

For a convalescing loved one, a caregiver provides personal care, manages the household, and manages daily life. It is a full-time job taken on out of love and devotion and also financial necessity. Many balance caretaking with a family and/or a full-time career, or a job may be given up in order to allow time for caretaking. Care in the home provides familiarity and family and is less expensive than hospital care or a nursing home. The costs of being a caregiver are often physical fatigue, mental stress, and financial burden. Caregivers who give up paid employment to provide care may even suffer economic hardships in their later years because they have been unable to make pension contributions.

Caregivers run into problems because long-term home care is a full-time job that leaves them with very little time for themselves. Due to the stress and the demands of the job, they run the risk of becoming patients themselves—secluded, or neglectful of their own needs. When they exhaust their physical and inner resources, they can be faced with **burnout,** the exhaustion of physical and emotional strength brought on by continuous stress and frustration.

Burnout manifests itself as:
- Sleeplessness
- Weight loss
- Loss of appetite
- Constipation
- Morning restlessness
- Weeping
- Social isolation
- Self-neglect

THE LOCAL AREA AGENCY ON AGING

Support to caregivers is provided by both professional and volunteer organizations through-

RECOVERING FROM BURNOUT

Burnout does not require medical treatment. Instead, the help of other people is needed to restore the inner resources of the caregiver. The first step in preventing or recovering from burnout is having realistic expectations of your abilities—realizing that you need to share the burden of caregiving with another person. There are several keys to finding help:

■ Establish a real partnership with a health-care professional. It is important to have access to the practitioner whenever it is needed, even late at night or during the weekends.

■ Seek emotional support from family and friends. Reluctance to look for help is very common, but you must be willing to accept assistance from others. Don't feel guilty because you can't do everything yourself.

■ Be knowledgeable about the illness or injury from which your loved one suffers. The more you know, the more you can act as an advocate on behalf of the patient and make appropriate decisions and referrals regarding medical care.

■ Find support groups with people who are having the same experiences dealing with the same circumstances. Members can help you understand the different stages and what may be the best ways to handle them. For support groups, call your state's Area Agency on Aging. They can help access family support groups in your area.

out the country. Every state has its own unique programs. The local Area Agency on Aging, which can be found listed in the human services section of the phone book, can provide a remarkable amount of information about legal issues, Meals on Wheels, and alternatives to full-time, in-home care, including:

■ Home health care: skilled nursing services under a physician's care

■ Respite care: provides relief to the principal caregiver of a terminally ill or chronically ill person. Care may be given at home or in a facility.

■ Adult day-care centers: daytime programs for older adults that provide health care and assessment, personal care, social programs, meals, and transportation

■ Foster care: a family other than the person's own assumes responsibility for that person's physical and mental well-being.

■ Residential care in a board-and-care home

■ Retirement communities

■ Hospice care: health care for the terminally ill that addresses the patient's physical and emotional needs and offers support to the family or caregiver

PLANNING FOR THE FUTURE

Since long-term and degenerative illnesses can be costly, financial planning is necessary. Sometimes a caregiver and a loved one are faced with a treatment or accident that requires more care and expense, and decisions must be made about what type of care will be provided and how it will be paid for. The caregiver and the patient should discuss the possible future, focusing on the special needs the illness or condition will bring about.

The patient, the practitioner, the attorney, and the caregiver may want to discuss the following measures, when they will be necessary, and how they will be carried out:

■ Power of attorney. This document gives someone else the authority to make decisions for the patient. It has a specified time frame and may be revoked.

■ Durable power of attorney. This gives a person other than the patient authority over health-care decisions for an unlimited period of time, though it may also be revoked.

■ Guardianship for an incompetent patient. This can only take place after a court rules that the patient is incompetent.

■ Living will. This is a declaration that expresses a person's desires as to the type of medical care she wants to receive if she becomes unable to make her own decisions.

■ Long-term care insurance policy

The patient should be included in the discussions and decision-making process before the progression of the illness or condition makes these issues urgent.

PROFESSIONAL LONG-TERM CARE

As the illness progresses, there may come a time when the patient needs more assistance than the caregiver is able to provide. It is a difficult decision, but there are definite indications of when it is time to move a loved one into a nursing home:

■ When the individual does not recognize his or her surroundings

■ When the individual is not able to cooperate or collaborate, for example, with tasks such as going to the bathroom with only a little assistance

■ When someone who has been assisting the caregiver must drop out

■ When the caregiver feels he or she has gone as far as possible in giving help

The *Barron's Dictionary of Insurance Terms* defines long-term care as day-to-day care that a patient receives following an illness or injury, or in old age. The patient cannot perform two or more of the five basic activities of daily life: walking, eating, dressing, using the bathroom, and mobility from one place to another. Professional long-term care is provided at home or in a nursing facility.

There are three basic types of long-term care. **Skilled-nursing care** is provided by skilled medical professionals, as prescribed by a physician. Medicare pays a limited amount of the costs. **Intermediate care** is provided by skilled medical professionals, as prescribed by a physician. In this case, the patient requires occasional nursing and rehabilitative assistance. **Custodial care** is provided by skilled medical professionals, as ordered by a physician. The patient requires personal assistance in order to conduct basic daily living activities.

NURSING HOMES

According to the Health Care Financing Administration, by the year 2000 almost 9 million older Americans will need long-term-care services, and many of these people will require nursing homes.

The time to consider a nursing home is before it is needed. In this way, the family can include the patient in the decision-making process, then thoroughly investigate which facilities would meet the patient's personality, illness, and specific needs. During the middle

BUYING A LONG-TERM-CARE POLICY

If you decide to buy a long-term-care insurance policy, there are several points you should consider:

■ Renewability. The policy should be a guaranteed renewable contract.

■ Waiting period. The length of time before benefits are paid should not exceed 90 days.

■ Age eligibility. The upper age limit (the age after which the company will not grant a policy) should be at least 80.

■ Length of time benefits are paid. The range should be five to 10 years. Ideally, a policy should pay benefits for life.

■ Inflation guard. The benefit level should be automatically adjusted annually according to the increase in costs charged by the long-term-care giver.

■ Premium waiver. After the patient has received benefits for at least 90 days, the patient is no longer required to make premium payments for as long as he or she is under long-term care.

■ No increase of premiums with age. Premiums should be based on the age at the time of application and should never increase as a result of age.

■ No limitations for preexisting conditions.

stage of disease, a caregiver should talk with a loved one's practitioner about the time to consider a nursing home. This is one of many points when knowledge of the illness can help greatly in making these decisions.

When people enter nursing homes, they don't leave their personalities at the door. Nor do they lose their basic human rights and needs for respect, encouragement, and friendliness. All individuals need to retain as much control over the events in their daily lives as possible. The patient should be involved in the search for a facility. It is also important to consider his or her personality, interests, and personal preferences.

Of course, it is also important to consider the characteristics of the illness or symptoms of old age. Someone who suffers only from the symptoms of old age, for example, would probably not benefit from a facility that specializes in Alzheimer's disease. On the other hand, a person with Alzheimer's has special needs that may not be met at a standard nursing facility. Many facilities do specialize; consider this when making a list of possible homes. A practitioner or the local Area Agency on Aging can be contacted for a list of specialized facilities.

Research should be done before visiting a nursing home. Each local Area Agency on Aging is required by federal law to have an Office of the Long-Term Care Ombudsman. Ombudsmen are officials who visit nursing homes on a regular basis, and they are often aware of what goes on in facilities in their communities. In addition, they receive and investigate complaints made by or on behalf of nursing home residents and work to resolve the problems. While they cannot advise an individual on any one particular nursing home, they can supply current information regarding local nursing homes. The local ombudsman should be asked about:

■ Information about the latest survey report on the facility

■ Any complaints against the nursing home you plan to visit

✓ SOME QUESTIONS TO ASK

The Health Care Financing Administration recommends that when you have chosen a facility you would like to visit, first contact them by phone and ask key questions, including:

■ Is the nursing home certified for participation in the Medicare or Medicaid program?

■ What is the "typical profile" of a resident in the facility? Be sure the profile matches your needs.

■ Does the nursing home require that a resident sign over personal property or real estate in exchange for care?

■ Does the facility have vacancies, or is there a waiting list?

When you decide to visit a nursing home, remember to consider whether it matches your health-care needs and the type of lifestyle you would like to lead. Also consider how close it is to family and friends, how easy it is for people to visit, and how near it is to other community contacts and resources that you may want to use in the future.

To ensure the quality of long-term care:

■ Ask about nursing accreditation. Nursing facilities can voluntarily apply for accreditation from the Joint Commission on Accreditation of Healthcare Organizations (JCAHO). The review includes a self-review, on-site visit by experts, and a written evaluation by JCAHO.

■ Assess the grounds and services. Take some time to sit in the lobby, eat a meal, check out planned activities, and chat with the nurses and their aides. Also talk to residents and family members about their experiences with the facility. Consider:

— Safety. Are the buildings fireproof? Are the sidewalks well maintained? Are there grip bars in the showers and the bathrooms?

— Livability. Are there wheelchair ramps? Is there access to public transportation? Is the neighborhood safe? Are the lobbies and recreation areas well maintained? Is there enough room for the residents?

— Comfort. Are the rooms neat and clean? Is there enough light? Is there air-conditioning? Is there an adjoining bathroom?

■ Observe the availability of the staff. Is there a physician on the premises each day? Is there a physician on call 24 hours a day? Is a registered nurse on duty 24 hours a day? Is there access to a pharmacist?

■ Ask about patient rights. Can a resident select her own practitioner? Her own hospital? Does the facility subscribe to a Patient's Bill of Rights?

■ The number and nature of complaints for the past year against the facility

■ The results and conclusions of the investigation into these complaints

■ What to look for as telltale signs of good care in facilities

Information should also be collected from several other sources, including:

■ Hospital discharge planners or social workers

■ Your family practitioner

■ Religious organizations

■ Volunteer organizations such as Meals on Wheels

■ State nursing home associations

■ Close friends or relatives

HOSPICE CARE

Hospices were developed solely to assist dying patients—typically cancer patients who have exhausted the various forms of curative treatment—and to help them live their remaining weeks or months as free of symptoms and as much in control as possible. For people who do not wish to receive further aggressive treatment for a terminal illness, or for whom only palliative care can be provided, a hospice offers an opportunity for the patient and family to help each other during the dying process.

Hospice care places emphasis on symptom control, preparation for death, and support for survivors. Care can be provided in the home or in professional facilities with a home-like setting, but the idea is to allow death with dignity and keep the family close to the person, away from the high-tech surroundings of a hospital. Medicare regulations now provide for hospice coverage both in and out of the home. A local Social Security office can provide more information. The Hospice Association of America can also help with Medicare questions.

CHANGING ROLES OF THE CAREGIVER

It is common for a caregiver to feel that no one else can provide care as well as he or she can. The caregiver may also feel a sense of guilt for not being able to provide the right kind of care anymore.

When placing a loved one in a nursing home, a family caregiver may experience separation anxiety. This is normal and occurs whenever a change in a relationship occurs. The feeling is very intense, yet it is short-term and part of the adjustment. A person should discuss feelings of anxiety with someone who will understand, yet not question his or her judgment. Some nursing homes provide a support person to talk to.

Remember that at this point, the caregiver still has an active role to play. It is important that the caregiver become visible to the staff of the nursing home to ensure that the best of care is provided. The caregiver should act as an advocate for the patient, but not adversary of the nursing home. In other words, she should be a voice for her loved one and act as a liaison between the patient and the staff. In this way, the staff will be able to understand their patient's background, former lifestyle, and idiosyncrasies. This helps the staff see the loved one as an individual.

The caregiver should also keep in contact with any support groups she attended. She may be able to help someone who is in the midst of making the same choices and decisions she had to make.

SEE death and dying; insurance; medical rights.

255

For more information on long-term care, contact:

American Association of Homes and Services for the Aging
901 E St., N.W., Suite 500
Washington, DC 20004-2037
202-783-2242

American Health Care Association
1201 L St., N.W.
Washington, DC 20005
202-842-4444

Children's Hospice International
700 Princess St., Lower Level
Alexandria, VA 22314
703-684-0330

Foundation for Hospice and Homecare
513 C St., N.E.
Washington, DC 20002
202-547-6586

Health Care Financing Administration
7500 Security Blvd
Baltimore, MD 21224
410-786-3000
http://www.hcfa.gov

Health Insurance Association of America
Public Affairs Department
555 13th St., N.W., Suite 600E
Washington, DC 20004
202-824-1600

Hospice Association of America
519 C St., N.E.
Washington, DC 20002
202-546-4759

National Academy on Aging
1275 K St., N.W., Suite 350
Washington, DC 20005
202-408-3375
http://www.geron.org

National Association of Meals Program
101 N. Alfred St., Suite 202
Alexandria, VA 22314
703-548-5558

National Council on Aging
409 Third St., S.W.
Washington, DC 20024
202-479-1200
info@ncoa.org

National Family Caregivers Association
9621 E. Bexhill Dr.
Kensington, MD 20895-3104
301-942-6430
caregiving@aol.com

National Hospice Organization
1901 N. Moore St., Suite 901
Arlington, VA 22209
703-243-5900
http://www.nho.org

LUPUS

Lupus erythematosus is a chronic, inflammatory disease that affects the connective tissue, the network of tissue that supports the organs and other tissues of the body. The condition, which flares up at intervals, causes the production of infection-fighting substances in the blood, called antibodies, which attack the body's own tissues rather than foreign organisms. There is no known cause for lupus, but there is evidence that it may have some genetic basis.

The most characteristic symptom of the disease is a butterfly-shaped rash across the cheeks and the bridge of the nose, which resembles the facial markings of a wolf. "Lupus erythematosus" means "red wolf" in Latin.

An estimated 500,000 individuals suffer from lupus each year, and the majority of them are women. Women are nine times more likely to develop lupus than men, and black women are more likely to develop it than white women. The risk of the disease is one in 700 for white women and one in 250 for black women.

The symptoms of lupus vary and tend to come and go. They include:

■ A butterfly-shaped rash across the cheeks and the bridge of the nose

■ A rash on the upper body

■ Sensitivity to the sun

■ Painful joints

■ Fingers and toes that become white and blue when exposed to cold (Raynaud's phenomenon)

■ Low-grade fever

■ Fatigue

■ Chest pain

In addition to arthritis-like pain, lupus can lead to inflammation of the membranes that surround the heart and the lungs and to problems with the central nervous system, such as seizures. Kidney disease is also a problem for at least half of all people with systemic lupus. Women with lupus are at higher risk for miscarriage, and the symptoms may flare up during pregnancy. Some women also experience a flare-up of the condition after delivery.

TYPES OF LUPUS

The three types of lupus are discoid lupus, systemic lupus erythematosus (SLE), and drug-induced lupus.

Discoid lupus is usually mild and affects only the skin, causing a rash on the face and on the upper body. **Systemic lupus erythematosus (SLE)** is more severe than discoid lupus, though the symptoms range from mild to severe. It spreads throughout the entire body and may affect the joints, kidneys, brain, heart, and lungs. SLE can be fatal if it is not kept under control. However, according to the Lupus Foundation of America, less than 10 percent of those with lupus die from the disease or its complications.

Lupus can also be caused by a reaction to medications. This condition, known as **drug-induced lupus,** is responsible for 10 percent of all lupus cases. It is most often triggered by procainamide (Pronestyl), used to treat heart irregularities. Other drugs that cause lupus are hydralazine (a blood pressure drug), isoniazid (used to treat tuberculosis), quinidine (used to treat heart irregularities), and chlorpromazine (used to treat psychosis and severe vomiting). Drug-induced lupus disappears when the individual stops taking the medication.

DIAGNOSIS

Discoid lupus can usually be identified by the presence of the butterfly rash across the face. Individuals with discoid lupus should also be tested for SLE.

To test for systemic lupus, an antinuclear antibody (ANA) test can be performed. This blood screening test can detect the presence of antibodies in 99 percent of people with SLE. However, because the antibodies may be produced in response to certain medications, viral infections, and types of arthritis, a positive ANA test does not necessarily mean lupus. A negative test, however, does rule out lupus. A blood test can also be done to detect antibodies to a person's genetic material, DNA. This antibody can be detected in 75 percent of people with SLE.

If drug-induced lupus is suspected, different drugs may be prescribed, or medications may be stopped, to see if the condition subsides.

TREATMENT

With the exception of drug-induced lupus, the disease cannot be cured. Discoid lupus may be very mild and may not even require treatment. When necessary, it is usually treated with topical steroid creams and sunscreens. For more severe discoid lupus, Plaquenil, a drug used to treat rheumatoid arthritis, may be prescribed.

SLE may be treated with aspirin, nonsteroidal anti-inflammatory drugs (NSAIDs),

PREVENTION AND SELF-CARE

Though there is no known cause for discoid lupus or SLE, experts have found that some activities and substances may trigger flare-ups of the conditions. To help avoid such attacks:

■ Avoid ultraviolet rays by staying out of the sun or by wearing sunscreen. For many people, ultraviolet rays bring on lupus symptoms.

■ Exercise. By strengthening muscles, you can ease joint pain.

■ Keep up an adequate nutritional program.

■ Avoid stress. It is also thought to spark lupus.

■ Avoid drugs that may trigger lupus flare-ups. These may include oral contraceptives. Avoid chemical and toxic exposure.

and antimalarial drugs. For flare-ups of the disease, steroid drugs, which reduce inflammation, may be used to prevent permanent damage to major organs. However, it has been found that long-term steroid use may lead to kidney disease and heart failure. SLE may also be treated with drugs that suppress the immune system; however, these drugs lower the body's defenses against serious infection and may cause nausea, anemia, or liver damage.

For more information on lupus, contact:

Arthritis Foundation Information Line
P.O. Box 19000
Atlanta, GA 30326
800-283-7800
404-872-7100 (Georgia)
http://www.arthritis.org

Lupus Foundation of America
4 Research Place, Suite 180
Rockville, MD 20850-3226
800-558-0121
301-670-9292
http://www.lupus.org/lupus

MALPRACTICE

The *Mosby Medical Encyclopedia* describes malpractice as a professional mistake that is a direct cause of injury or harm to a patient. It may result from a lack of professional knowledge, experience, or skill that can be expected in others in the profession. It may also result from a failure to use reasonable care or judgment in applying professional knowledge, experience, or skill.

Four standards of care, according to the *Columbia University College of Physicians and Surgeons Complete Home Medical Guide* (New York: Crown, 1989), constitute a practitioner's legal obligations toward his or her patients; any one of these obligations, if violated, can be grounds for a lawsuit:

■ The practitioner must obtain the patient's informed consent before treatment. This means that a patient must understand the risks involved in a procedure before consenting to it; it does not mean that a practitioner must detail every remote possibility or that a consent form must be signed every time a patient is treated. A signed consent form, however, is required by law before surgery or an invasive diagnostic test is done. If informed consent is not obtained properly—if, for example, a patient is asked to agree to "any or all" procedures, or the consent is obtained when the patient is sedated just prior to surgery—the practitioner is technically open to a charge of assault and battery.

■ In treating a patient, the practitioner must use reasonable skill and care in accordance with accepted medical practice, and within the limits of his or her competence. The key words

here are "reasonable" and "accepted." Both may be difficult to define, and it has sometimes proved to be extremely difficult to establish in court that this standard has been violated, except in cases of extreme negligence.

■ A practitioner must adequately supervise those aspects of a patient's care that he or she delegates to others. Doctors, for example, customarily delegate to nurses and other health-care personnel; this is acceptable legally as long as the practitioner assumes responsibility for those who are helping. (Under certain circumstances, hospital nurses and aides, although not in the practitioner's employ, are considered to be under the practitioner's supervision.)

■ A patient, once accepted by a practitioner, cannot be abandoned. A practitioner is not under any obligation to accept a patient, but once treatment has begun, he or she must continue to care for that patient until treatment is no longer needed, until the patient voluntarily leaves the practitioner, or until the practitioner has properly notified the patient that he or she will no longer be responsible for the patient's care and has given the patient appropriate alternative referrals. This should not take place in the middle of treatment.

THE PRACTITIONER'S VIEW

Practitioners who view patients as potential lawsuits practice what is called defensive medicine. **Defensive medicine** is the ordering of a battery of diagnostic tests and procedures to guard against overlooking something that could

(continued on page 262)

FILING A MALPRACTICE SUIT

You may decide to file a malpractice suit if your injuries are severe and you have a strong desire to get satisfaction from a clearly inadequate practitioner or institution. This is a matter for you and a qualified malpractice attorney to review. A malpractice suit may take years to resolve and end in an out-of-court settlement.

Alternatives to Litigation

Arbitration is an alternative to litigation. A patient who signs an arbitration agreement before treatment gives up the right to a jury trial if there is a later claim of malpractice and a lawsuit. Instead, the case is presented to a neutral panel consisting of one arbitrator chosen by the patient, one chosen by the practitioner, and one disinterested arbitrator. The panel decides all questions of fault and sets an award. Several states sanction arbitration as an alternative dispute-resolving forum for medical malpractice claims.

Many practitioners and patients choose arbitration because it can be less costly and speedier than a full trial.

How to Select a Malpractice Attorney

Find someone you know who can refer you to a personal-injury lawyer. Ideally, the person will have worked with that lawyer in a medical malpractice situation. There are also a number of reference books in law libraries that might help you. The *Martindale-Hubbell Law Directory* and *Markham's Negligence Counsel* are two such references.

Schedule appointments with the lawyer or lawyers who seem best suited to your needs. When you meet with them, you'll want to ask some key questions, including:

■ What sorts of medical malpractice cases have they handled? How much experience do they have, and what were the outcomes of some of the cases?

■ Who will actually try the case? Many successful personal injury attorneys frequently divide responsibility for a case among staffers. Be sure that the staff is competent and the attorney you hired is involved in the case, especially in the courtroom.

■ Is your lawyer competent to handle your type of case? In most instances, an experienced medical malpractice attorney will be able to handle it—unless your case involves pharmaceuticals, in which case an expert may be your best bet. Usually, there are one or two attorneys who have done the exhaustive research necessary to litigate such cases, and it might be wise to contact them.

Beware of legal firms that extensively advertise or otherwise aggressively prospect for victims of medical treatment.

Fees

The standard contingency-fee contract calls for an attorney to receive one-third of all monies awarded to a client. However, that percentage can vary. In medical malpractice cases, the amount can be as high as 40 or 45 percent because of the amount of time and costs such cases require. Your state may also mandate graduated percentages based on award amounts.

According to the attorney's code of professional responsibility and the laws of every state, clients are responsible for costs. Those costs can be high, easily topping $10,000 in many cases. What are you to do if you don't have the thousands of dollars required? Here are some options:

■ Suggest to a lawyer that he or she advance you the money to pay for costs and subtract that "advance" from the final settlement or judgment. This is a fairly common practice, and many lawyers will suggest it to clients. What happens if you lose the case and there is no settlement? Most lawyers will offer verbal assurances, such as, "I've never sued a client for costs," or something to that effect.

■ Put a clause in your contract with the lawyer that limits costs. If, for instance, you have some available cash, you might want to insert a clause that stipulates that any costs over a certain amount ($7,500, for instance) will be deducted from the lawyer's fee. Again, this is an accepted practice that many lawyers will agree to.

■ Consider an advance on cases the attorney is reluctant to take on. If you believe your case has merit, you might persuade an attorney to review the case by offering an advance ($2,500 is a typical amount). That will enable the attorney to spend sufficient time to determine whether you have a chance of winning and will also limit your costs.

Preparing a Case

The more information your attorney has and the faster it's provided, the easier it will be to plan a strategy.

Here's what you should bring:

■ All records available to you: medical history, hospital and office visits

■ A written chronology of events that led up to your problem. Dates, times, places, and people involved should be clearly listed.

■ Copies of relevant prescriptions

■ Bills received from practitioners, hospitals, and other health-care facilities

Settlements

In many medical malpractice suits, defendants wish to settle out of court. At some point during the legal process, you might be confronted with a settlement decision. Here are some things you should consider:

Remember it's your decision, not your lawyer's, the defendant's, or the judge's. A settlement can't be imposed upon you, unless you are a minor.

Before making the decision, be sure you have all the facts. Be sure to ask:

■ What, if any, limitations does the state law impose on the amount of money that is recoverable?

■ Is there a likelihood that more money might be offered?

■ Is it likely that additional money will be offered before, or during, the trial?

■ How long will the settlement offer be on the table? In many instances, the offer will change or be withdrawn depending on what develops as the case evolves.

■ If you reject the settlement, what are your chances of losing the case and receiving nothing?

lead to a lawsuit. Defensive medicine is more expensive, and extensive testing may lead to unnecessary treatment.

Many people believe that changing the laws surrounding malpractice litigation may help protect health-care providers from costly lawsuits. Proponents of tort reform (a tort is a wrongful act) believe it to be the only way to discourage inappropriate lawsuits. Major components of tort reform legislation generally include:

■ Limits on awards for pain and suffering

■ Limits on attorney's fees

■ Reducing the statute of limitations (the time period in which legal action must be taken) to two years

■ Requiring periodic payment of awards

■ A collateral source rule: the reduction of a monetary award by the amount of any other payment a plaintiff may receive from a source other than the defendant

■ Imposing penalties for groundless lawsuits

Supporters of tort reform legislation claim that these changes would allow practitioners to practice medicine free from the threat of unwarranted legal action. Opponents feel that the restrictions will make it more difficult for a consumer to bring about a lawsuit.

THE PATIENT'S VIEW

While some people believe that patients are ready to sue a practitioner at the drop of a hat, studies show that most people involved in malpractice litigation see unconcerned, uncaring, and unqualified practitioners as the primary reasons for malpractice. Several myths surround the reasons a suit is brought to court:

■ Myth: A malpractice suit is usually an attempt to get rich quick. A Harvard University study of hospital discharge records in New York State shows just the opposite is true. A review of more than 30,000 medical records revealed that about 4 percent of all hospitalized patients experienced some form of adverse occurrence. Yet fewer than 50 of the patients whose records were reviewed filed a malpractice claim. When the researchers applied these figures to statewide hospitalizations, they determined that some 5,000 patients received serious and disabling injuries as a result of hospitalization. However, a review of malpractice claims revealed only slightly more than 3,500 patients had filed suit.

■ Myth: Malpractice victims always win their day in court. This myth was dispelled when a study, published in the *Annals of Internal Medicine,* found that physicians win 76 percent of the time—which means that plaintiffs prevail in only 24 percent of the cases. This study also revealed that the overwhelming majority of these court cases are truly warranted: most of the cases were tried after the practitioner's own insurance company had reviewed the facts and determined that the care provided was questionable.

■ Myth: There will be a "million-dollar payday" for plaintiffs who win suits. According to Jury Verdict Research, a firm that tracks malpractice awards, the latest figures reveal that the average award, in a case involving a physician, is around $375,000. While this may appear to be a sizable award, it should be remembered that at least one-third goes to cover attorney's fees. Limitations on attorney's fees are now in effect in more than 20 states in order to guarantee that the plaintiffs receive the majority of the awards.

SEE medical records; medical rights.

MAMMOGRAPHY

Mammograms are x-rays of the breast that can detect growths that are too small to be felt during breast examinations. Because they can find cancer at an early stage, mammograms can be lifesavers for women. A routine mammogram is known as a **screening mammogram.** A **diagnostic mammogram** is done when a suspicious lump has been detected.

When having a mammogram, a woman stands before an x-ray machine. One at a time, each breast is placed onto a plastic platform and then gently compressed by another plastic plate as the x-rays are taken. For most women, the procedure is not painful, but it may be uncomfortable. Mammograms should not be scheduled the week before a woman's period, when the breasts may be tender. Deodorant powders and lotions should not be used the day of a mammogram because they may show up in the x-ray.

The American College of Radiology accredits mammogram facilities based on the credentials of the technicians who do the testing and the medical specialists called **radiologists** who interpret the results. These radiologists must complete special training requirements and are usually board-certified.

WHAT DOES A MAMMOGRAM SHOW?

The radiologist who interprets the mammogram compares the images of the breasts with each other, or with the images from a mammogram done at a previous time, looking for changes in the density of breast tissue as well as calcifications and nipple changes. Mammograms do not show cancer *per se,* but they do show abnormal or suspicious areas and help to decide if further tests need to be done. If an abnormality is cancerous, its borders tend to be irregular or its shape poorly defined or spindle-shaped. A benign (noncancerous) abnormality usually has well-defined, clear borders that are not irregular. The mammogram also provides information about the size, location, and possible spreading of a growth. If a suspicious area is found, a biopsy (removal of tissue for microscopic analysis) or other diagnostic test is done to diagnose or rule out cancer.

WHO SHOULD HAVE A MAMMOGRAM?

Experts do not agree on the age at which a woman should begin to have annual screening mammograms. For women between the ages of 50 and 65, the benefits of mammography seem to be clear. Studies done around the world show that regular screening mammograms can cut the death rate from breast cancer by 30 percent or more in these women. Few experts dispute those findings.

Practitioners also agree that mammograms can be helpful in other situations. A mammogram may be recommended:

■ As early as age 25 for women who have a grandmother, mother, father, brother, or sister who developed breast cancer at a young age

■ For women with noncancerous breast lumps, to be sure cancer is not hidden among benign, fluid-filled cysts

■ For women with noncancerous breast lumps, if new lumps that do not fit the normal cyclical pattern of lumpy breasts are discovered through self-examination

Among most women aged 40 to 49 or younger, however, the benefits of regular screening mammograms are much less clear.

In 1993 the National Cancer Institute (NCI) revised its recommendation for routine screening mammograms for women between 40 and 49, saying that there was no evidence that such screening saved lives. According to the NCI panel, which reviewed research from the preceding 20 years, mammography reduced deaths by 30 percent for women over 50 but made no statistical difference in women between 40 and 49. However, the NCI is currently taking another look at the issue, and may soon revise its guidelines once again to include women ages 40 to 49.

Those who oppose routine mammograms for women under 50 maintain that the screenings cannot accurately detect an abnormality in the dense breast tissue of younger women. As a result, they say, a woman under 50 is more likely to undergo a biopsy based on the inaccurate findings of a mammogram.

On the other hand, many organizations, including the American Cancer Society, say there is no evidence that annual mammograms for women between ages 40 and 49 cannot save lives. They believe that mammograms should be recommended even if only a small number of women benefit. The groups also fear that the opposition's stand will discourage women from

THE RISK OF DEVELOPING CANCER FROM THE RADIATION OF X-RAYS

Most experts agree that the risk of developing breast cancer as a result of being exposed to the radiation of the mammogram is minimal.

However, no one knows a woman's lifetime risk of developing cancer as a result of regular radiation exposure from yearly mammograms starting at age 40. It is thought that younger women's breasts are more sensitive to radiation exposure than older women's breasts, but no one knows what that means in terms of an increased risk of radiation-induced cancer. It has been estimated that about one in 25,000 women who begin mammography screening at age 40 will develop radiation-induced breast cancer sometime during her life, but this has not been proved.

Radiation dosages can vary widely among mammography centers, and among different kinds of breast x-ray techniques, which include **xeromammography,** where

an image is produced as a positive image on paper; **film-screen with grid,** a device that improves image quality when x-raying large breasts; and **film-screen without grid.**

It is important to ask the radiology technician (who takes the x-rays) what your "radiation absorbed dose" (rad) will be. Compare that figure with those below, which the National Council on Radiation Protection says provide good image quality at low dosage:

Xeromammography	.8 rad per two-view exposure
Film-screen with grid	.8 rad per two-view exposure
Film-screen without grid	.2 rad per two-view exposure

having needed mammograms and discourage insurance companies from covering mammogram costs.

THE ACCURACY OF MAMMOGRAMS

There is a possibility that the results of the mammogram will not be accurate. A **false-positive** mammographic result means the mammogram detects an abnormality that, on biopsy, proves to be nonmalignant. While confirming a possibly inaccurate biopsy means undergoing a breast biopsy, the smaller a cancer, the more it may resemble a benign, noncancerous lump. In other words, there is a trade-off between finding early cancer and tolerating a certain number of benign biopsies. The rate of false-positive results varies according to a woman's age and the physician's diagnostic skill. A woman having yearly mammograms from ages 40 to 50 has a 33 percent chance of a false-positive result. For a woman 55 to 65 years old, there is a 20 percent chance. Women younger than age 40, because the breast tissue is denser, have a very high rate of false-positive results.

A **false-negative** mammographic result means the mammogram finds no signs of cancer when cancer is actually present. It can lead to a delay in treatment and possibly lead the woman to disregard self-exams and ignore new lumps. They also can create anxiety. Studies show that in 10 to 15 percent of all cases, there is a false-negative result. For mammograms performed on women under 40 years of age, false-negative results occur 60 to 70 percent of the time; in other words, abnormalities that are present are not detected by a mammogram in 60 to 70 percent of the cases.

The American College of Radiology warns practitioners not to rely on mammograms alone when making a diagnosis. Mammogram results should be combined with a physical examination of the breast and, if necessary, another diagnostic test.

CONFIRMING MAMMOGRAM RESULTS

A **biopsy** is the surgical removal of tissue which is then analyzed for cancerous cells. Eighty percent of biopsied tissue turns out to be noncancerous. While biopsy is the most common diagnostic test used to confirm or rule out cancer, there are other options.

A **core-needle biopsy** is a nonsurgical procedure that removes a tiny piece of the tissue for analysis with a hollow needle. While the nonsurgical biopsy is less expensive and less invasive than a surgical biopsy, some experts believe such a small sample is inadequate for testing. Fine needle biopsy is the minimum testing required to diagnose what is happening in a defined mass.

Another option is **ultrasound,** which uses echoes from sound waves to visualize lumps. An ultrasound is 96 to 100 percent accurate at distinguishing fluid-filled cysts from solid tumors; however, it can miss small, solid lumps and cannot help with the diagnosis of a solid mass.

Both **thermography,** which supposedly shows abnormal areas as "hot spots," and **trans-illumination,** which consists of shining a bright light through the tissue of the breast, are considered unreliable at detecting abnormal areas.

SEE breast biopsy; breast—fibrocystic conditions; breast lumps, benign; breast self-examination; cancer, breast.

MASSAGE THERAPY

Massage therapy is the healing art in which manual manipulation of the body is employed to create a feeling of relaxation, ease mental and physical tensions, alleviate aches and pains, improve circulation, and generally reinvigorate and stimulate the body's systems. A massage therapist is trained in one or more of the following forms of massage therapy: Swedish massage, shiatsu, acupressure, Rolfing, reflexology, polarity, and bioenergetics.

Archaeological evidence indicates that prehistoric healers rubbed their patients' bodies with oil to produce a healing effect. The ancient Chinese included massage in their regimen of exercise, martial arts, and meditation. Ancient Greeks and Romans discovered that massage could be used to relieve headaches, improve joint function and circulation, and ease pain and muscle fatigue.

While massage was once used in the United States primarily to condition athletes (usually to limber up joints and relieve pain), today there is more interest in the use of massage therapy for a myriad of health-care problems. Massage thera-

pists claim it is effective in treating stress and fatigue, headaches, insomnia, lower back pain, and pregnancy and postpartum problems as well as in aiding digestion and circulation. Medical practitioners such as osteopaths and chiropractors manipulate joints in the skeletal system to treat certain conditions. Erotic massage techniques are used to alleviate sexual dysfunction and enhance orgasm for women and men.

Massages often begin at the head or feet, then gradually work toward the heart to replicate the body's natural circulatory path. Each massage is composed of a series of strokes or movements done with different pressure. The basic massage strokes are kneading, tapping or striking, and gliding. Swedish massage makes use of two additional motions: vibration and friction. Shiatsu and acupressure rely almost exclusively on the application of pressure. There are a great many massage techniques available that are used to relieve physical and mental discomfort.

Since massage therapy is noninvasive and involves no drugs, just about anyone can enjoy its benefits.

SEE Chinese medicine.

For more information on different types of massage, or to find a qualified therapist in your area, contact:

American Massage Therapy Association
820 Davis St., Suite 100
Evanston, IL 60201-4444
708-864-0123

MEDICAL
ABBREVIATIONS

Health-care professionals use abbreviations for medical terms and everyday words. Understanding the language is an important key to complete participation in many aspects of medical care, from reading a medical chart to completely understanding a condition and prognosis.

The following list is a collection of abbreviations frequently used in charts and records, on forms and prescriptions, and even in everyday conversation. If an abbreviation you encounter doesn't appear on this list, ask your practitioner, nurse, hospital patients' representative, or some other professional for a translation.

a = before
aa = of each
a.c. = before meals
Ad. = to, up to
ADL = activities of daily living
ad lib. = as needed; as desired
A.F. = auricular fibrillation
agit = shake, stir
AM = morning
AMA = against medical advice
Ap. = appendicitis
Aq. = water
ASHD = arteriosclerotic heart disease
B.E. = barium enema
b.i.d. = twice a day
Bl. time = bleeding time
B.M. = bowel movement
B.M.R. = basal metabolic rate
BP = blood pressure

BRP = bathroom privileges
Bx = biopsy
C = centigrade
c̄ = with
CA = cancer
CAD = coronary-artery disease
cap(s) = capsule(s)
CBC = complete blood count
CBD = common bile duct
cc = cubic centimeter(s)
CC = chief complaint
CCU = coronary-care unit
CHD = coronary heart disease or congenital heart disease
CHF = congestive heart failure
Chol = cholesterol
Cl. time = clotting time
cm = centimeter
CNS = central nervous system
comp = compound
cont rem = continue the medicine
COPD = chronic obstructive pulmonary disease
CSF = cerebrospinal fluid
CV = cardiovascular
CVA = cardiovascular accident
CVP = central venous pressure
CXR = chest x-ray
d = give
D&C = dilation and curettage
D&E = dilation and evacuation
dd in d = from day to day
dec = pour off
dexter = the right

dil = dilute
disp. = dispense
div = divide
DM = diabetes mellitus
DNR = do not resuscitate
dos = dose
dur dolor = while pain lasts
D/W = dextrose in water
Dx = diagnosis
ECG or EKG = electrocardiogram
EEG = electroencephalogram
emp = as directed
ER = emergency room
ext = for external use
F = Fahrenheit
FBS = fasting blood sugar
febris = fever
FH = family history
Fx = fracture
GA = general anesthesia
garg = gargle
GB = gallbladder
GC = gonorrhea
GI = gastrointestinal
GL = glaucoma
gm = grams
gr. = grains
grad = by degrees
gravida = pregnancies
gtt = drops
GTT = glucose tolerance test
GU = genitourinary
GYN = gynecology
h = hour
Hb or Hgb = hemoglobin
HCT = hematocrit
HHD = hypertensive heart disease
HOB = head of bed
h.s. = at bedtime, before retiring
Hx = history
ICU = intensive-care unit

I&D = incision and drainage
IM = intramuscular
I.M. = infectious mononucleosis
ind = daily
I&O = intake and output (measure fluids going into and out of body)
IPPB = intermittent positive pressure breathing
IV = intravenous
IVP = intravenous pyelogram
L = left
liq = liquid
LLE = left lower extremity
LLQ = left lower quadrant
LMP = last menstrual period
LOL = "Little Old Lady" (a passive, unquestioning female senior citizen)
LP = lumbar puncture
LPN = licensed practical nurse
LUE = left upper extremity
LUQ = left upper quadrant
(m) = murmur
M = mix
m et n = morning and night
mg = milligram(s)
MI = heart attack (myocardial infarction)
ml = milliliter(s)
mor dict = in the manner directed
M.S. = morphine sulfate
NA = nursing assistant
neg. = negative
N-G = nasogastric
no. = number
noct. = at night
non rep; nr = do not repeat
non repetat = no refill
NPO = non per os (nothing by mouth)
NS = normal saline
NSR = normal sinus rhythm (heart rate)
N&V = nausea and vomiting
o = none
O = oxygen

oc = oral contraceptive
OD = right eye (oculus dexter)
O.D. = once a day
OL = left eye
OOB = out of bed
OPD = outpatient department
OR = operating room
OS = left eye (oculus sinister)
OT = occupational therapy
OU = both eyes
P; $\overline{P}$ = after
Para = number of births
Path. = pathology
pc = after meals
PE = physical examination; pulmonary
  embolus
PI = present illness
PID = pelvic inflammatory disease
pil = pill
PM = evening
p.o. = per os (by mouth)
Post. = posterior
post-op = postoperative, after the operation
pr = per rectum (by rectum)
PR = pulse rate; rectally
prn = as needed, as often as necessary
Prog. = prognosis
pt = patient
PT = physical therapy
PTA = prior to admission
Px = prognosis
q = every
qd = once a day
qh = every hour (q4h = every four hours;
  q8h = every eight hours; and so on)
q.i.d. = four times a day
qn = every night
qod = every other day
qs = proper amount, quantity sufficient
qv = as much as desired
R = right

rbc = red blood cells
RBC = red blood cell count
rep = repeat
RHD = rheumatic heart disease
RLE = right lower extremity
RLQ = right lower quadrant
RN = registered nurse
ROM = range of motion
RR = respiratory rate; recovery room
RT = radiation therapy
RTI = reproductive tract infection
rub = red
RUE = right upper extremity
RUQ = right upper quadrant
Rx = prescription; therapy
$\overline{s}$ = without
S&A = sugar and acetone (a urine test)
sc = subcutaneous
scop. = scopolamine
SH = social history
SICU = surgical intensive-care unit
sig = write; let it be imprinted; label;
  directions
sig ut dict = take as directed
sing = of each
SOB = shortness of breath
sol = solution
solv = dissolve
SOP = standard operating procedure
SOS = can repeat in emergency
ss = half
S&S = signs and symptoms
SSE = soapsuds enema
stat = right away, immediately
STD = sexually transmitted disease
STI = sexually transmitted infection
suppos = suppository
Sx = symptoms
T&A = tonsillectomy and adenoidectomy
tab = tablet
TAT = tetanus antitoxin

tere = rub
TIA = transient ischemic attacks
t.i.d. = three times a day
tinc. or tinct. = tincture
top = apply topically
TPR = temperature, pulse, and respiration
Tx = treatment
ung = ointment
URI = upper respiratory infection
ut dict = as directed
UTI = urinary tract infection
VD = venereal disease
VS = vital signs

wbc = white blood cells
WBC = white blood cell count
WC = wheelchair
x = times
y.o. = year-old
↑ = increase
↗ = increasing
↓ = decrease
↙ = decreasing
→ = leads to
← = resulting from
♂ = male
♀ = female

SEE medical language (appendix A); medications.

MEDICAL RECORDS

The medical record is one of the most important aspects of good care. It contains a woman's medical history, complaints, questions, practitioner's notes on visits and health, laboratory results, x-ray reports, medications, descriptions of procedures, treatments, other practitioners' findings, and any relevant communications.

Most people assume that the health-care provider keeps the medical record and, should they require a copy, they merely request it. However, this is not always true.

Some practitioners and hospitals restrict an individual's access to his or her medical records, reasoning that he or she will not understand the information or could be frightened away from a particular procedure. While the American Hospital Association's Patient's Bill of Rights includes the right to see medical information, the bill is a guideline, not a rule.

The laws governing access to medical records are enacted at the state level, resulting in a confusion of laws, court decisions, and health department regulations. While there is no state where it is illegal to obtain medical records, only 25 states have some form of legislation that permits direct access to them. These states are:

Alaska	Louisiana	Oklahoma
Arkansas	Maryland	South Carolina
California	Michigan	South Dakota
Colorado	Minnesota	Virginia
Connecticut	Montana	Washington
Florida	Nevada	West Virginia
Georgia	New Hampshire	Wisconsin
Hawaii	New Jersey	
Indiana	New York	

✓ ACCESSING YOUR MEDICAL RECORDS

State Laws

Even if a state has no regulation covering direct access to medical records, there is nothing to preclude asking a practitioner or facility for copies of your records.

As with any administrative request, knowing the formalities and going about the request in the proper way help guarantee the best outcome. Here is how to go about getting your medical records:

1. Contact the practitioner or facility that has your records and ask for a copy. If they have a specific procedure for release, ask for the details.

2. If your state is one of those with access laws and you run into a problem, let the contact person at the office or the facility know that you are aware of the rights of access. Some office managers and other clerical personnel claim that it is illegal for an individual to have copies of his or her records, but there is no state where it is illegal to obtain copies of medical records.

3. Always put your request in writing. This documents your efforts and proves that you are working through normal channels. Name, address, patient identification number (if known), and the specific entry or file requested should be included in the letter. Indicate your willingness to pay reasonable copying fees (anything less than 50 cents a page).

4. If the initial request is denied by the office manager or records administrator, ask that person to put the denial in writing and cite the reasons why access to your records is being denied—for example, state law, health department regulation, or office policy. Then ask for the statute number or specific regulation. To verify the statute or regulation, contact your state's Attorney General's Office.

5. Learn about any appeals process that permits you to resubmit your request for specific parts of your record.

6. Contact a hospital patients' representative if there are problems obtaining hospital records. You may consider asking your practitioner to request copies of your records on your behalf.

7. When all else fails, contact a lawyer familiar with your state's laws. You may be able to obtain a court order from a magistrate or civil court judge if you can show good cause for needing your medical records.

Federal Laws

Access to medical records from federal hospitals—including military, Veterans Administration, and prison hospitals—is covered under the federal Privacy Act and the Freedom of Information Act. A person still in active duty must write to the hospital at his or her post or at the previous duty station. Retirees and anyone else no longer in active duty must write the National Archives Record Center, 9700 Page, St. Louis, MO 63132. Military identification number, branch of service, and dates of service must be included.

Practitioners in Maine, Massachusetts, and Texas have the option of providing a summary of the patient's records if they choose not to release the entire record.

PRIVACY ISSUES

Most people assume that their medical records are confidential, seen only by their personal practitioners. In reality, health and life insurance carriers, employers, and company medical directors may have access to medical records. If a company is self-insured, employers have access to the medical information on the claim. Confidentiality is compromised when these reports are read by unauthorized managers or employees. Computer databases and on-line networks also make it easier for anyone with a modem and computer skills to access medical records.

Individuals can inadvertently compromise the confidentiality of their records by signing blanket consent forms allowing the release of their medical history. An individual should carefully read the release form to determine the nature and extent of the information requested. The language of the release form should be modified to limit the scope of the request, so that only appropriate information is released.

There is also the chance that an error could occur within a medical record. If a woman does not know the contents of her own medical record, the information could be incorrect without her knowledge. An inaccuracy could become the basis for denial of coverage or benefits. By keeping track of her medical record, a woman can note and correct any misinformation.

MEDICAL INFORMATION BUREAU

The Medical Information Bureau (MIB) is an association established by the insurance industry of the United States through which member companies share health information about clients. The information is provided when individuals complete health or life insurance applications and forms. Most people answer the many detailed questions about their present and past medical history, and the chances are excellent that the information provided has found its way to the MIB.

Health and life insurance companies contact the MIB to verify that the information provided on insurance applications is correct. Because these companies rely upon the information stored at the MIB to determine whether or not they will insure an individual, it is very important that the file be accurate. A woman's right to inspect her file is limited to all nonmedical information, such as the names of insurance companies that reported information to the MIB and the names of insurance companies that received a copy of the information within the last six months.

However, the MIB will release medical information to an individual through a medical professional. A helpful practitioner can be enlisted to assist in obtaining the medical information contained in the file. A disclosure-of-information form can be requested by writing the MIB and asking for a copy of the "Request for Disclosure of MIB Record Information": Medical Information Bureau, P.O. Box 105, Essex Station, Boston, MA 02112; 617-329-4500.

SEE medical rights.

MEDICAL RIGHTS

Under a variety of state and federal laws, consumers have rights. This is true for health care as well. Medical rights guarantee an individual's complete participation in his or her own health care.

Hospitals and health-care professionals once assumed authority to make choices about treatment and care for their patients. The patients, accepting the judgment of the practitioner, generally trusted that the recommended procedures were the best course of action. The arrangement left patients unaware of the details about their health and possible treatments. At the worst, it led to unnecessary surgery or experimental procedures performed without the patient's knowledge.

INFORMED CONSENT

The basis of a consumer's medical rights is the principle of **informed consent.** It is a legal doctrine that requires that an individual be given all of the relevant information about a treatment before he or she consents to undergo the procedure or treatment. The information should include not only what the procedure or treatment is and what it is designed to accomplish but also risks and benefits, possible complications, side effects, and alternative procedures available. An individual should also be told what could happen if he or she decides to forgo the recommended treatment.

 ## BEFORE YOU SIGN

Make sure your procedure has been fully explained, as well as the risks, benefits, and alternatives. Any confusing details should be explained before signing. Ask for statistics, survival rates, the practitioner's success rate, or written information on the procedure—whatever it takes to answer the question.

Review the consent forms to make sure all of the information is correct. The name of the practitioner who is performing the procedure, and a description of the procedure, should be included. If a procedure other than the one you are aware of is listed, get clarification before signing. The form may also have clauses that are unfamiliar, such as asking for your permission to have observers in the operating room.

A consent form is not law; it is designed by the hospital and can be revised. If the consent form includes a phrase or clause which you do not agree with, discuss the possibility of amending the form with your practitioner. Specific requests can be added to the form, and troublesome phrases can be deleted. An individual can specify, for example, that the hospital cannot dispose of any tissue that may be removed during the procedure (so that it may be used to confirm diagnosis or used for study) or that only a particular physician may perform the surgery.

A PATIENT'S BILL OF RIGHTS

Hospitals that belong to the American Hospital Association (AHA) often post or provide a copy of AHA's Patient's Bill of Rights for their patients. The bill is a guideline, not a rule, for patients' rights, and as such may not be strictly enforced in every hospital. Consumers should use the bill as a starting point in their negotiations for patients' rights.

The American Hospital Association presents "A Patient's Bill of Rights" with the expectation that observance of these rights will contribute to more effective patient care and greater satisfaction for the patient, her physician, and the hospital organization. Further, the association presents these rights in the expectation that they will be supported by the hospital on behalf of its patients as an integral part of the healing process. It is recognized that a personal relationship between the physician and the patient is essential for the provision of proper medical care.

The traditional physician-patient relationship takes on a new dimension when care is rendered within an organizational structure. Legal precedent has established that the institution itself also has a responsibility to the patient. It is in recognition of these factors that these rights are affirmed.

1. The patient has the right to considerate and respectful care.

2. The patient has the right to obtain from her physician complete current information concerning her diagnosis, treatment, and prognosis in terms the patient can be reasonably expected to understand. When it is not medically advisable to give such information to the patient, the information should be made available to an appropriate person on her behalf. She has the right to know, by name, the physician responsible for coordinating her care.

3. The patient has the right to receive from her physician information necessary to give informed consent prior to the start of any procedure and/or treatment. Except in emergencies, such information for informed consent should include, but not necessarily be limited to, the specific procedure and/or treatment, the medically significant risks involved, and the probable duration of incapacitation. Where medically significant alternatives for care or treatment exist, or when the patient requests information concerning medical alternatives, the patient has the right to such information. The patient also has the right to know the name of the person responsible for the procedures and/or treatment.

4. The patient has the right to refuse treatment to the extent permitted by law and to be informed of the medical consequences of her action.

5. The patient has the right to every consideration of her privacy concerning her own medical-care program. Case discus-

A survey undertaken by the President's Commission for the Study of Ethical Problems in Medicine and Biomedical and Behavioral Research found that 96 percent of patients said they wanted to know everything. That number included 85 percent who said they would even want to hear facts about imminent death. Furthermore, studies have shown that people who

sion, consultation, examination, and treatment are confidential and should be conducted discreetly. Those not directly involved in her care must have the permission of the patient to be present.

6. The patient has the right to expect that all communications and records pertaining to her care should be treated as confidential.

7. The patient has the right to expect that within its capacity a hospital must make reasonable response to the request of a patient for services. The hospital must provide evaluation, service, and/or referral as indicated by the urgency of the case. When medically permissible, a patient may be transferred to another facility only after she has received complete information and explanation concerning the needs for and alternatives to such a transfer. The institution to which the patient is to be transferred must first have accepted the patient for transfer.

8. The patient has the right to obtain information as to any relationship of her hospital to other health-care and educational institutions insofar as her care is concerned. The patient has the right to obtain information as to the existence of any professional relationship among individuals, by name, who are treating her.

9. The patient has the right to be advised if the hospital proposes to engage in or perform human experimentation affecting her care or treatment. The patient has the right to refuse to participate in such research projects.

10. The patient has the right to expect reasonable continuity of care. She has the right to know in advance what appointment times and physicians are available and where. The patient has the right to expect that the hospital will provide a mechanism whereby she is informed by her physician or a delegate of the physician of the patient's continuing health-care requirements following discharge.

11. The patient has the right to examine and receive an explanation of her bill, regardless of source of payment.

12. The patient has the right to know what hospital rules and regulations apply to her conduct as a patient.

No catalog of rights can guarantee for the patient the kind of treatment she has the right to expect. A hospital has many functions to perform, including the prevention and treatment of disease, the education of both health professionals and patients, and the conduct of clinical research. All these activities must be conducted with an overriding concern for the patient, and, above all, the recognition of her dignity as a human being.

are told all of the facts ahead of time make better postoperative adjustments to stress and pain. However, women should be aware that while most practitioners agree patients should be given all the facts, others believe that they should use their best judgment regarding the timing for sharing information they believe may jeopardize the patient's health.

CONSENT FORMS

A consumer usually gives his or her informed consent by reading and signing a consent form. At some facilities, the form is a "blanket" consent form which gives the facility the right to treat the condition for which the person was admitted. At others, another type of consent form is requested for each individual procedure. Some hospitals have created consent forms that are releases against negligence on the part of the hospital, or forms that require the individual to waive his or her right to a lawsuit in the event of malpractice. However, these forms may not be legally binding because the hospital has a tremendous bar-gaining advantage which places consumers in an unequal position.

PATIENT ADVOCATES

Individuals can have a relative or friend accompany them to the hospital or practitioner's office. This person, acting as a patient advocate, can help with communication, provide general support, and make sure that the patient's rights are upheld. Many hospitals now have a representative on staff to act as a patient advocate. The advocates handle patient concerns and complaints and make sure that rights are respected. However, because the representatives work for the hospital, some people say there is a built-in conflict of interest.

SEE death and dying; malpractice; medical records; second opinion.

MEDICATIONS

Because women, on average, live longer than men, they often find themselves taking more medications for longer periods of time. There is also concern about which drugs are safe for a woman to take during pregnancy and breast-feeding. As a result, the safety and effectiveness of medications are important issues for women. Different women react differently to different drugs, and the reactions may vary according to age and dosage. Dosage may need to be adjusted (usually downward) as a woman grows older. Medications may also react with other medications, or even with food, to cause harmful side effects. By being aware of her medications and their properties, a woman can be sure she is receiving safe, proper treatment.

THE PHARMACIST

The pharmacist is the professional who is charged with dispensing the medications for which a practitioner has written a prescription. A pharmacist must have at least a bachelor's degree in pharmacy and must pass an examination administered by a state board in order to receive a license to practice. Some states require the individual to take continuing-education courses to retain the license.

Pharmacists are a valuable source of health information, providing advice on how to use medications and answering any questions the consumer may have. Pharmacists also keep records of allergies and of other medications

QUESTIONS TO ASK

To take all factors into account and provide the proper medication, a medical practitioner should ask you the following questions before writing a prescription:

■ Have you ever had an allergic reaction to any drug?

■ Are you currently taking any other medications? This includes everything from nonprescription, over-the-counter drugs to vitamins.

■ Do you have any medical conditions (such as diabetes, high blood pressure, or pregnancy)?

■ Are you following any special diets?

■ How much alcohol do you consume?

To find out more about the medications being prescribed, ask your practitioner:

■ What is the name of the drug? What is it supposed to do?

■ How and when do I take it, and for how long?

■ What foods, drinks, or other medicines or activities should I avoid while taking this drug? What can the drug negatively react with?

■ Are there any side effects? What should I do if they occur?

■ Is there any written information available about the drug? The *PDR Family Guide to Prescription Drugs* (Medical Economics Data, 1993) or the *Complete Drug Reference* (Consumer Reports Books, 1995) may be a good place to start.

being taken to prevent the wrong medications from being dispensed. In addition, they are excellent sources for information on over-the-counter (OTC) drugs. A woman should have only one pharmacist handle her prescriptions so that he or she will be able to keep a complete record, known as a patient medication profile, and accurately monitor medications. Pharmacists may now use computers to generate drug and patient information.

A pharmacist should:

■ Reference a patient's medication profile to determine whether the practitioner has ordered the right medication or discontinued the use of a therapy at the appropriate time.

■ Double-check the practitioner's directions for use.

■ Check for concurrent use of similar drugs.

■ Look for potentially harmful drug interactions, which may occur from a mixture of chemicals in the body.

■ Look for under- or overdosages and notify the practitioner of the appropriate adjustments.

■ Determine whether any allergies were taken into account.

HOW TO READ A PRESCRIPTION

A standard prescription, written by a health professional and subsequently filled by a pharmacist, contains several basic facts: the practitioner's name and address; the patient's name and address; the name of the drug, its strength, and its dosage; special instructions that the patient must be aware of (whether the drug should be taken with food, at bedtime, etc.); the practitioner's signature; and authorization for (or against) any generic substitutions of a brand name drug.

The information on most prescriptions, however, is usually coded and may be puzzling to the untrained eye. Here are some phrases and terms that are frequently noted on prescription sheets:

a.c. = before meals
ad lib. = freely; as needed
AM = morning
b.i.d. = twice a day
c̄ = with
cap = capsule
cc or cm = cubic centimeter(s)
disp. = dispense (number of tablets or amount of medicine to dispense)
ext = for external use
h.s. = at bedtime
mg = milligram(s)
ml = milliliter(s)
noct. = at night
non repetat = no refill
OD = right eye
OS = left eye
OU = both eyes
pc = after meals
PM = evening
p.o. = by mouth
prn = as needed
qd = once a day
qh = every hour
q.i.d. = four times a day
qtt = drops
rep = refill
s̄ = without
sig = label; directions
sig ut dict = take as directed
stat = at once
tab = tablet
t.i.d. = three times a day
top = apply topically
x = times

MEDICATION AND SAFETY IN THE HOME

If prescription and OTC drugs are not used correctly, they can become dangerous. Drugs should be stored in a cool, dry place in their original containers. Excessive heat and cold may change the chemical composition of the drug, which could lower its effectiveness or cause it to become harmful. Medications should also be disposed of properly after they have expired because they may lose effectiveness or become harmful. If a pill appears discolored or unusual—or a liquid or salve has become cloudy or lumpy—it should be discarded.

FIND A PHARMACIST WHO:

■ Keeps important family medication records and uses them to help prevent allergic reactions to drugs, dangerous interactions, duplicate medications, and drug abuse.

■ Advises how to use prescription and nonprescription medications: how and when to take medication; what the possible side effects are; what the shelf life is; how to store the medication; and whether there is potential for dangerous interactions with food and/or other medications.

■ Answers your questions about the staggering variety of medicines, tonics, pills, capsules, and powders on the market.

■ Advises you, when necessary, to seek a medical practitioner's help.

■ Offers generic alternatives to brand name medications when appropriate.

✓ MEDICATIONS AND THE HOSPITAL

In a hospital, keeping track of your medication can be difficult, as nurses and physicians monitor how doses are administered to a variety of patients. In a hospital setting, too, several new drugs may be prescribed for a patient at one time. As a result, medication errors often occur. These errors are defined as (1) being given the wrong medications; or (2) being given the wrong dose (or missing a dose); or (3) being given medication at the wrong time.

Several studies have shown that 2 to 10 percent of all hospital drug doses are administered incorrectly depending on the dispensing method used. However, by being alert about the medications you take—while at home and in the hospital—you can avoid potentially dangerous mix-ups.

The American Society of Hospital Pharmacists (ASHP) has developed a series of guidelines to prevent medication errors during a hospital stay. Their recommendations are:

■ Inform all your health-care providers (physicians, nurses, pharmacists) of your known allergies, sensitivities, and current medications.

■ Ask questions about any recommended procedures and treatments.

■ Learn the names of all drug products that are prescribed and administered to you.

■ Keep track of the medications. Record all drug therapy, including prescribed drugs, nonprescription drugs, home remedies, and medical foods (special diets high in nutrients).

■ Be assertive if something seems incorrect or different from the norm. (For example, if a red pill was given with the last meal, and now a green one has been given, ask why. Also ask when you have not been given medication you are expecting.)

■ Take prescription medication as prescribed. If possible, bring your prescription medications to the hospital with you and make arrangements with your practitioner and the nursing station to take them according to schedule. The hospital may request that you sign a release form.

A woman should always check the label of the medication, and the dosage, before taking it. If other individuals in the household also have medications, the bottles can be color-coded to avoid mix-ups. Children should never be left alone where medication is kept; child-resistant containers should be used whenever practical.

If there are no children in the household, day-of-the-week pillboxes may be used to organize and keep track of medications. If necessary, a family member or friend can be enlisted to double-check a pillbox to be sure it holds the correct types and doses of medicine. If any medications are taken accidentally, the poison control center, a practitioner, or a pharmacist may be contacted for help.

SEE antibiotics; hormone replacement therapy; medical abbreviations; medical language (appendix A).

MENOPAUSE

Menopause is the time at "midlife" when a woman's last menstrual period ends. It happens when the ovaries stop releasing eggs. The average age for natural menopause is 51 years, and the process can be gradual or sudden. Women who undergo a bilateral oophorectomy (surgical removal of both ovaries), or whose ovaries are damaged by chemotherapy or radiation, immediately begin menopause when the ovaries stop functioning. This sudden, induced menopause is known as **surgical menopause.**

Perimenopause, also known as the climacteric, is the gradual period of change leading into menopause. During perimenopause, the ovaries produce increasingly less estrogen and ovulation can become infrequent. Hormones fluctuate, causing irregular periods and physical and emotional changes similar to those of puberty, though they are often more intense. For most women, perimenopause lasts only a few years, although for some women, it can last up to 12 years.

Menopause may be confirmed through a blood test for hormone levels, which can indicate whether a woman is approaching, or has already experienced, menopause. The symptoms of menopause usually begin before the menstrual periods stop and continue for a short time afterward. However, the symptoms may continue, off and on, throughout a woman's life.

SYMPTOMS

Some 10 to 15 percent of American women experience no symptoms of menopause, while another 10 to 15 percent are physically or emotionally disabled for various lengths of time during menopause. While there are no sure signs that a woman is approaching menopause, common indicators include:

■ Hot flashes. These sudden, unpredictable, and uncontrollable changes in body temperature are the most common signs of menopause. Women experiencing hot flashes usually feel a tingling sensation followed by intense warmth rising to the upper half of their bodies. Hot flashes are often accompanied by uneasiness, redness of the skin, rapid heartbeat, extreme sweating, and chills. They last from 30 seconds to five minutes and can occur anytime, day or night. Hot flashes are often the cause of insomnia in menopausal women.

Although the severity of hot flashes varies, nearly 75 percent of menopausal women in the United States experience hot flashes to some degree. During menopause, 50 percent of American women have one hot flash each day, while 20 percent have more than one a day. In 10 percent of women, hot flashes still occur up to five years after menopause. They are very uncommon after five years.

■ Vaginal atrophy (thinning and dryness of the tissue lining the vagina). During and after menopause, the layers of the vaginal epithelium (tissue lining the vagina) become thin due to lower estrogen levels. As a result, the vagina may become dry and irritated, making sexual intercourse and masturbation uncomfortable. Slowly through the years after menopause, the vagina also becomes shorter and narrower, and its elasticity is reduced. Regular sexual intercourse or masturbation may prevent these changes.

■ Mood swings and depression. Medical experts do not know the precise cause of sudden mood swings and depression that some women experience during menopause. Many believe they are psychological responses to changes that menopausal women are going through—especially sleep deprivation due to nocturnal hot flashes. It is important to remember that during menopause many women are simultaneously experiencing other milestone changes in their lives—children leaving home, divorce, widowhood, and retirement, to name a few—that can

SELF-CARE DURING MENOPAUSE

Women may help to alleviate symptoms of menopause by adopting a healthful lifestyle and following a few simple rules of thumb:

Tips for relieving and preventing hot flashes:

■ Exercise regularly. Physically active women report fewer hot flashes than those who are sedentary.

■ Take a cold shower or splash cold water on yourself to help cool down.

■ Try to alleviate stress. Tension may trigger hot flashes.

■ Keep rooms cool. While warmth doesn't cause hot flashes, it can make them seem worse than they are.

■ Reduce your intake of tea, alcohol, hot beverages, and spicy foods.

■ Try herbal or homeopathic remedies, which may help relieve hot flashes.

■ Drink eight glasses of water daily.

■ Maintain a healthful diet and be sure to get the recommended dietary allowance of vitamins and minerals, perhaps through a daily multivitamin supplement.

■ Wear thin layers of all-cotton clothes. If a hot flash strikes, remove layers until you are more comfortable.

■ Keep a hot-flash diary to learn what triggers them. By keeping track of what triggers hot flashes, you may be able to learn what foods and activities you should avoid.

Tips for alleviating vaginal dryness and sexual discomfort:

■ Try over-the-counter vaginal lubricants. Some women find that yogurt inserted into the vagina, alone or with vegetable or safflower oil, prevents drying and helps regulate the acidic balance of the vagina.

■ Consider estrogen replacement creams, available by prescription. These creams make the lining of the vagina softer and more flexible and trigger lubrication.

■ Have sex more often. Frequent sexual intercourse helps keep the vagina flexible and helps promote lubrication.

Tips for strengthening vaginal muscles, enhancing sexual sensation, and alleviating loss of urine:

■ Practice Kegel exercises to strengthen the muscles of the pelvic floor, which can help intensify orgasm and prevent urinary incontinence in women *and* men. (For instructions on Kegel exercises, see "Strengthening the Pelvic Floor" on p. 228.)

■ Try to get one hour a day of full-frequency daylight, either outdoors or through full-frequency electric bulbs.

■ Be sure that you are including 1 1/2 grams of absorbable calcium a day along with the bone minerals magnesium and boron.

influence their menopausal experiences. Distress over aging and the loss of fertility, combined with feelings of loneliness and helplessness, may lead some women to depression. However, most experts believe that menopause alone does not cause depression.

Some women may face loss of secondary sex characteristics, such as breast tissue, buttock shape, and pubic fat. Some hair growth may appear on the upper lip, around the nipples, or on the abdomen. Other possible effects of menopause are:

- Anxiety
- Headache
- Vaginal infections
- Insomnia
- Dry skin
- Frequent urination
- Difficulty concentrating

Menopause may also be seen as a new freedom—from concerns about pregnancy and premenstrual syndrome—and thus be enthusiastically embraced. Margaret Mead coined the term "postmenopausal zest" to describe the new vitality many women feel after menopause.

EFFECTS OF MENOPAUSE

OSTEOPOROSIS

Loss of estrogen during perimenopause causes osteoporosis, or gradual loss of bone mass, in many women. Peak bone density occurs at age 25 to 30 and then decreases over the years, during which time bones become more brittle and more easily broken. Over 250,000 hip fractures, the most significant result of osteoporosis in women, occur each year in the United States, generally in women over 65. Fewer than one-half of women who suffer a hip fracture regain normal function. Some 15 percent die shortly after the injury, and 30 percent die within one year. In most cases, the deaths are not a direct result of the fracture itself, but of complications such as pneumonia, blood clots, and fat embolism (bone marrow fat trapped in the lungs)—results often due to confinement to bed.

A woman can determine if she is losing bone mass through a bone-density test. Measurements of the hip, spine, and wrist can give an indication of bone health. New urine tests for rate of calcium loss are also now available.

Once bone mass has been lost, it is very difficult to replace. Therefore, it is important for women to build bone mass early in life and continue activity through menopause. Weight-bearing exercise, such as walking, running, and weight lifting, and diets rich in calcium and vitamin D will build bone mass essential to the prevention of osteoporosis. In addition, lost estrogen can be replaced through hormone replacement therapy for those who are at high risk of osteoporosis.

HEART DISEASE

Heart disease in women appears most often after menopause, when the body loses the natural protection of estrogen, which helps to lower blood pressure and cholesterol levels. In fact, studies show a marked increase in the risk of heart disease for menopausal women. Hormone replacement therapy (HRT) is often prescribed to replenish the level of estrogen in the blood. Progestin is generally prescribed with estrogen to offset the risks of endometrial cancer; however, some experts believe that progestin limits the cardiovascular benefits of the HRT.

SEXUALITY AND MENOPAUSE

Though menopause signals the end of the child-bearing years, it does not mean the end of sexual activity. Many women enjoy sex more than ever after menopause, since they no longer have to worry about unintended pregnancy. However, menopause does not protect from sexually transmitted infections. Women with multiple sex partners, or who have sex with people whose sexual histories they do not know, should always use condoms or the vaginal pouch. Sexual desire often decreases during perimenopause, but it usually returns during postmenopause. Vaginal atrophy, which may make sex uncomfortable, may be relieved with topical hormones, lubricants, or HRT.

PREPARING FOR AND COPING WITH MENOPAUSE

It's never too early to prepare for perimenopause and menopause. All women—pre- or post-menopausal—should get annual gynecologic examinations, including Pap tests and mammograms. Bone-density screening is also recommended for those prone to osteoporosis. It is important for a woman to find a practitioner with whom she is comfortable. If a woman has questions about menopausal changes she is experiencing, she may want to set up an appointment to meet with her practitioner just to talk, without a physical examination.

Although some health-care providers and medical researchers tend to treat menopause as an illness, it is a natural occurrence that all women must experience. Women going through menopause should keep in mind that they are not alone. Many women form self-help support groups to talk about the psychological, emotional, spiritual, social, and physical changes that accompany menopause. It is also important to educate men about menopause, so they are able to offer support, too.

SEE estrogen; heart disease; hormone replacement therapy; incontinence, urinary; menstrual cycle and ovulation; osteoporosis; reproductive system and sex organs of the woman.

For more information on menopause, contact:

National Osteoporosis Foundation
1150 17th St., N.W., Suite 500
Washington, DC 20036
202-223-2226
http://www.nof.org

National Women's Health Network
514 10th St., N.W., Suite 400
Washington, DC 20004
202-347-1140

North American Menopause Society
c/o University Hospitals of Cleveland
Department of OBGYN
11100 Euclid Ave.
Cleveland, OH 44106
216-844-3334
http://www.menopause.org

Planned Parenthood Federation of America, Inc.
810 Seventh Avenue
New York, NY 10019
For the Planned Parenthood nearest you, call:
    800-230-PLAN
http://www.ppfa.org/ppfa

A Friend Indeed **Newsletter**
Box 515
Place du Parc Station
Montreal, Canada H2W 2P1

Hot Flash: Newsletter for Midlife and Older Women
Jane Porcini and the National Action Forum for
    Midlife and Older Women
Box 816
Stony Brook, NY 11790-0816

MENSTRUAL CYCLE AND OVULATION

The menstrual cycle is the process that takes place in a woman's body as it prepares for pregnancy. The menstrual cycle lasts from 21 to 35 days, and its duration varies from woman to woman, and, in each woman, from month to month. Girls begin their menstrual cycle during puberty, usually between ages 10 and 16. The start of a girl's first menstrual cycle, called **menarche,** marks the beginning of her reproductive years. The menstrual cycle ends when a woman reaches menopause, around age 50. After menopause, she no longer ovulates.

HOW THE MENSTRUAL CYCLE WORKS

There are three phases of the menstrual cycle: the menstrual phase, the proliferative phase, and the secretory phase.

The **menstrual phase** begins with the first day of menstruation, the shedding of uterine lining built up in preparation for a pregnancy that did not occur. This menstrual bleeding, called the menstrual period, lasts from two to seven days. While the amount of menstrual discharge varies greatly among women, only three to four tablespoons of it are blood. The rest is fluid and tissue. Women manage the menstrual flow using pads that attach to the underwear, or with tampons that fit inside of the vagina.

As menstruation ends, the levels of estrogen and progesterone are at their lowest. These low levels cause the hypothalamus and pituitary gland (the parts of the brain that control hormone production) to produce follicle-stimulating hormone (FSH) and luteinizing hormone (LH). The levels of these hormones continue to rise throughout this **proliferative phase** (also known as **preovulatory,** or **follicular, phase**), approximately days five to 13 of the cycle, and cause the maturation of a new egg to be released at ovulation.

Estrogen levels also rise during the proliferative phase, causing many of the follicles in the ovary to grow. Only one (or sometimes two, which could develop into twins) actually develops to where an egg is shed. The endometrium (uterine lining) thickens in preparation for the implantation of a fertilized egg from this developing follicle, called the **Graafian follicle.**

At the end of the proliferative phase, the high estrogen level causes the pituitary gland to release a large amount of LH, causing the mature Graafian follicle to release an egg, or eggs. This release is called **ovulation.**

The egg travels through one of the two fallopian tubes to await fertilization. If it is fertilized by a sperm cell, the egg travels down the tube into the uterus, where it matures into a fetus. When fertilization does not occur, the egg passes with the menstrual flow out of the uterus through the cervix, the narrow neck of the uterus, then to the vagina and out of the body. Ovulation takes place about 14 days before menstruation begins. It is the stage between menstruation and ovulation—the proliferative phase—that is most variable and irregular for most women.

Ovulation marks the end of the proliferative

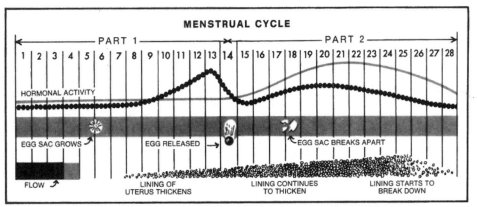

MENSTRUAL CYCLE

PART 1 —————————————→|←————————————— PART 2 —————————————→

| 1 | 2 | 3 | 4 | 5 | 6 | 7 | 8 | 9 | 10 | 11 | 12 | 13 | 14 | 15 | 16 | 17 | 18 | 19 | 20 | 21 | 22 | 23 | 24 | 25 | 26 | 27 | 28 |

HORMONAL ACTIVITY

EGG SAC GROWS →   EGG RELEASED →   ← EGG SAC BREAKS APART

FLOW →   LINING OF UTERUS THICKENS   LINING CONTINUES TO THICKEN   LINING STARTS TO BREAK DOWN

Sequence of major changes if a woman's menstrual periods always occurred exactly 28 days apart.

phase and the beginning of the **secretory phase** (also called **postovulatory,** or **luteal, phase**), which lasts approximately 14 days. Once it has released the egg, the empty Graafian follicle is transformed into the **corpus luteum,** a small, yellow lump on the surface of the ovary that secretes both estrogen and progesterone. The endometrium continues to thicken, and the uterine glands begin producing substances to prepare the uterus for a pregnancy.

If fertilization does not occur, the high levels of estrogen and progesterone secreted by the corpus luteum cause a decrease in the production of FSH and LH. This causes the corpus luteum to stop producing estrogen and progesterone. Without the necessary estrogen, the endometrium (lining of the uterus) can no longer thicken, so it is shed as menstrual bleeding, and the cycle begins again.

AMENORRHEA

Nearly every woman misses a few menstrual periods in her lifetime. The absence of menstrual periods is known as amenorrhea, a sign that hormone patterns have been disrupted. Stress and illness can temporarily disrupt hor-

mone levels, so one or two missed periods is usually nothing to worry about. Failure to start menstruation or a long time between periods may indicate a more serious problem that should not be ignored. For example, it could indicate irregular estrogen levels. Too little estrogen production in the ovaries can lead to osteoporosis, while too much can put women at a higher risk of endometrial and breast cancer.

Persistent physical stress can cause amenorrhea, often accompanied by weight loss. Women who suffer from anorexia nervosa, and women athletes who train seriously for competition, often have amenorrhea. No matter what the cause is, amenorrhea must always be evaluated and treated properly.

Pregnancy is the most common cause of amenorrhea. It is also caused by absence of ovulation. Lack of ovulation is also fairly common and not directly harmful; however, it is a major obstacle for women trying to become pregnant. Practitioners can prescribe drugs to induce ovulation in order to increase a woman's fertility.

For women who are not trying to conceive, practitioners may prescribe synthetic progestin pills to interrupt the steady estrogen level and reduce the risk of uterine cancer. Ovulation can

285

occur unpredictably at any time in women with amenorrhea, so birth control must be used at all times to prevent pregnancy.

Missed periods are often caused by a problem in the hypothalamus. When the hypothalamus and the pituitary gland do not produce follicle-stimulating hormone and luteinizing hormone, the ovaries do not produce normal estrogen and progesterone. Illness, weight loss (especially to the point where little body fat is present), and stressful activities and events, either physical or mental, can suppress hormone production by the hypothalamus. If hypothalamic amenorrhea persists for more than a few months, hormone replacement therapy is essential to protect bone density. Oral contra-ceptives are also a sufficient source of estrogen for women who want contraception as well.

Other causes of amenorrhea are low hormone production by the thyroid gland, structural abnormalities, problems with the endometrium, a pituitary gland tumor, head trauma, shock following blood loss, menopause or premature menopause, delayed puberty, and abnormal chromosome structure.

Women who miss three or more periods should see a practitioner to determine the cause of amenorrhea and prescribe treatment to reduce the risk of later complications. Some alternative therapies that may be effective in treating amenorrhea are acupuncture and herbal and homeopathic remedies.

PERSPECTIVES ON MENSTRUATION

Menstruation is a sign that you are healthy. A girl who is anticipating getting her first period should ask her mother, older sister, or another woman she trusts about what menstruation is like. A woman with a daughter should be open about the facts—every healthy adult woman menstruates, and it is nothing to be shy or embarrassed about. A woman should answer a girl's questions and explain the use of pads, tampons, and other ways to manage the menstrual flow. The more a girl knows about menstruation, the more positive the experience will be. In some parts of the world, menarche is celebrated with gifts and parties to honor the new young woman.

Keep in mind:

■ Women can enjoy sex during their menstrual periods. Orgasm can help promote blood flow, which may relieve cramps.

■ It is possible to become pregnant before your first period.

■ It is possible to become pregnant while bleeding. Bleeding may be spotting at ovulation instead of the menstrual flow.

■ Exercise can be beneficial during menstruation. Usually, there is no need to stay in bed. Activities such as swimming and bathing can be continued as usual.

■ A woman should consider using the least absorbent tampon appropriate for her menstrual flow. Tampons should not be left in place for long periods of time. The use of high-absorbency tampons has been linked to toxic shock syndrome, a rare condition that causes rash, fever, and possibly death if left untreated.

■ Any unusual symptoms, delayed periods, or severe menstrual cramps should be reported to a health-care provider.

DYSMENORRHEA

Dysmenorrhea, or severe menstrual cramping, can make menstrual periods painful, if only for a day or two. Cramps are primarily caused by excessive levels of a prostaglandin hormone: too much prostaglandin turns a normal muscle contraction into a strong, more painful spasm. When a spasm constricts the uterine blood vessels, blood flow to the uterine muscle is reduced, and pain results. Besides cramps, dysmenorrhea may be associated with backaches, leg pain, diarrhea, nausea, headaches, dizziness, and vomiting.

Although dysmenorrhea is common—at least 70 percent of women suffer from cramps to some extent—its symptoms can be debilitating in some women. Because severe pain may indicate an underlying problem such as endometriosis, uterine fibroid tumors, or a pelvic infection, women with dysmenorrhea should have a gynecologic examination.

If the practitioner determines that there is no other medical problem causing cramps, over-the-counter pain relievers, such as ibuprofen, may offer relief. A healthful diet can help prevent constipation, which exacerbates cramps. Many women are helped with supplements of magnesium, vitamin B$_6$, and unprocessed vegetable oils, especially primrose or borage oil. Oral contraceptives usually lessen dysmenorrhea. Other suggestions are back massage, herbal and homeopathic medicines, a heating pad, soaking in a tub, exercise (to stimulate endorphins, the brain's natural pain relievers), orgasm, and rest. Acupuncture treatment is another option.

If cramps still persist, women may want to consult their practitioner about prescribing antiprostaglandin medicine, which decreases the body cells' production of prostaglandin.

FLUID RETENTION

Many women gain weight and experience bloating in the 14 days between ovulation and menstruation. During this time, fluid seeps into cells, and only part of the water that is absorbed is passed out. Some water remains and gradually accumulates in cells and body tissues, contributing to weight gain. Fluid retention may also make fingers and ankles swell. Excessive weight gain or bloating premenstrually may occur in women with or without PMS. To minimize fluid retention, women should eat a low-salt diet and drink more chemically free water.

CHARTING MENSTRUAL CYCLES: FERTILITY AWARENESS METHODS

Because the menstrual cycle follows a regular pattern with noticeable signs, most women can learn how to chart their cycle with reasonable accuracy. Charting enables a woman to predict when her menstrual periods are expected and note changes in her body's patterns. These fertility awareness methods can be used to predict a woman's fertile days, either for contraception or to maximize the chances of planned pregnancy. Charting can also aid in the diagnosis and treatment of impaired fertility and premenstrual syndrome.

Generally speaking, women are fertile for approximately a week during each cycle, about halfway between two menstrual periods, up to six days before ovulation. An egg lives only about 24 hours after leaving the ovarian follicle, but sperm can survive five or more days in the woman's reproductive tract.

Although the length of the menstrual cycle differs among women, one consistency exists: ovulation nearly always occurs 14 days (give or take two days) before the next menstrual period begins, regardless of the cycle's total length. With this fact in mind, a woman can observe and record changes in her body during ovulation. Fertility awareness methods include the calendar method, the cervical mucus method, the basal temperature method, and the symptothermal method (which combines the other three methods). For more information on these methods (which are described in more detail in the section in this book on contraception), a woman should ask her practitioner for instruction.

SEE contraception; endocrine system; premenstrual syndrome; reproductive system and sex organs of the woman; toxic shock syndrome.

For more information on menstruation and ovulation, contact:

American College of Obstetricians and Gynecologists
409 12th St., S.W.
Washington, DC 20024
202-863-2518
http://www.acog.com

American Society for Reproductive Medicine
[formerly the American Fertility Society]
1209 Montgomery Hwy.
Birmingham, AL 35216-2809
205-978-5000
http://www.asrm.com

National Women's Health Network
514 10th St., N.W., Suite 406
Washington, DC 20004
800-772-9100
202-347-1140

Planned Parenthood Federation of America, Inc.
810 Seventh Avenue
New York, NY 10019
For the Planned Parenthood nearest you, call:
800-230-PLAN
http://www.ppfa.org/ppfa

MIGRAINE HEADACHE

Migraine headache attacks are severe headaches characterized by throbbing pain, often on one side of the head (although the pain may switch sides), that can last from a few hours to a few days. Approximately 10 percent of Americans, some 25 million, experience varying degrees of migraine attacks. They affect three times more women than men. Migraines can occur as frequently as three to four times a week, or as rarely as once every few years. In almost all cases, headaches establish a pattern of locations and duration. They are often preceeded by an aura, a warning with visual disturbances such as bright or flashing lights.

SYMPTOMS

In addition to head pain, migraines can also cause:

- Nausea
- Vomiting
- Diarrhea

- Nasal congestion and sinus pain
- Hypersensitivity to light and sounds
- Aversion to visual stripes
- Sleep disturbances
- Mood disorders
- Neurologic symptoms, such as dizziness, mood changes, and irritability

TYPES OF MIGRAINES

Two main types of migraines have been identified: **migraine without aura** (once labeled **common migraine**) and **migraine with aura** (once labeled **classic migraine**). An aura is a group of neurologic symptoms that signals oncoming migraines. Auras can include dizziness, numbness, language difficulties, mood changes, hyperactivity, extreme fatigue or irritability, flashing lights, and micropsia (when all objects appear to be very small).

Except for the presence or absence of an aura, the two major types of migraines are virtually the same. An estimated 6 percent of the general population have migraines without aura in one year, and 9 percent have them at some time in their lives. For migraines with aura, the numbers are 4 percent and 6 percent.

Migraine headaches can also take other forms. **Hemiplegic migraine** causes temporary paralysis on one side of the body (known as hemiplegia). Symptoms include vision problems and vertigo—the feeling that everything is spinning.

An **ophthalmoplegic migraine** causes pain around the eye, often accompanied by a droopy eyelid, double vision, and other sight problems.

The **basilar artery migraine** is the result of the disturbance of a major brain artery. It is often preceded by vertigo, double vision, and poor muscular coordination. Adolescent and young adult women are most prone to basilar artery migraine attacks, which are often associated with the menstrual cycle.

A **benign exertional headache** is caused by running, lifting, coughing, sneezing, or bending. The headache starts at the onset of activity and usually does not last long.

A **headache-free migraine** includes symptoms such as visual problems, nausea, vomiting, constipation, and diarrhea—but not head pain. Headache experts believe unexplained pain in certain parts of the body, fever, and dizziness may also be types of headache-free migraine attacks.

CAUSES OF MIGRAINES

Migraine attacks were once thought to be exclusively psychosomatic illnesses, physical illnesses caused or influenced by emotional factors. Research has since proved otherwise; migraines, like other headaches, are in fact neurobiologic disorders, although exactly what causes them is still not clear.

A major factor is thought to be blood flow changes in the brain. One theory suggests that the nervous system responds to a trigger and creates a spasm in the nerve-rich arteries at the base of the brain. The spasm constricts several arteries supplying blood to the brain, reducing the flow of blood to the brain.

Simultaneously, platelets clump together, releasing a powerful chemical called serotonin. Serotonin constricts the arteries even more, further reducing blood supply, and consequently oxygen, to the brain. To compensate for the reduced oxygen supply, arteries in the brain expand, as do those in the neck and scalp. The widening of these arteries prompts the release of prostaglandins and other pain-increasing substances. These substances and the dilation of the scalp arteries stimulate pain-sensitive nerves, resulting in a throbbing migraine headache.

Some headache experts believe migraine sufferers have an inherited abnormality in the regulation of blood vessels. While it is true that many sufferers have a family history of migraine attacks, their exact hereditary nature is not known.

Migraines are often associated with clinical depression. A 1994 study provided the first evidence that the two share underlying mechanisms, rather than the previous popular theory that depression results from debilitating migraine attacks. According to the new study, each disorder increases the likelihood of onset for the other.

A recent Harvard University study suggests that migraine sufferers may be twice as likely to have a stroke as nonmigraine sufferers. Possible reasons for the increased risk are changes in blood flow in the brain and an increase in platelet clumping, which can form a blood clot. However, when examining the results of earlier studies, no definitive conclusions could be drawn between migraine headaches and a propensity for stroke. While medical experts disagree on the exact nature of the risk, it would be prudent for women who have migraine headaches to discuss their individual risk.

MIGRAINE TRIGGERS

Several conditions are thought to bring on or be associated with migraines in some women:

- Changes in hormone levels. Sixty percent of women migraine sufferers report that menstrual migraines occur just before and during menstruation, and sometimes at ovulation, as a result of fluctuating hormone levels. The relationship between female sex hormones and migraines is unclear. During pregnancy, some women develop migraines for the first time, while others report less frequent attacks. The Pill may worsen migraines in women who already have them. The good news is that most migraines decrease or come to a halt after menopause.

- Food. Some scientists believe food allergies trigger migraines. Others believe they are caused by chemical compounds within food that constrict arteries in the brain. Regardless of which theory is correct, people prone to migraines may find relief by staying away from certain foods, including wheat, corn, milk, chocolate, caffeine, alcohol, aged cheese, and seafood. Food additives, such as monosodium glutamate (MSG), nitrite, and aspartame (Nutrasweet), may also cause migraines.

- Stress. Like many other headaches, migraines are often the result of too much stress.

- Fatigue

- The weather

- Scents, such as tobacco smoke, perfume, paint, and diesel or gasoline fumes

- Bright lights. Sensitivity to light is a common symptom of migraines with and without aura.

- Changes in atmospheric pressure

- Smoking

- Hunger or fasting

- Epidural anesthesia, often used during childbirth

- Environmental pollutants

TREATMENT

For years, women who suffered from migraines were apt to do just that—suffer. In the past five years, however, new treatments have brought relief to many people plagued by migraines. The safest, most effective treatments are those designed by an experienced practitioner, since medications may have side effects, especially if they are combined with other drugs. Medica-

SELF-CARE FOR MIGRAINES

The treatment of migraines involves knowing how to prevent attacks as well as how to relieve their pain, should preventive measures fail.

Here are some things you can do to lessen the occurrence of your migraine attacks:

■ Keep a record of the foods you eat and note which ones precede migraines—these could be migraine triggers.

■ Avoid possible migraine triggers—foods, scents, undue stress, etc.

■ Establish a regular routine—wake up, eat meals, and go to bed at approximately the same times every day.

■ Exercise regularly to boost circulation and reduce stress.

■ Visit a chiropractor, who may be able to provide treatment or preventive therapy.

■ Use monophasic oral contraceptives or continue combined hormone replacement therapy so that hormone levels are kept constant.

■ Try an ice pack on the affected site.

■ Try an alternative medical therapy. Massage, yoga, homeopathic remedies, and acupuncture are often used to treat migraines.

■ Try herbal medicines, such as the herb feverfew, which British research has found is effective in reducing migraines' frequency, if not their duration. Keep in mind that herbs are drugs that may have side effects. Follow your practitioner's guidelines for their use.

tions should never be taken without a practitioner's supervision.

The most recent and the best available treatment for acute migraine attacks is **sumatriptan succinate,** marketed as **Imitrex.** Unlike other medications, it can be administered at any stage of a migraine and will provide almost immediate pain relief in 70 percent of sufferers. Currently, Imitrex is available as an injection and in pill form. Practitioners can teach patients how to give themselves an injection. Imitrex has relatively few side effects, usually limited to tightness in the chest or jaw and a tingling sensation immediately following the injection.

Another commonly used drug is **ergotamine tartrate,** which constricts arteries, counteracting the painful dilation stage of a migraine. In order for it to be effective, ergotamine tartrate must be taken during the early stages of an attack. It can cause nausea and vomiting and should not be taken excessively or by people with angina pectoris, severe hypertension, or vascular, liver, or kidney disease. **Cafergot** is a mixture of caffeine and ergotamine. It is effective only if taken in the first hour of a migraine (and even then, it works only 50 percent of the time).

If prescription drugs are not available, **aspirin** or **ibuprofen** will help alleviate migraine pain, although complete relief is improbable. **Applying pressure** to the temples can also provide temporary relief—in fact, one practitioner designed an elastic headband with rubber disks to wear specifically for this purpose. Small amounts of **caffeine** may also help if taken in the early stages of an attack.

Preventive treatment is also available for women who have recurring migraines. Preventive drugs include **methysergide maleate,** which reverses blood vessel constriction, **propranolol,** which halts blood vessel dilation, and **amitriptyline,** an antidepressant. A study conducted by the Houston Headache Clinic found that migraine sufferers improved most on a combination of propranolol and **biofeedback,** an alternative therapy used to train the mind to influence the involuntary systems of the body—heartbeat, blood circulation, and the digestive system. Another study reported that propranolol may prevent migraines even after patients stop taking it, which suggests that long-term propranolol therapy could be beneficial.

Antidepressant drugs called **MAO inhibitors** also prevent migraine attacks by blocking an enzyme that helps nerve cells absorb serotonin, the artery-constricting chemical. However, MAO inhibitors can have serious side effects, especially if mixed with food or beverages containing tyramine, such as aged cheese, processed meats, red wines, figs, and foods with monosodium glutamate. The combination can produce dangerously high blood pressure.

Women who have recurring headaches should see a practitioner for a diagnostic workup and proper subsequent treatment, if needed. It is important to find a practitioner who is knowledgeable about migraine attacks and up-to-date on their treatment. Too many patients are told, "It's all in your head."

For more information on headaches, contact:

American Council for Headache Education
875 Kings Hwy., Suite 200
West Deptford, NJ 08096
800-255-ACHE

Association for Applied
Psychophysiology and Biofeedback
[formerly the Biofeedback Society of America]
10200 W. 44th Ave., Suite 304
Wheat Ridge, CO 80033
303-422-8436
http://www.aapb.org

National Headache Foundation
428 W. St. James Place
Chicago, IL 60614-2750
800-843-2256

New England Headache Treatment Program
778 Longridge Rd.
Stamford, CT 06902
800-245-0088
203-968-1799 (Connecticut)

MISCARRIAGE

Miscarriage, or loss of an early pregnancy, is the expulsion of a fetus from the uterus before it has developed sufficiently enough to survive. Known medically as **spontaneous abortion,** miscarriage occurs in 15 to 20 percent of recognized pregnancies in the United States. Some 90 percent of miscarriages occur within the first trimester of pregnancy, between the sixth and 12th weeks.

CAUSES OF MISCARRIAGE

At least half of all miscarriages are caused by an anatomic or genetic abnormality in the fetus. When the fetus is not developing normally, the hormone levels drop, and the uterine lining often begins to shed. The pregnancy separates from the uterus and passes out of the body. A miscarriage may also be caused by an immunological reaction in which the woman's body rejects the fetus as foreign tissue.

There are also several maternal risk factors that may cause miscarriage, including:

■ A weakened cervix

■ Chromosomal abnormality. These disorders cause some 60 percent of miscarriages in the first half of the first trimester; 15 to 20 percent in the second half of the first trimester; and 10 percent in the second trimester.

■ An age of 35 or older. Studies show that the risk of miscarriage doubles between the 20s and the 30s, then doubles again between the early and late 30s.

■ Maternal illnesses, such as sexually transmitted infections, hypertension, and diabetes

■ Obesity (a weight of 20 percent above the average body weight). Excess weight may lead to high blood pressure and diabetes and may mask symptoms of other disorders.

■ Hormonal insufficiency. Inadequate production of progesterone, needed to sustain the pregnancy, may cause miscarriage.

■ A history of infertility, previous miscarriage, or premature birth

■ Uterine abnormalities, such as a retroverted (backward-tilted) uterus, a double or divided uterus, uterine scar tissue, or fibroids

Illegal drug and alcohol use by the pregnant woman increases the risk of miscarriage. Exposure to environmental toxins has been linked to miscarriage as well. DES daughters—women whose mothers took the synthetic hormone **diethylstilbestrol** (DES) to prevent miscarriage during pregnancy—are at increased risk for miscarriage and should report this information to their practitioner. There is also a slight risk of miscarriage associated with some prenatal testing, including chorionic villus sampling and amniocentesis.

Ultrasound, a prenatal test that creates an image of the fetus using sound waves, may be used to determine early on whether the pregnancy is developing normally or whether there is an anomaly that will result in spontaneous abortion.

Miscarriage is not caused by the activities of a healthy pregnant woman, such as jumping, vigorous exercise, and frequent vaginal intercourse; trauma causes miscarriage only very rarely. Stress and emotional shock do not cause miscarriage either.

SIGNS OF MISCARRIAGE

Typical signs of possible miscarriage include:

- Slight vaginal bleeding or spotting
- Severe abdominal pain
- Severe cramps
- Dull, lower back ache, pressure, or pain
- Intermittent lower abdominal or thigh pain
- A change in vaginal discharge

If any symptoms occur during pregnancy, or anything unusual occurs, a health-care professional should be contacted immediately. Some miscarriages may be prevented if action is taken quickly. Not all miscarriages are painful, and some women miscarry without being aware of the fact.

TYPES OF MISCARRIAGE

Miscarriage may be categorized by medical professionals as threatened, inevitable, missed, or septic. When symptoms occur that indicate a pregnancy may end prematurely, a **threatened miscarriage** is diagnosed. To determine if a miscarriage is threatened, a three-step evaluation is done. An internal pelvic exam is performed to determine the condition of the uterus

PREVENTING MISCARRIAGE

To prevent miscarriage or preterm delivery (labor before 36 weeks of pregnancy, when it is unlikely the fetus will be able to survive on its own):

- Get proper prenatal care. Talk with your practitioner about weight gain, lifestyle, stress, and any other concerns you may have.
- Take folic acid. Studies show that folic acid, when taken in the first six weeks of pregnancy, may help prevent birth defects, such as spina bifida, which could trigger miscarriage. Leafy green vegetables, eggs, and orange juice contain folic acid.
- Avoid both smoking and drinking during the pregnancy.
- Refrain from heavy lifting and strenuous tasks if you are at high risk. Women who are at low risk of complications, and who are accustomed to physical work, may continue as usual until the second half of pregnancy.
- Exercise carefully. If you are at risk for miscarriage, don't overexert yourself. Also avoid any exercises done on your back after the fourth month because they decrease the blood flow to the placenta. The best exercises for pregnant women are swimming, walking, and relaxation exercises.
- Ask your practitioner which sexual activities you are allowed to continue and which you should avoid.
- Contact your practitioner immediately if you have any unusual symptoms, particularly vaginal discharge with a strong odor. Many women dismiss early signs of miscarriage.

Various levels of bed rest may be prescribed for women with previous miscarriage, preterm labor, or premature birth. Some women may engage in a minimum of activity, while others must stay in bed all of the time.

and cervix; a blood test is taken to measure the level of human chorionic gonadotropin (HCG), a hormone secreted by the placenta; and ultrasonography (the creation of an image using sound waves) is done to determine if the fetus is alive, developing normally, and the expected age for this time in pregnancy.

When threatened miscarriage occurs early in pregnancy (after one or two missed periods), a miscarriage usually follows. If a miscarriage does occur, a **dilation and curettage (D&C),** the scraping of the uterine lining with an instrument called a curette, may be performed to remove any remaining products of the pregnancy.

An **inevitable miscarriage** occurs when there is a rupture of membranes, severe vaginal bleeding and/or cramps, indicating that no medical treatment can avert a miscarriage. In this stage, the amniotic membranes have ruptured, the cervix is dilating, and the fetus and placenta are in the process of being expelled.

A **missed miscarriage** occurs when a dead embryo or fetus remains inside the uterus. Symptoms are barely noticeable, and there may be no vaginal bleeding. If the fetal tissue remains in the uterus, dilation and curettage may be necessary because the pregnancy tissue can become attached to the uterus and bleeding complications may occur.

A **septic miscarriage** is any miscarriage that involves infection of the uterus and/or the placental tissues. Symptoms include marked tenderness of the uterus and lower abdomen, chills, fever, and an elevated white blood count, in addition to vaginal bleeding. Septic miscarriage is treated with antibiotics. If the fetus is not spontaneously expelled, a D&C is performed.

MULTIPLE MISCARRIAGE

In general, miscarriages are due to factors that do not recur in future pregnancies. While the cause of a miscarriage should be investigated to see if future instances can be avoided, a full-scale

THE EMOTIONAL RESPONSE TO MISCARRIAGE

Miscarriage can produce strong feelings of grief and disappointment. Women who have suffered a miscarriage should remember:

■ Grief is a normal response to the loss of a pregnancy and should not be downplayed or denied.

■ Communication is an important part of the recovery process. Discussing the loss with a partner, family member, friend, and support group may help to ease the feelings associated with miscarriage.

■ A new pregnancy cannot take the place of one that has been lost. Emotional and physical healing needs to take place before future pregnancy plans are made. If you are anxious about the possibility of another miscarriage, discuss with your practitioner the suspected or known causes of the miscarriage and the chances of having a successful pregnancy.

■ Practitioners can recommend local support groups that help women and their partners cope with the aftermath of a miscarriage. In addition to many local hospitals, some community centers and religious organizations have support groups.

workup is generally not recommended until after the third consecutive miscarriage, called **habitual miscarriage.** Tests are done to detect hormonal imbalances, genetic abnormalities, blood antibodies, and infections such as chlamydia, toxoplasmosis, and cytomegalovirus. An x-ray of the abdominal cavity, known as a **hysterogram,** may be done. An **endometrial biopsy,** in which a sample of the uterine lining is taken and examined under a microscope, may also be done.

SEE death and dying; pregnancy—prenatal concerns.

For more information about miscarriage support groups, contact:

A.M.E.N.D. (Aiding Mothers & Fathers Experiencing Neo-Natal Death)
c/o Maureen Connelly
4324 Berrywick Terr.
St. Louis, MO 63128

Compassionate Friends
National Office
P.O. Box 3696
Oak Brook, IL 60522-3696
708-990-0010
tzht72a@prodigy.com

Unite, Inc.
Jeanes Hospital
7600 Central Ave.
Philadelphia, PA 19111
215-728-2082

NUTRITION

Poor nutrition has been linked to disease, especially heart disease, colon and rectal cancer, and breast cancer. With proper nutrition that includes a diet high in minerals, vitamins, and protein and low in fat and salt, Americans can look forward to longer, healthier lives.

The Departments of Health and Human Services and Agriculture provide dietary guidelines for Americans. It includes the following points:

- Eat a variety of foods.
- Maintain healthy weight.
- Choose a diet low in fat, saturated fat, and cholesterol.
- Choose a diet with plenty of vegetables, fruits, and grain products. Eat at least 20 to 30 grams of fiber per day.
- Use sugar and salt (sodium) only in moderation.
- If you drink alcoholic beverages, do so in moderation.
- Drink at least eight glasses of chemically free water each day.

These guidelines are designed to include all Americans, but women have special nutritional needs. Poor nutrition has been linked to breast cancer, osteoporosis, iron deficiency, weight gain, and complications in pregnancy—all issues that are unique to, or more prevalent in, women.

WOMEN AND NUTRITION

In addition to following the federal nutrition guidelines, women should pay particular attention to calcium and iron. Experts agree that it is important for a woman to build on her calcium intake before the age of 30 in order to decrease her risk of osteoporosis. The body is adequate at making bone up to age 30. After that, it slacks off. If the bones are fortified before 30, as evidence shows, a woman can reduce her postmenopausal bone-mass loss by 43 percent. Adequate calcium intake, at least one gram per day, is thus very important for young women.

Women need more iron than men do because they lose 15 to 20 milligrams every month during menstruation. Without enough iron, an iron-deficiency anemia can develop, manifesting in pallor, fatigue, and headaches. Postmenopausal women who are experiencing iron-deficiency symptoms should be examined by a health-care practitioner. The loss of iron in women is usually associated with menstruation; postmenopausal women should be checked for another source of iron loss. Women need more magnesium for the same reasons.

THE FOOD PYRAMID

Nutritional information has been made easier to understand and more accessible to the American public. Food labels are easier to read, and the new

READING FOOD LABELS

The new food labels are designed to help you make sound nutritional choices. They can help you monitor your intake of fat, cholesterol, and sodium. On the front of the label, manufacturers use descriptors such as "free," "low," or "reduced" if the product is low in a certain dietary component that is linked to disease, perhaps fat, cholesterol, or sodium. On the back of the label, the serving size and the number of servings per container are listed at the top.

When reading all labels, remember to consider the serving size. The calories and calories from fat are listed just below. Based on a 2,000-calorie diet, the percentage of the daily recommended amounts of total fat, saturated fat, cholesterol, sodium, total carbohydrates, including dietary fibers and sugars, and protein are provided. The percentages do not represent the percentage of each component in the product itself, but how a single serving stacks up against the daily recommended intake. For example, if a soup label lists total fat at 40 percent per serving, that represents 40 percent of your total daily intake, not 40 percent of the soup.

The gram amounts of total fat, saturated fat, cholesterol, sodium, total carbohydrates, and protein are also listed. This information is particularly useful when used with the recommended dietary value for each of these components listed at the bottom of the label. There, you will find recommended intakes for a 2,000-calorie diet and a 2,500-calorie diet. Compare the listed grams of each component for the product with the recommended daily intake provided on the label.

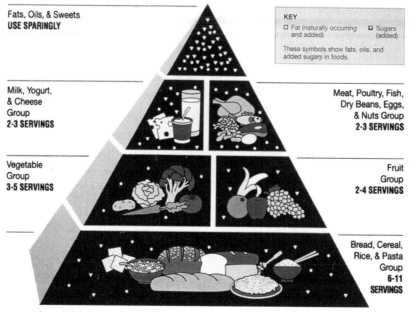

Fats, Oils, & Sweets
USE SPARINGLY

KEY
☐ Fat (naturally occurring and added)   ☐ Sugars (added)
These symbols show fats, oils, and added sugars in foods.

Milk, Yogurt, & Cheese Group
2-3 SERVINGS

Meat, Poultry, Fish, Dry Beans, Eggs, & Nuts Group
2-3 SERVINGS

Vegetable Group
3-5 SERVINGS

Fruit Group
2-4 SERVINGS

Bread, Cereal, Rice, & Pasta Group
6-11 SERVINGS

Source: U.S. Department of Agriculture/U.S. Department of Health and Human Services

Source: U. S. Department of Agriculture

USDA food pyramid makes nutritional guidelines easier to follow. Gone are the days of the four basic food groups. Today, experts agree that the Food Guide Pyramid, which illustrates six food groups and is based on the food guidance developed by the U.S. Department of Agriculture, is a better representation of a healthful diet.

The pyramid is based on "servings" that are defined by experts for each food group as the following, starting at the pyramid's base:

■ For bread, cereal, rice, and pasta group, one serving equals: 1 slice of bread, 1 ounce of ready-to-eat cereal, or $1/2$ cup cooked cereal, rice, or pasta.

■ For fruit group, one serving equals: 1 medium apple, banana, or orange, $1/2$ cup chopped, cooked, or canned fruit, or $3/4$ cup fruit juice.

■ For vegetable group, one serving equals: 1 cup raw, leafy vegetables, $1/2$ cup other vegetables (cooked or chopped raw), or $3/4$ cup vegetable juice.

■ For meat, poultry, fish, dry beans, eggs, and nuts group, one serving equals: 2 to 3 ounces of cooked lean meat, fish, or poultry; 1 to $1 1/2$ cups cooked dry beans; 2 to 3 eggs; or 4 to 6 tablespoons of peanut butter.

■ For milk, yogurt, and cheese group, one serving equals: 1 cup of milk or yogurt, $1 1/2$ ounces of natural cheese, or 2 ounces of processed cheese.

FAT

According to the Food and Drug Administration, there is a strong link between high-fat diets and breast cancer. For example, in the United States, 27 out of 100,000 women die of breast cancer each year, while in Japan, breast cancer deaths are fewer than seven out of 100,000. The key, some scientists believe, is the different amount of fat in the average diet: Japanese women consume a diet that averages

20 percent fat, while American women consume a diet that averages 40 percent. High-fat diets are also linked to heart disease and certain cancers, particularly colon and rectal cancer.

NUTRITION FOR PREGNANCY

A woman has special nutritional needs during pregnancy. After all, a fetus relies strictly on the pregnant woman's intake of the nutrients it requires to grow and develop. While the fetus requires only 300 extra calories a day—hardly "eating for two" (later in pregnancy, a little over 300 may be necessary)—it does need extra nutrients, notably folic acid, protein, and calcium. The ideal diet during pregnancy makes every calorie count. In this way, the woman provides her fetus with all the necessary nutrients while avoiding the empty calories that would

FINDING OUT THE FAT

Experts agree that no more than 30 percent of your total calories should come from fat. However, your average intake of fat over a few days is what is important, not necessarily the amount you consumed in one meal. If you eat a meal high in fat, try to balance it with low-fat foods, such as fish and vegetables, for the rest of the day or the next day.

Food labels list fat in grams. To find out what your total daily intake should be limited to, multiply your daily calories by .3 and divide by 9 (the number of fat calories in a gram of fat). For example, a woman who is maintaining her weight at 2,200 calories will have the following equations:

2,200 calories x .3 = 660 calories from fat

660 calories from fat ÷ 9 = 73 grams of fat

What type of fat you consume is as important as how much. The three types of fats are saturated, polyunsaturated, and monounsaturated. Saturated fat is the culprit for heart disease and raising blood cholesterol levels. The main sources of saturated fat are foods that come from animals, such as meat, butter, cream, ice cream, and cheese. And while polyunsaturated fat does not increase LDL cholesterol levels, it may actually lower good HDL levels. In addition, polyunsaturated fats may be associated with an increase in free radicals (highly reactive molecules, formed by oxygen), which may cause cellular injury by damaging the fatty outer membranes of cells. Monounsaturated fat reportedly helps LDL levels drop while maintaining HDL levels, so at this time, it is considered the best choice for those concerned with heart disease and cholesterol levels.

Polyunsaturated fat's best sources are plant-based oils, such as sunflower, corn, soybean, cottonseed, and safflower. Monounsaturated fats are found in olive, canola, and peanut oils.

To help reduce fat in your diet, broil, bake, or microwave food rather than frying or deep fat frying. Use little butter and margarine, and avoid margarine containing partially hydrogenated oils. Instead of cream or mayonnaise, substitute plain low-fat yogurt, blender-whipped low-fat cottage cheese, or buttermilk.

HOW TO PREPARE VEGETABLES AND KEEP THEIR NUTRIENTS HIGH

Vegetables begin to lose nutrients as soon as they are picked. If it has been a long time since they were harvested, chances are their nutrients have plummeted.

Prepare vegetables as soon as possible after picking. Cook them in as little water as possible; steam them instead of boiling them. If cooking them over the stove, use a steamer basket to hold the vegetables away from the water so their nutrients won't be washed away. If microwaving them, use only a very small amount of water (usually enough to cover the bottom of the dish) and cook on high for only a few minutes. Do not overcook them. Steam them until they present a bright, vibrant color, then season them with fresh or dry herbs instead of salt, creams, butters, or sauces.

only help her in gaining extra weight that she will have to lose after pregnancy. A good diet also helps the woman in other ways: anemia and preeclampsia are more common among poorly nourished women; fatigue, morning sickness, constipation, leg cramps, and other pregnancy symptoms can be reduced through diet; well-nourished women are less likely than women on poor diets to deliver too early; and a healthful diet can also help control mood swings.

Every pregnancy requires protein, vitamin C, calcium, vitamin A, vitamin E, riboflavin, folic acid, B vitamins, and iron, and plenty of fluids:

■ Protein, found in yogurt, cheese, eggs, fish, red meat, and tofu, is especially important in building the cells of a healthy baby. A daily intake of 60 to 75 grams of protein is more than enough.

■ Vitamin C, found in citrus fruits, strawberries, blackberries, raspberries, tomatoes, vegetable juice, raw cabbage, red or green pepper, and broccoli, is needed for proper development of strong bones and teeth. This is a nutrient the body cannot store, so a new supply is needed every day.

■ Calcium, found in milk, yogurt, and cheese, is not only important to a fetus's developing bones and teeth but also vital for the development of its heart, muscles, and nerves as well as for blood clotting and enzyme activity. Magnesium is also very important.

■ Yellow and green leafy vegetables supply vitamin A in the form of beta-carotene, a necessary nutrient for cell growth. These foods also provide essential vitamin E, riboflavin, folic acid, and B_6 as well as minerals. They also provide fiber, which helps prevent the constipation that affects many pregnant women. Folic acid has been shown to reduce the risk of some birth defects.

■ Experts recommend women get 20 to 30 grams of fiber a day.

■ B vitamins, found in whole grains and legumes, are necessary to the total development of the fetus.

■ Iron, found in beef, sardines, spinach, and soybeans, is a nutrient that is vital to blood supply, both of the woman and of the fetus.

■ At least two quarts of fluids, preferably chemically free water, every day help reduce constipation, water retention, and the risk of urinary tract infection. It is important, however, to be sure that the drinks do not have excessive calories, which can add up quickly.

CHOOSING A NUTRITIONIST

A health-care provider is usually the first person a woman turns to with questions about nutrition. Although many are well versed, most health-care providers have limited backgrounds in nutrition because the majority of medical schools do not emphasize education in nutrition. Professionals trained in nutrition are called nutritionists, and there are many schools providing certification in the field.

Many of these schools, however, are not accredited by an agency recognized by the U.S. Secretary of Education or the Council on Post-Secondary Accreditation. Here are some important points to remember when choosing a nutritionist. Does the nutritionist:

■ Ask a lot of questions about your medical history, lifestyle, and current eating habits?

■ Ask you to keep a detailed diet diary to establish a "baseline" before she recommends major changes?

■ Formulate an individualized diet plan that includes your special needs and individual lifestyle?

■ Monitor your progress with follow-up visits, answer your questions, and boost your morale?

■ Involve your family members in your diet plan?

■ Refrain from promoting and selling nutritional supplements?

The American Nutritionists Association can be contacted for the name of a certified nutritionist in a local area.

SEE pregnancy—preconception concerns; pregnancy—prenatal concerns; weight reduction.

For more information on nutrition, contact:

American Dietetic Association
216 W. Jackson Blvd., Suite 800
Chicago, IL 60606
800-366-1655
http://www.eatright.org

American Nutritionists Association
P.O. Box 34030
Bethesda, MD 20817

Food and Drug Administration
5600 Fishers Ln., HFE88
Rockville, MD 20857
301-443-3170

Food and Nutrition Information Center
National Agricultural Library (USDA)
10301 Baltimore Blvd., Room 304
Beltsville, MD 20705-2351
301-504-5719
http://www.nal.usda.gov/fnic/

Vegetarian Resource Group
P.O. Box 1463
Baltimore, MD 21203
410-366-8343
http://www.envirolink.org/arrs/VRG/home.html

OOPHORECTOMY

An oophorectomy, also called an ovariectomy, is the surgical removal of an ovary. If both ovaries are removed, the procedure is known as a **bilateral oophorectomy.**

Removal of one ovary reduces a woman's chance of becoming pregnant but does not make her infertile. Removal of both ovaries results in infertility, the end of menstrual cycles, and menopause, since these organs are the source of both ova (eggs) and most of the body's estrogen.

Removal of the ovaries is often accompanied by a **salpingectomy,** removal of one or both fallopian tubes. If one tube is removed, it is called a **unilateral salpingectomy.** If both are removed, it is a **bilateral salpingectomy.** When an ovary and fallopian tube are removed, it is known as a **salpingo-oophorectomy.**

While a fallopian tube is usually removed with its adjoining ovary, ovaries are generally left in place if the condition is confined to the fallopian tube, because the ovary produces necessary hormones. This is usually necessitated by an ectopic pregnancy, a potentially life-threatening condition that occurs when a fertilized egg implants in the fallopian tube rather than in the uterus.

REASONS FOR SALPINGO-OOPHORECTOMY

A salpingo-oophorectomy is done primarily in the treatment of the following conditions:
- Cancer of the ovaries
- Cancer of the fallopian tubes
- Cancers of the uterus that have a tendency to spread to and recur in the tubes and ovaries
- Benign ovarian tumors that are too large to be removed without taking the ovary
- Hormone-dependent breast cancer (affected by the level of hormones, estrogen, or progesterone in the blood)
- Infections of the ovaries that do not respond to antibiotics, such as those secondary infections resulting from pelvic inflammatory disease

An oophorectomy and the accompanying removal of the fallopian tubes are necessary in the treatment of certain cancers and when organs are damaged beyond repair. However, in other circumstances, the use of the procedures is debated. In women of childbearing age, salpingo-oophorectomy should be considered only when more conservative treatment is not effective, since the procedure results in infertility. In postmenopausal women, removal of both ovaries and fallopian tubes should also be a last resort, since even after menopause the ovaries continue to produce a small amount of a number of hormones. A salpingo-oophorectomy should not be done as part of hysterectomy, removal of the uterus, unless the condition specifically necessitates the procedure. Prior to surgery, a woman should have a clear understanding with her doctor regarding which organs will be removed and why. It is a good idea to record the date and details of the surgery in a medical record for future use by subsequent practitioners.

PROCEDURE

The surgeon can remove the ovaries and fallopian tubes with **laparoscopic surgery** (during laparoscopy, a long, narrow optical instrument is inserted through a small incision in the abdominal wall just below the navel) or with an **open procedure,** which involves cutting into the abdomen. In either case, the patient is under general anesthesia. Ovarian remnant syndrome is a condition that causes pelvic pain and can lead to obstruction of the ureters (the tubes bringing urine from the kidneys to the bladder). To avoid this, the surgeon should be careful to remove all of the tissue of the ovaries.

SIDE EFFECTS AND RISKS

Removal of both ovaries in premenopausal women causes "surgical" menopause. The chief side effects are all those assigned to "natural" menopause: flushing, hot flashes, increased risk of cardiovascular disease, and depression. In surgical menopause, however, symptoms are often abrupt and severe due to the rapid drop in levels of hormones. Medical treatment of premenopausal women who have had both ovaries removed is controversial, but medical opinion seems to increasingly favor the use of hormone replacement therapy to counteract the effects of surgical menopause. Relatively high doses may be prescribed at first, but gradually the hormone doses should be decreased.

ALTERNATIVES TO SALPINGO-OOPHORECTOMY

Alternatives to salpingo-oophorectomy should be sought whenever possible. Except in cases of infections that cannot be eradicated with antibiotics, or injury so severe that repair is impossible, there seems to be no compelling reason to remove the ovaries or fallopian tubes. Even when surgery is deemed necessary, it may be possible to save one of the ovaries and fallopian tubes in order to preserve fertility and/or the natural hormone balance of the body.

In the case of hormone-dependent breast cancer, the medication tamoxifen (Nolvadex) can be used to suppress the growth of hormone-dependent breast cancers. Therefore, there is an alternative to salpingo-oophorectomy for breast cancer alone.

Normal ovaries do not need to be removed as a part of hysterectomy, removal of the uterus, either, even when uterine cancer is present. A study of 1,000 women who had hysterectomies—some with and some without removal of the ovaries—showed that the rate of undiagnosed cancer present in the removed ovaries was zero. This lends support to the idea of leaving the ovaries in place if they appear normal during a hysterectomy.

Despite these findings, some surgeons continue to remove both ovaries when only one is diseased or damaged. Some routinely remove both during a hysterectomy. These practices perpetuate the controversy surrounding hysterectomy.

SEE hysterectomy; hormone replacement therapy; laparoscopy; menopause; second opinion.

For more information on salpingo-oophorectomy, contact:

HERS Foundation (Hysterectomy Educational Resources and Services)
422 Bryn Mawr Ave.
Bala Cynwyd, PA 19004
610-667-7757
tzht72a@prodigy.com

Society of Gynecologic Oncologists
401 N. Michigan Ave.
Chicago, IL 60611
312-644-6610
http://www.sgo.org

OSTEOPOROSIS

Osteoporosis is a bone-thinning disease that makes bones brittle and easily broken. One fourth of American women—and one-eighth of American men—are afflicted by osteoporosis. By the time they are 75 years old, nearly 90 percent of women have the disease. Spinal osteoporosis is four times more common in women than in men, hip fractures are 2 $\frac{1}{2}$ times more common, and forearm and wrist fractures 10 times more common.

Osteoporosis, which means "porous bones," is often characterized by a humped back and loss of height as vertebrae fracture and become compressed. Those with osteoporosis are also prone to hip fractures. Of the women who suffer hip fractures because of osteoporosis, 50 percent do not regain normal function. In addition, 15 percent die shortly after the hip fracture, while 30 percent die within a year. The deaths do not result from the injury itself, but rather from blood clots, pneumonia, or a fat embolism (fat trapped in the lungs)—all possible results of being confined to bed.

CAUSES OF OSTEOPOROSIS

Throughout a woman's life, bone mass constantly changes, as cells called **osteoclasts** break down existing bone while cells called **osteoblasts** create new bone. In a healthy person, the two balance each other. Osteoporosis occurs when there are insufficient amounts of calcium and other vitamins and minerals for absorption into bone mass. At this point, the osteoblasts cannot keep up with the osteoclasts, and the bones are weakened. The exact cause of osteoporosis remains a mystery, although it is believed to be at least partially genetic.

WOMEN AND OSTEOPOROSIS

In both women and men, bone density usually peaks at around age 35. After this point, bone mass either stays constant or decreases, as more bone tissue is lost than is replaced. Women lose bone mass more rapidly than men (nine times as quickly at the highest rate) because their bones are less dense. By age 80 the rates of loss are the same for both genders. Another reason for the unequal rate of bone loss is that women tend to exercise less frequently than men, and exercise is believed to slow bone loss. In addition, estrogen helps to maintain bone mass, and the decline in the body's production of estrogen after menopause makes women's bones less capable of absorbing needed calcium from the diet.

SYMPTOMS

Symptoms of osteoporosis include:
- Gradual loss of height
- Lower back pain
- Rounded shoulders
- Stooped posture (and subsequent protruding abdomen)
- Frequent bone fractures
- Periodontal disease. (This may be the earliest sign of bone loss.)

RISK

Several factors increase a woman's risk for osteoporosis:
- Family history of osteoporosis
- Fair complexion, blond or red hair, and freckles
- Race. White and Asian women are at the highest risk for osteoporosis. Black women have denser bones and are less susceptible.
- Petite stature, small boned. Obese women's bodies produce more estrogen, which combats osteoporosis.
- Not enough weight-bearing exercise
- Excessive amounts of alcohol, soft drinks (which have a high phosphorus content), coffee, or tea

- Use of certain over-the-counter and prescription drugs, especially systemic steroid medications such as Prednisone
- Smoking
- Bilateral oophorectomy (surgical removal of both ovaries) without hormone replacement therapy. This procedure results in a decrease in the body's production of estrogen, which helps to protect against osteoporosis.
- Natural menopause before age 40
- History of prior bone fractures
- Endometriosis (growth of uterine lining tissue outside the uterine cavity)
- Scoliosis (curvature of the spine)
- History of anorexia nervosa
- Amenorrhea (absence of menstrual periods)
- Gastrointestinal disease, which can cause poor calcium absorption

DIAGNOSIS

Practitioners can measure bone mass using several bone-density scan techniques, including **single-beam** and **dual-beam densitometers** and **dual-energy x-ray absorptiometry (DEXA).** These tests simply involve placing the hip, lower spine, or wrist underneath the scanner, which passes over the bone several times to measure its density. The tests are painless, and there is little exposure to radiation. One should request a DEXA scan because it is the most accurate of the techniques. However, it is expensive, and many insurance companies do not cover the cost of bone-density testing.

While these tests are often used to diagnose osteoporosis when symptoms are present, they are also recommended for all women to help prevent osteoporosis. The National Osteoporosis Foundation recommends having bone density tested:

✓ WHAT YOU CAN DO TO PREVENT—OR SLOW—BONE LOSS

■ Exercise regularly. Exercise should be consistent and weight-bearing, like walking, jogging, dancing, and weight lifting, in order to increase bone density. Optimally, women should exercise for 45 to 60 minutes four days a week.

■ Get enough vitamins: a diet rich in calcium, magnesium, boron, and vitamins D and C. Vitamin D, magnesium, and vitamin C enhance calcium's absorption. Young women should be sure to build bone mass by getting enough calcium in their diets. Sufficient daily calcium intake is:

Children and young adults	800 to 1,000 mg
Adults and postmenopausal women taking estrogen	1,000 mg
Pregnant and breast-feeding women	1,300 to 1,500 mg
Postmenopausal women not taking estrogen	1,500 mg

Since the average woman obtains only about 500 mg calcium in her diet, supplementation is generally recommended to make up the rest of the required amount. Careful reading of calcium supplement packages is important. The amount of calcium in the supplement is usually listed in fine print on the back of the bottle.

■ Eat right. Cut down on alcohol, sugar, fats, processed meats and cheeses, soft drinks, chocolate, and caffeine. Instead, try soy products, whole grains, beets, peas, green peppers, nuts, fish, bananas, apples, and nectarines. This diet will improve the body's calcium levels.

■ Know your personal and family health history. Some women are more prone to bone loss than others. If you take a calcium-depleting drug or have a history of anorexia nervosa, you may have had premature or excessive bone loss and should adjust your diet and exercise patterns to increase bone strength.

■ Don't smoke.

Once bone mass begins to decrease around age 35, it is difficult to stop completely; however, women can slow it down considerably. Women under 35 should follow the same steps in order to prevent osteoporosis.

■ After menopause (surgical or natural)

■ In the event of spinal abnormalities or a loss of height

■ If steroids are being taken for other medical conditions, because they can cause rapid bone loss

■ If hyperparathyroidism has been diagnosed, and the parathyroid gland has not been removed. This can lead to bone loss.

■ If osteoporosis has been diagnosed

Other ways to measure bone loss are **CAT scans** (cross-sectional x-rays), **bone biopsies** (usually used to distinguish between osteoporosis and osteomalacia, abnormal bone mineralization associated with vitamin D deficiency), and traditional **x-rays.** In addition, **blood and urine tests** can be done to measure the levels of calcium in the body. A new urine test that reveals excreted metabolic components of bone holds promise as a less expensive way of screening for bone loss.

TREATMENT

Once osteoporosis has resulted in significant bone loss, no known treatment can undo its damage, but treatment can prevent further deterioration. Painkillers like aspirin, heat, massage, and orthopedic supports can provide some relief from physical discomfort. Herbal and homeopathic remedies are also used.

For postmenopausal women with the beginning stages of osteoporosis and women who are at risk for the condition, **hormone replacement therapy** (HRT) is one solution. The estrogen component of HRT helps bones absorb calcium and can maintain—but not build more—bone mass. However, estrogen therapy alone holds an increased risk of endometrial cancer, so it is combined with progestin in the HRT regimen to offset that risk. Estrogen therapy may also increase the risk of breast cancer; however, for most women, the benefits of HRT outweigh the risks. Once a woman begins HRT to treat osteoporosis, she must continue it for the rest of her life to avoid the bone loss that would result if she stopped taking it.

Calcitriol, an activated form of vitamin D, combats osteoporosis by allowing calcium to be absorbed through the intestines. However, use of the vitamin D hormone for osteoporosis can result in excess calcium in the blood and a reduction in kidney function. It is considered toxic in the United States pending further testing by the Food and Drug Administration (FDA) and may be only prescribed for rickets and those on chronic kidney dialysis.

Calcitonin, a calcium-regulating hormone given by tablet, injection, or nasal spray, can also be used to treat osteoporosis. Calcitonin slows the breakdown in bone and in some cases appears to increase bone density. In addition, the drug **etidronate,** used to treat Paget's disease (a condition in which the bones become enlarged and weak), has been used to treat those with moderate to severe osteoporosis who cannot take estrogen.

Recently, the FDA approved another treatment for osteoporosis. The drug **Fosamax,** which does not contain hormones, increases bone strength and reduces fractures in older women. The drug works by stopping osteoclasts from dissolving new bone formed by osteoblasts. An FDA advisory committee reported that Fosamax poses seemingly fewer risks than estrogen; so far, the only identified side effect is mild stomach discomfort.

Another drug, **slow-release sodium fluoride,** is awaiting FDA approval (at time of publication). Studies have shown the drug may help to actually reverse bone loss.

SEE estrogen; hormone replacement therapy; menopause; nutrition.

For more information on osteoporosis, contact:

National Health Information Center
U.S. Department HHS
P.O. Box 1133
Washington, DC 20013
800-336-4797
http://nhic-nt.health.org

National Osteoporosis Foundation
1150 17th St., N.W., Suite 500
Washington, DC 20036
800-223-2226
http://www.nof.org

OVARIAN CYSTS

Ovarian cysts are small, fluid-filled sacs that form on one or both ovaries. They are common, usually benign (non-cancerous), and do not always cause symptoms. However, ovarian cysts may become painful if they grow very large or rupture. During a routine pelvic exam a practitioner may discover an ovary enlarged with a cyst.

TYPES OF OVARIAN CYSTS

Functional cysts, which are benign or non-cancerous, are the most common ovarian cysts and consist of two types: follicle and luteum cysts. A **follicle cyst** forms when a follicle (a small group of cells surrounding an egg) grows large in preparation for ovulation but then fails to rupture and release an egg. A **corpus luteum cyst** occurs when the structure the follicle forms, the corpus luteum, does not shrink after ovulation and instead forms a cyst. A luteum cyst may delay a menstrual period or make the flow light.

Dermoid cysts (teratoid tumors), also benign, most often occur in younger women. The cysts contain pieces of hair, teeth, or bone and are thought to be remnants of abnormal embryo development. They generally need to be removed. A condition known as **polycystic ovary syndrome** occurs when many small cysts form in the ovaries. Women with this syndrome also may have more facial hair and irregular periods. Ovarian cysts sometimes become very large and rupture, causing severe pain. Ruptured cysts are often difficult to diagnose.

SYMPTOMS

The cysts often have no symptoms, though they may include:

- Abdominal swelling and pain
- Painful intercourse
- Irregular or painful periods

TREATMENT

If there is no severe pain, if the woman is premenopausal, and if the cyst is less than five centimeters in diameter, a practitioner will usually wait to see if the ovarian cyst disappears on its own. **Oral contraceptives** may reduce the growth and symptoms.

If the cyst does not go away, if the woman is postmenopausal, or if the cyst is larger than five centimeters, the practitioner should test to see if the cyst is benign or cancerous. An x-ray or ultrasound (a procedure in which sound waves are used to create an image of the pelvis) may be used or a **laparoscopy** (a procedure in which a small viewing scope is inserted through an incision in the abdomen) may be done. A **biopsy,** in which a portion of the tissue is removed for diagnosis, may also be done. Cancerous cysts are rare.

Benign cysts may not need treatment if they are causing no symptoms. However, if the cysts become large, rupture, or cause severe pain, a **cystectomy,** in which the surgeon removes only the cyst and preserves as much of the normal ovarian tissue as possible, is usually recommended. However, sometimes with a large cyst, the ovary cannot be saved.

SEE cancer, ovarian; laparoscopy; oophorectomy.

PAP TEST

A Pap test, often called a Pap smear or cervical smear, named for its inventor, Dr. George Papanicolaou, is a method of cancer screening that can diagnose cell changes in the cervix that may indicate cancer or precancerous changes. In the test, the practitioner gently rotates a wooden spatula (like a popsicle stick) and then a small brush called a cytobrush across the cervix to collect random cells. The sample is smeared on a glass slide to be examined under a microscope. A Pap test is generally done in a clinic or a practitioner's office as part of a pelvic examination.

Cervical cancer is one of the most preventable of all cancers because Pap tests can detect cell changes long before they progress to cancer. However, an estimated one-fourth of women do not have annual Pap tests. The rate of cervical cancer among women who do not have Pap tests is 50 to 60 per 100,000; experts believe that 90 percent of deaths from cervical cancer could have been prevented if more women had Pap tests.

The American Cancer Society (ACS) recommends that all women who are sexually active or have reached age 18 should have an annual Pap test and pelvic exam. If a woman has three or more consecutive normal Pap tests and is at low risk of developing cervical cancer, they can be performed less frequently, as determined by the woman and her practitioner. There is no age limit on the recommendations.

It is recommended by the ACS that women who were younger than age 18 at first sexual intercourse, who have a history of genital herpes or human papilloma virus (HPV), who smoke, or who have more than one sex partner continue with annual exams because their risk of cervical cancer is increased.

Lubricants, contraceptive foams and jellies, semen, and blood can interfere with the cells taken during a Pap test. For maximum accuracy, a woman should avoid using these products and should use a condom or vaginal pouch during intercourse for one or more days before the Pap test. Douching should also be avoided because it can wash away the cells the practitioner needs to sample. If possible, a Pap test should be scheduled when the woman is not menstruating. The practitioner should be encouraged to use a cytobrush, rather than a cotton swab, along with the wooden stick, because it allows for better results.

CLASSIFICATION OF RESULTS

The results of a Pap test are classified according to the degree of cell changes that exist. Cytopathologists (experts in the study of abnormal cells) use a classification system with categories ranging from normal to cancerous.

There have been several systems used to classify Pap test results. The older, which is generally considered obsolete, uses categories ranging from Class I to Class V:

Class I. Normal smear. Repeat at intervals suggested by your practitioner.

Class II. "Atypical" cells indicative of inflammatory changes (such as infection), but no evidence of cancerous changes. Any infection should be treated, and the Pap test should be repeated in six to 12 months.

Class III. "Suspicious" cells are present indicating dysplasia (abnormal development of cells that may or may not be cancerous) and sometimes carcinoma-in-situ (surface cancer that has not yet spread further into the cervix). Inflammation, if present, should be treated and the Pap test repeated after the next menstrual period.

Class IV. Positive. Cells strongly suggest cancer. A biopsy is always taken to confirm or rule out cancer.

Class V. Positive. Cancer cells are present. Following biopsy, surgery or other treatment is carried out immediately.

Other terms that have been frequently used are mild, moderate, or severe **dysplasia** (abnormal development of cells); and **cervical intraepithelial neoplasia** (CIN), a term used to indicate a combination of dysplasia and early **carcinoma-in-situ,** surface cancer that has not yet spread. The severity of CIN is indicated by the numeral I, II, or III.

In 1988 a new method of classifying Pap tests, known as the Bethesda System, was developed by the National Cancer Institute, in Bethesda, Maryland, to create better uniformity and accuracy in reporting results. The Bethesda System has largely replaced the older classification system, although the latter is still in use. The elements of the Bethesda System are:

1. A statement of whether the specimen is adequate for diagnosis. (Under the previous system, "inadequate" samples were referred to as Class 0 and were repeated.)

2. A general categorization of the diagnosis as "normal" or "other." The latter category can include anything from a bacterial or viral infection to cell abnormalities.

3. A descriptive diagnosis detailing the findings under "other"

The newer system separates all degrees of dysplasia and CIN into two categories:

a. Low-grade squamous intraepithelial lesions, or SIL (referring to mild dysplasia as well as CIN I, the least severe form of CIN)

b. High-grade squamous intraepithelial lesions (referring to moderate dysplasia, CIN II, severe dysplasia, carcinoma-in-situ, and CIN III)

Using the terms of the Bethesda System, Pap tests can be rated as low- or high-grade SIL; or invasive cancer.

UNDERSTANDING THE RESULTS

Usually an abnormal Pap test does not mean a woman has cancer; instead, it may indicate a precancerous condition or inflammation. Pap tests are not always 100 percent accurate. A false-negative result means that abnormal cells are present in the cervix but were not scraped off during the procedure. A false-positive result means suspicious cells are found that are not actually cancer.

A Pap test revealing abnormal but noncancerous cells (classified as Class II in the older system) means that there is no indication of cancer, though some cell changes exist. A woman should have her practitioner explain the abnormality. It could be due to a vaginal infection, inflammation associated with use of an IUD, fetal exposure to the drug diethylstilbestrol (DES), or a viral infection, such as one of the human papilloma viruses (HPV). If an infection is present, it can make identification of precancerous cells difficult. A second Pap test may be done after the infection has been treated, no sooner than one month after the first.

Mild dysplasia (CIN I, or a low-grade squamous intraepithelial lesion, as categorized in the Bethesda System) is not treated by some practitioners; instead, a Pap test is done every three to six months to monitor the condition.

THE ACCURACY OF PAP TESTS

Pap test screening is not perfect. Fifteen to 30 percent of those who are tested are found to have normal results when in fact there are abnormal cells present. Some of the errors are attributed to the practitioner taking the sample, some to the cytologists interpreting it, and some because the cells may not have shed from the surface of the cervix at the time the Pap test was obtained.

A 1987 *Wall Street Journal* article investigated some Pap screening laboratories and found overworked, undersupervised technicians, many paid on a piecework basis that encouraged them to rush the analysis. Partly because of this investigation, the Clinical Laboratory Improvement Amendments (CLIA) were enacted in 1992. The federal legislation put caps on the number of tests that could be processed per day and regulated record keeping and the storage of specimens. Some experts say that Pap test interpretation has improved as a result; others feel it is too soon to tell.

The introduction of the Bethesda method of classification in 1988 was also intended to improve the accuracy of Pap testing. While the method standardized the reporting of results, some believe it has opened the door for overdiagnosis and overtreatment with its yes/no approach to classification.

Women should be sure to get the results of their Pap tests explained to them, and keep a record of the dates and category of any abnormal results.

To ensure that a Pap test is accurate, you should ask practitioners the following questions:

■ Where will my sample be sent? Laboratories can be certified by the College of American Pathologists and the American Society of Cytology. Experts say these certifications tend to indicate reliability.

If the results of a Pap test show it to be abnormal, make sure you understand the situation completely. Find out:

■ How has my Pap test been classified, and what does it mean?

■ What are my options for further diagnosis and treatment?

Others believe that a diagnostic procedure, such as cervical biopsy by **colposcopy** (a procedure where a magnifying instrument called a colposcope is used to visualize lesions to be sampled), may be more conclusive.

On the other hand, some experts feel it is important to treat even mild dysplasia if a Pap test indicates a condition that may be associated with HPV. Some forms of HPV increase the risk of cancer of the cervix, vulva, vagina, and penis. The HPV virus associated with cancer is transmitted through sexual intercourse and often accompanies another type of HPV that causes genital warts.

A Pap test that shows high-grade squamous intraepithelial lesions, according to the Bethesda method (moderate or severe dysplasia; CIN II or III; or Class III of the older method), indicates that cell abnormalities may be present that could progress to invasive cancer unless there is treatment. Colposcopy and biopsy, two diagnostic tests, are necessary to determine the need for treatment and to select the best type of treatment. While some cases regress without treatment, there is no way of knowing when or if that will occur.

If invasive cancer is indicated by a Pap test, action should be taken immediately. A woman should discuss with her practitioner her options. If invasive cancer is present, surgical removal of the uterus, called hysterectomy, may be necessary.

WHAT IS INVOLVED IN DIAGNOSIS AND TREATMENT?

Once the results of a screening have been confirmed, there are several post-Pap test diagnostic procedures that can be used to determine if an abnormality is actually cancer.

Most health-care professionals follow a clearly abnormal or suspicious Pap test with a **cervical biopsy,** a test in which bits of suspicious tissue are removed from the cervix for microscopic examination. A cervical biopsy should be done in conjunction with **colposcopy.** During the colposcopy—in which a magnifying instrument called a **colposcope** is used to view the abnormalities that need to be sampled—

cells may also be scraped from the cervical canal, a procedure called **endocervical curettage.** Both the biopsy and curettage samples are sent for microscopic examination. They are highly accurate in diagnosing cervical cancer.

If the biopsy confirms that cervical cell abnormalities require treatment, there are several choices available. Most forms of dysplasia on the surface of the cervix can be removed in a simple, in-office procedure that usually requires no anesthesia. The abnormal sections are destroyed by freezing, in a procedure called **cryosurgery.** Other methods of removing a lesion are **cauterization** (burning lesions away), **laser therapy** (use of a laser to vaporize lesions), and **electrosurgery** (use of an electric wire to remove abnormal tissue). Electrosurgery is used with a local anesthetic.

If abnormal cells extend into the cervical canal, a **cone biopsy** (or **conization**), a surgical procedure in which a cone-shaped piece of tissue is removed from the center of the cervix and analyzed, may be recommended. Conization can interfere with fertility and a woman's ability to carry a child to term. Electrosurgery has replaced many cone biopsies.

If invasive cancer is present, surgical removal of the uterus, called a hysterectomy, may be necessary.

SEE cancer, cervical; gynecologic exam.

PELVIC INFLAMMATORY DISEASE

Pelvic inflammatory disease (PID) is a bacterial infection of the uterus (endometritis), the fallopian tubes (salpingitis), or the ovaries (oophoritis). The infection causes inflammation of the organs and may cause the formation of scar tissue and abscesses (collections of pus surrounded by inflamed tissue). In the United States, more than 1 million women have PID each year. Of these women, 25 percent are hospitalized as a result of the disease.

The sexually transmitted infections chlamydia and gonorrhea are the two most common causes of PID. Organisms that normally inhabit the vagina and bowel may also cause PID, entering the body through the vagina, usually when the cervix is dilated and more open to infection, such as after childbirth, abortion, a dilation and curettage procedure, or during the insertion of an intrauterine device (IUD). In some parts of the world, tuberculosis is a common cause of PID.

Symptoms of PID include:
- Lower abdominal pain
- Fever
- A pus-filled cervical discharge
- Vaginal bleeding
- Painful urination
- Pain during intercourse
- Nausea
- Heavy menstrual flow and severe cramping

Most commonly in PID, scar tissue forms and blocks the fallopian tubes, causing infertility. Women who have had one episode of PID have a 13 percent chance of infertility, while women who have had PID three times have a 75 percent chance. PID also increases the risk of ectopic pregnancy, a potentially life-threatening condition in which a fertilized egg implants in the tube or elsewhere outside of the uterus.

Prompt treatment reduces the risks of infertility, scarring, and the formation of abscesses. If PID goes untreated, it may result in serious complications. If an abscess forms, then ruptures, it can spread bacteria throughout the abdominal cavity, which may result in infection of the lining of the abdomen. This condition, known as **peritonitis,** is life-threatening and can cause death in a matter of hours. PID can also result in the enlargement of the fallopian tubes, which may also rupture. Septicemia, or blood poisoning, may occur in cases where the infection entered through the cervix after childbirth, abortion, or miscarriage.

DIAGNOSIS

PID is often difficult to identify because the symptoms resemble those of other conditions, such as appendicitis, urinary tract infections, ovarian cysts, and endometriosis. Mild cases of PID may have no symptoms at all. To diagnose PID, a pelvic examination is done, along with a culture of any vaginal discharge. A blood test may be done to detect high levels of white

PREVENTING PELVIC INFLAMMATORY DISEASE

The following measures can be taken to reduce the risks of PID:

■ Practice safer sex. Because PID can be sexually transmitted, using a condom or vaginal pouch can reduce the risk of the disease.

■ Don't douche. Though douching does not cause PID, it can spread infections from the vagina into the uterus and fallopian tubes, increasing the risk of PID.

■ Don't smoke. Studies show that a woman who smokes more than 10 cigarettes a day increases her risk of PID.

■ If you think you may have been exposed to gonorrhea or chlamydia, have a vaginal culture done to detect the bacteria. Most women with these sexually transmitted infections have no symptoms and may unknowingly have PID.

■ For several weeks after childbirth, abortion, miscarriage, or dilation and curettage, avoid inserting anything (finger, tampon, penis) into the vagina. The cervix remains partially dilated after these circumstances and is open to infection.

■ If you are at risk for sexually transmitted infections, use a form of birth control other than an IUD. If you use an IUD, have it checked annually and be alert to the symptoms of PID.

■ When choosing a contraceptive, consider that oral contraceptives are thought to offer some protection against PID by thickening cervical mucus and preventing organisms from reaching the uterus, fallopian tubes, and ovaries. However, keep in mind that the Pill does not protect against sexually transmitted infections of the lower genital tract.

blood cells, indicating infection. If an abscess is suspected, **ultrasound**—a noninvasive procedure that uses sound waves to create an image of the abdominal cavity—may be used to determine its location. To confirm the diagnosis, a **laparoscopy** may be done. This procedure involves the use of a thin, tubelike viewing scope inserted through a small incision in the abdomen.

TREATMENT

Early treatment of pelvic inflammatory disease is the most effective way to prevent infertility and other complications. Once PID is diagnosed, antibiotics are given to combat infection.

If an IUD is being used, it should be removed during treatment. If the case is severe, the woman may be hospitalized and the antibiotics given intravenously. In addition to medications, bed rest is recommended because it speeds the healing, and sexual intercourse should be avoided. Several courses of different types of antibiotics are given in order to be sure the disease has been eradicated and will not recur. If PID persists despite three or more courses of antibiotics (about a month of treatment), the condition is categorized as chronic, or persistent.

Because it can be sexually transmitted, a woman's partner must be treated for PID as well in order to prevent reinfection. Though it is unlikely, PID can be transmitted from woman to woman, so sexually active lesbians should undergo routine gonorrhea testing.

There are also several surgical treatments for PID. Because abscesses do not always respond to antibiotics, surgery may be necessary to drain them. Scar tissue caused by PID may be removed surgically during **laparoscopy** or through **laser surgery,** which vaporizes scar tissue, or **cauteri-** **zation,** which burns adhesions away. Laser surgery and cauterization may also be used to remove scar tissue from the fallopian tubes to restore fertility. For severe, chronic symptomatic PID, a **hysterectomy** (removal of the uterus) or a **salpingo-oophorectomy** (removal of a fallopian tube and ovary) may be performed as a last resort to provide relief from symptoms.

SEE laparoscopy; sexually transmitted infections.

PHYSICAL FITNESS

Physical fitness is the ability to complete everyday tasks without becoming overly tired. It is an important part of every woman's health, regardless of her age. Exercise helps to maintain weight, aerobic fitness, and muscle tone and can help fight the effects of osteoporosis after menopause. Along with physical fitness come added energy, strength, and even self-esteem.

The four components of physical fitness are cardiorespiratory (or aerobic) fitness, muscular fitness, flexibility, and body composition. **Cardiorespiratory fitness** is the heart's ability to pump blood and oxygen throughout the body. **Muscular fitness** refers to muscles' strength and endurance. **Flexibility** is the range of motion of a specific joint and its corresponding muscles. **Body composition** deals with the portion of body weight consisting of fat.

People attain physical fitness through exercise, and most women today do not get enough of it. In a Centers for Disease Control and Pre-vention (CDC) survey of over 50,000 women, three out of four reported that they do not get the amount of exercise needed to prevent heart disease, breast cancer, and osteoporosis. Thirty percent of the women said they had no leisure-time exercise in the previous month, and another 40 percent exercised, but not up to the levels recommended by the CDC.

Exercise has many benefits, both physical and psychological. They include:
- Cardiovascular fitness
- Improved muscle tone
- Weight maintenance and prevention of obesity
- Increased energy
- Improved self-image
- Increased social sphere
- Outlet for frustration and stress
- Prevention against high blood pressure and diabetes
- Lowered risk for heart attacks, osteoporosis, stroke, and some cancers

GETTING STARTED

For many women, the hardest part of becoming physically fit is getting started. Finding time—not to mention motivation—to exercise is often difficult, but it can be done. Typical forms of exercise are walking, jogging, aerobics, swimming, weight training, and other sports. Public health officials also recommend a wide range of activities, including gardening.

EXERCISE AND WEIGHT REDUCTION

Exercise is an important part of losing weight and keeping weight off. When combined with a proper, nutritious diet, exercise works to burn calories and boost metabolism. When the number of calories a person burns through exercise exceeds the amount of calories taken in through food, the body turns to its reserves of fat for energy, promoting weight loss. Exercise also builds muscle, which requires more calories to maintain than other types of tissue.

Most experts recommend exercising at least three times a week. The exercise should get the heart rate up to between 60 and 90 percent of its maximum level and keep it up for at least 20 minutes. (To find maximum heart rate, subtract age from 220.) Good cardiovascular exercises are walking, running, and swimming. (Keep in mind that cardiovascular exercise strengthens the heart and lungs, while weight-bearing exercise protects against osteoporosis.) Though a regular program of exercise is necessary to reap its full benefits, experts say that even a walk around the block now and then will make a difference.

A weight-loss plan of exercise, diet, and nutrition should be developed with the help of a practitioner and tailored to meet individual needs. This ensures that the plan is safe and that the woman will get the most benefit from it. Women who are pregnant or who have osteoporosis, for example, can benefit greatly from exercise, but some positions and activities may need to be avoided.

PREGNANCY AND PHYSICAL FITNESS

Many women curtail exercise while they are pregnant and following childbirth. Reasons for this include fatigue, fear of harming the fetus, preoccupation, and lack of sleep (the result of caring for a newborn infant). However, moderate exercise during and after pregnancy has many benefits. It improves muscle tone and prevents some problems associated with the weight gain and weight loss of pregnancy. It helps to alleviate pregnancy-related discomforts like backache, bloating, constipation, and swollen hands and feet. Exercise can also help pregnant women psychologically by allowing them to relax and providing them with a sense of control over their constantly changing bodies.

Although moderate exercise does not harm the fetus, experts say that after the fourth month, women should not do calisthenics lying on their backs, full sit-ups, double leg raises, or toe touches with knees straight, all of which can strain the back.

The key to exercising while pregnant is moderation, which is different for each woman, depending on her level of physical fitness before pregnancy. Each woman should talk to her obstetrician about the best exercises for her. Walking and swimming are usually well tolerated. As a general rule, pregnant women should stop exercising when they become tired, breath-

✓ MAKING THE MOST OF EXERCISE

Regardless of which activities you choose, here are a few tips to help you make the most of your exercise:

■ Develop an exercise plan, complete with goals. Incorporate the plan into a regular routine that will help you stay committed to the plan.

■ Always warm up and cool down as the first and last phases of your exercise program. Stretching before and after a workout will increase flexibility and help prevent injuries.

■ Don't push too hard too fast. Becoming physically fit takes time. Moderation is the key to success—don't strain yourself.

■ Don't give up. Even on days you just don't feel like working out, stick with your program. The longer you stick to it, the more it becomes a habit.

■ Don't let your menstrual period interrupt your routine. Many women think they cannot exercise while they have their period, when, in fact, the opposite is true. Exercise can help relieve menstrual cramps and other discomforts women experience during menstruation. However, too much vigorous exercise may interfere with hormone levels and the menstrual cycle, which can result in amenorrhea (absence of menstrual periods) or even a loss in bone density. Again, use moderation and see your practitioner if problems arise.

■ Have fun! An exercise program should not be all work and no play. Try different activities until you find one or two you really enjoy.

■ Drink plenty of fresh water to replace what you lose in sweat. One should drink at least eight glasses of water a day.

■ Wear well-fitting and correctly sized athletic shoes. Poor footwear can result in injuries.

---

less, or dizzy or experience pain in the chest, back, hip, or pubic area.

Women with pregnancy-induced hypertension, premature labor, persistent bleeding, or an incompetent cervix should not exercise.

EXERCISE FOR OLDER WOMEN

Although our society often associates physical fitness with youth, the menopausal and post-menopausal years are a time when exercise is crucial to a woman's health. Regular exercise—as little as 30 minutes three times a week—helps reduce the risk of heart attacks, diabetes, and bone fractures resulting from osteoporosis. Recommended aerobic exercise includes brisk walking, running, bicycling, cross-country skiing, and swimming.

A recent study presented to the American Heart Association found that physical activity reduces the risk of heart attack in post-menopausal women by up to 60 percent. According to the study, women who walked 30 to 45 minutes three times a week lowered their risk of heart disease to half that of inactive women.

Another recent study suggests that a home-based high-intensity strength training program, using dumbbells and ankle weights or milk jugs filled with water, can reduce postmenopausal women's risk for bone fractures. The program includes the following exercises: side shoulder raise, biceps curl, overhead triceps, knee extension, hip extension, and knee flexion. Women should do eight to 12 repetitions of each exercise, rest, then repeat, and each exercise should be done slowly, with three seconds for the lift, a one-second hold, and three seconds for the release. Weight lifting will not only strengthen muscles but also improve bone density, flexibility, and balance.

WOMEN AND SPORTS

More and more women are becoming involved in sports, participating in activities ranging from tennis to softball to basketball to bodybuilding, and more. Besides physical benefits, sports give women an opportunity for fellowship, a way to meet new people and spend time with old friends. Some women meet their spouse or partner through sports. Studies have found that women who are athletes have more positive self-images and tend to be more assertive, self-sufficient, independent, intelligent, and achievement-oriented than nonathletes. However, one cannot draw simple conclusions from these findings because whether sports participation results in these positive effects or whether women who have these positive characteristics are drawn to sports is uncertain. Nevertheless, women can reap many benefits—both physical and psychological—from sports.

RISKS

Physical activity can cause injuries if not done properly, or if overdone, but in most cases the benefits greatly outweigh the risks. Some forms of exercise are riskier than others, especially for women with health conditions. Exercise programs should be tailored for each individual woman, taking into account her age and physical health. All women should see their practitioner for a physical examination before beginning an exercise program. They can also discuss exercise options with their practitioner.

There are also serious risks involved with steroid use. Anabolic steroids, derived from testosterone, are commonly used illegally by men and women to increase muscle size and strength. Anabolic steroid use can cause definite and irreversible masculine changes in a woman's body, including voice-deepening, menstrual irregularities, and liver disease.

SEE nutrition; weight reduction.

For more information on physical fitness, contact:

Aerobic and Fitness Association of America
15250 Ventura Blvd., Suite 310
Sherman Oaks, CA 91403
800-466-2322

Women's Sports Foundation
Eisenhower Park
East Meadow, NY 11554
800-227-3988
http://www.lifetimetv.com/WoSport

PRACTITIONERS,
HOW TO CHOOSE

When it comes to choosing a health-care provider, there are a number of options available. In addition to the traditional primary-care practitioner, the physician who handles a wide range of medical needs, there are specialists and subspecialists. There are also physician assistants and advanced-practice nurses, such as nurse-practitioners and midwives, who have additional training and qualifications. The challenge for a woman is to find the right practitioner for her particular needs.

For routine medical care, many women visit a primary-care physician. While not exclusively devoted to women's health issues, there are several traditional types of primary-care physicians from which a woman can choose: family practitioners, internists, and gynecologists and obstetricians.

General practitioners are physicians who have completed medical school and have had only one year of internship experience.

Family practitioners have been recognized by the American Medical Association (AMA) as specialists since 1969. Any doctor wishing to qualify must complete a three-year residency that covers certain aspects of internal medicine, gynecology, minor surgery, obstetrics, pediatrics, orthopedics, psychiatry, behavioral science, and preventive medicine, and pass a comprehensive examination.

Internists, specialists in internal medicine, do not normally take training in pediatrics, orthopedics, and child delivery, but instead have more advanced training in the diagnosis and management of problems involving such areas as the gastrointestinal system, heart, lungs, kidney, liver, and endocrine system.

Gynecologists and **obstetricians,** who are also used by women as primary-care physicians, specialize in the medical and surgical care of the female reproductive system and associated disorders. These physicians are also trained in general medicine and preventive medicine. They must pass a comprehensive written examination and after two years of active practice pass an oral comprehensive examination.

Nontraditional sources of primary care include the nurse-practitioner and the nurse midwife. **Nurse-practitioners (N.P.'s),** registered nurses with advanced training, are being used more often as primary health-care providers. N.P.'s can perform the basic functions of a physician, though serious medical conditions are referred to a physician. N.P.'s specialize in many areas, including family practice, gynecology, and obstetrics. **Nurse-midwives,** nurses with special training in gynecology and obstetrics, are also being used more often for routine primary care. They, too, are required to refer potentially serious cases to physicians. Both nurse-practitioners and nurse-midwives are described more fully later in this entry.

M.D.'S AND D.O.'S

A physician can be licensed in allopathic or osteopathic medicine. An allopathic physician holds a degree of doctor of medicine (M.D.), while an osteopathic physician is known as a doctor of osteopathy (D.O.). Both allopathy and osteopathy claim scientifically accepted methods of diagnosis and treatment as their basis. Except for a notable difference in philosophy and, to a lesser extent, practice habits, M.D.'s and D.O.'s are essentially the same.

An **allopathic physician (M.D.)** is the most common type of physician in the United States. Allopathy is founded on scientific principles in which diseases are treated with lifestyle changes or medications to counteract what is going on within the body. An allopathic physician begins with a medical history, then conducts an examination and diagnostic tests, which may include blood tests, x-rays, ultrasound, and other technologies. Once the diagnosis is determined, the allopath may administer medications or use treatments including chemotherapy, surgery, and ionizing radiation.

An **osteopathic physician (D.O.)** holds that the body is an interrelated system. These practitioners are called osteopaths (osteo means "bones") because they emphasize the role of bones, muscles, and joints of the body—the musculoskeletal system—in a person's well-being. D.O.'s use manipulation and palpation as an aid to the diagnosis and treatment of various illnesses. This hands-on philosophy and holistic approach are what distinguish D.O.'s from M.D.'s., although they also utilize all the recognized procedures and modern technologies, including drugs, radiation, and surgery.

Whether one becomes a D.O. or an M.D., the route of complete medical training is basically the same. In matters of licensing, D.O.'s hold the same unlimited practice rights as M.D.'s in all 50 states and the District of Columbia and can admit and treat patients in both osteopathic and allopathic hospitals and clinics. Osteopaths also participate in federal Medicare and Medicaid programs on an equal basis with their allopathic counterparts.

Most D.O.'s are generalists, but some have additional training and qualifications and work in specialized fields. Osteopathic specialties resemble allopathic ones. The American Osteopathic Association (AOA), a trade organization similar to the American Medical Association, recognizes 17 areas of specialty certification. The American Board of Medical Specialties recognizes 24 different areas of specialty certification.

SPECIALISTS

A **specialist** is a physician who concentrates on a specific body system, age group, or disorder. After obtaining an M.D. or D.O. degree, the doctor then undergoes two to five years of supervised specialty training (called a **residency**). Many specialists also take one or more years of additional training (called a **fellowship**) in a **subspecialty,** a specific area of their specialty. If the doctor goes on to complete training and education requirements and takes a national examination, he or she is **board-certified.** It is not necessary for a physician to have board certification in order to call himself or herself a specialist.

Though specialists usually treat specific illnesses and disorders, a woman often seeks preventive and routine care from an obstetrician-gynecologist, a specialist who deals with the health of a woman's reproductive system—care that includes routine Pap tests and breast exams, prescriptions for contraceptive pills and devices, fertility counseling, and hormone replacement

WOMEN'S HEALTH AS A SPECIALTY

Many women see just one health-care provider for their primary-care needs, whether it be a gynecologist, internist, or family practitioner, an arrangement that can leave gaps in medical care. Some professionals have suggested creating a women's health specialty to fill those gaps. They believe a certified women's health specialist would be able to provide a woman with well-rounded primary care as well as gynecological services, such as Pap tests and breast exams. The specialist would be able to provide care to meet the unique social and physical needs of a woman in a way that other primary-care givers could not.

Such a specialist, they argue, would be an expert in the needs of women, just as a pediatrician is an expert in the needs of children. Because some conditions, such as heart disease, manifest themselves differently in women than in men, training for the specialty would focus on women alone. In addition, offering board certification in the specialty would provide a standard for women's care; currently, there is no way of knowing, for example, if practitioners at a "women's center" have specialized training in women's health.

While it is generally agreed that care for women needs to be improved, some believe that a separate medical specialty for women's health is not the way to do it. First of all, some opponents say, a new specialty could spark the growth of more of what they feel are unnecessary fields. Another fear is that a specialty would take women's health further out of the mainstream, making all other physicians less accountable for learning about the particular health-care needs of women.

Instead, opponents of the specialty say, all practitioners should become more sensitive to women's health concerns and address the needs of women. The role of nurse-practitioners, physician assistants, and certified nurse-midwives—professionals trained in whole-woman care—could be expanded in a general practice to provide well-rounded care for women. Most important, communication could be fostered between practitioners and their patients, a step that would without a doubt improve care for women.

therapy. Physicians who have successfully completed a certified four-year training program in obstetrics and gynecology (called a residency training program), have practiced as a gynecologist or obstetrician on their own for two years or more, and have passed an extensive written and oral test given by experts can be board-certified in obstetrics and gynecology by the American Board of Obstetrics and Gynecology.

During pregnancy, a woman may also seek an obstetrician-gynecologist for routine care.

Obstetrics is a branch of gynecology that concentrates on all aspects of pregnancy and childbirth, including prenatal care and fetal testing and monitoring.

OTHER OPTIONS IN HEALTH CARE

Practitioners who often work alongside licensed physicians include advanced practice nurses—

nurse-practitioners and certified nurse-mid-wives—and physician assistants. They can work in a variety of settings, including private practices, hospitals, clinics, health maintenance organizations, and student health services.

The **nurse-practitioner** (N.P.) is a professional registered nurse, usually with a four-year degree in nursing, who has taken an extra year of training to learn to perform some of the basic functions of a physician. Nurse-practitioners can receive additional training in other areas, including family planning and fertility-related services, obstetrics and gynecology, family practice, pediatrics, and general adult care. They must hold a valid state license and practice under the rules

and regulations of the Nurse Practice Act of the state in which they work. This act spells out the degree of autonomy permitted and defines the privileges N.P.'s are permitted.

N.P.'s provide basic medical services with the approval of a consulting physician and are good resources for information on diet, exercise, and preventive care. In some states, they prescribe prescription drugs. While N.P.'s can treat a variety of conditions, they refer women with potentially serious medical problems to physicians. Depending upon the state in which they are licensed, N.P.'s may be considered independent practitioners, able to see patients, diagnose conditions, and prescribe treatment independently.

✔ THE SEARCH FOR THE PERFECT PRACTITIONER

Begin your search by getting a few good recommendations from family members, friends, and neighbors. Word of mouth is still one of the best methods of finding out which practitioners are taking new patients and what others think of them. Don't overlook your present health-care provider, especially if your relationship is ending because he or she is leaving practice or retiring. Other sources to consider are:

■ Physician referral services operated by the local medical society (usually county-based) and local hospitals. However, such services will refer only those practitioners who are members and will not comment on the ability of providers other than to perhaps mention their board certifications.

■ Newspaper advertisements of practitioners announcing the opening of a new practice. Ask yourself why the practitioner is advertising. To attract patients because he

or she is just out of medical school? Or has he or she just moved in from a state where his or her license was revoked?

■ The company personnel office. Companies sometimes use certain practitioners for employment physicals and disability claims.

■ Health insurance companies, which can sometimes be helpful when you require a specialist for a second opinion.

■ Listings in the telephone directory. Practitioners' names are usually arranged according to practice or specialty, but remember that a doctor can practice in any specialty area he or she chooses, whether or not he or she has had any advanced training. Look for board certification.

■ Nurses or other medical professionals

■ Senior centers. Some have lists of practitioners either affiliated with or recommended by the center.

The state board of nursing or the state health department can provide more information on the exact privileges granted to N.P.'s. Information is also available from:

American Academy of Nurse-Practitioners
P.O. Box 12846
Austin, TX 18711
512-442-4262

Certified nurse-midwives are registered nurses who have received additional training in obstetrics and gynecology. They are certified through a national examination administered by the American College of Certified Nurse-Midwives and must hold a valid nursing license in the state where they work. Though they generally provide prenatal and postpartum care for women with low-risk pregnancies, some midwives also offer routine gynecologic care. Information on nurse midwives can be obtained by contacting:

American College of Nurse-Midwives
818 Connecticut Ave., Suite 900
Washington, DC 20006
202-728-9860

A **physician assistant (P.A.)** is trained to carry out some functions of a licensed physician. A candidate must complete two years of college before qualifying for a P.A.-approved program, which can last from 15 months to four years and usually consists of academic and clinical (hands-on) experience. After graduation, the person must pass a national examination administered by the National Commission on Certification of Physician Assistants to become certified. A P.A. must also hold a valid state license and work within the practice guidelines established by a supervising physician. P.A.'s are qualified to take patient medical histories, complete physical examinations, counsel patients and families on health and disease, assist in surgery, and perform other therapeutic proce-

dures as directed. Some states also permit physician assistants to write prescriptions. To find out the limits of authority for P.A.'s, contact your state medical licensing board or the board of occupational and professional licensing.

GLOSSARY OF MEDICAL SPECIALTIES

The following is a list of some of the specialties designated by the American Medical Association, used by physicians to describe themselves and their primary and secondary fields of practice.

To verify the credentials of a certified specialist or subspecialist, contact the American Board of Medical Specialties at 800-776-2378.

A licensed physician may practice any specialty and call himself or herself a specialist in a particular field, whether or not the physician is actually board-certified or trained in that specialty.

Abdominal Surgery. Subspecialty of surgery involving the abdominal organs. These are usually specialists in general surgery.

Allergy and Immunology. Subspecialty of internal medicine or pediatrics involving the diagnosis and treatment of all forms of allergy and allergic disease and other disorders potentially involving the immune system

Anesthesiology. Involves the administration of drugs (anesthetics) to prevent pain or induce unconsciousness during surgical operations or diagnostic procedures. Anesthesiologists may further specialize in critical-care medicine as practiced in critical-care and intensive-care units, postanesthesia recovery rooms, and other settings.

Cardiovascular Diseases (Cardiology). Subspecialty of internal medicine that deals with the heart and blood vessels

Cardiovascular Surgery. Subspecialty of general surgery involving surgery on the heart and associated vascular system. Cardiovascular surgeons perform open-heart surgery, which may include heart transplants.

Colon and Rectal Surgery (Proctology). Diagnosis and treatment of diseases of the intestinal tract, rectum, and anus

Cosmetic Surgery. Surgery to reshape normal structures of the body in order to improve a person's appearance and self-esteem. A number of the various surgical specialties may refer to themselves as cosmetic surgeons (such as ear, nose, and throat).

Dermatology. Diagnosis and treatment of benign and malignant disorders of the skin and related tissues. The dermatologist can also diagnose and treat a number of diseases transmitted through sexual activity.

Diagnostic Radiology. Specialty of radiology employing the use of ionizing, electromagnetic, or sound wave imaging devices to diagnose medical problems

Emergency Medicine. Focuses on the immediate decision making and action necessary to prevent death or further disability. It is primarily hospital emergency department based.

QUESTIONS TO ASK

Once you've decided what type of practitioner you would like to visit, and found a few in your area, the next step is a face-to-face meeting. Call the office for an appointment and mention that you would be a new patient, then ask to arrange a get-acquainted visit, a 15-minute meeting where you can ask questions and find out a little more about the practitioner. Be aware that some practitioners charge for these appointments.

During the visit, evaluate the office and staff. Ask a receptionist about the procedures for making appointments, telephoning the practitioner, getting prescription refills, and obtaining copies of medical records.

Because the meeting with the practitioner is short, have your questions ready. You will want to know the practitioner's medical degree, board certification, and hospital affiliations. (Each practitioner only works out of one or two hospitals, so be sure your practitioner has privileges at one you prefer.) Ask about fees and payment plans.

This is also an opportunity to discover the philosophy and attitude of the practitioner and the value placed on preventive health measures, the attitude toward alternative therapies, and whether or not the patient is seen as a full partner in health care.

You will also want to consider:

■ Is the practice solo or group? If group, are the practitioners the same specialty or different specialties?

■ If solo, who covers for the practitioner on nights and weekends?

■ Does this practitioner publish or make available a list of fees and current charges?

■ Does the office appear neat and clean? Are there current magazines?

■ Is your insurance coverage accepted? Will the office file all insurance claims?

■ Does the staff maintain a professional, friendly attitude?

■ Was your get-acquainted appointment kept on time?

Endocrinology. Subspecialty of internal medicine that deals with disorders of the internal (or endocrine) glands such as the thyroid and adrenal glands. Endocrinology also deals with disorders such as diabetes, pituitary diseases, and menstrual, reproductive, and sexual problems.

Family Practice/General Practice. Concerned with continuing and comprehensive health care for the individual and the family. The scope of family practice is not limited by age, sex, organ system, or disease entity.

Gastroenterology. Subspecialty of internal medicine that involves disorders of the digestive tract: stomach, bowels, liver, gallbladder, and related organs

General Surgery. Surgery of the parts of the body that are not in the domain of specific surgical specialties (some areas do overlap, however). The standard residency program is five years of training after graduation from medical school.

Geriatrics. Subspecialty of family practice and internal medicine that deals with the diseases of the elderly and problems associated with aging

Gynecology. Diagnosis and treatment of problems associated with the female reproductive organs and general female medicine

Hematology. Diagnosis and treatment of diseases and disorders of the blood and blood-forming parts of the body. This is a subspecialty of internal medicine.

Immunology. Study and treatment of problems of the body's immune system, which may include allergies and life-threatening infections such as the human immunodeficiency virus (HIV) that can cause AIDS (acquired immune deficiency syndrome)

Infectious Diseases. Subspecialty of internal medicine involving the diagnosis and treatment of life-threatening infectious illnesses

Internal Medicine. Diagnosis and nonsurgical treatment of diseases, especially those of adults.

While internists may set up practices in which they act as highly trained family doctors, they often continue training to subspecialize in a specific area.

Maxillofacial Surgery. Subspecialty of dentistry that deals with problems of the mouth and jaw

Neonatal-Perinatal Medicine. Subspecialty of pediatrics that deals with disorders of newborn infants, including premature infants

Nephrology. Subspecialty of internal medicine concerned with disorders of the kidney

Neurological Surgery (Neurosurgery). Diagnosis and surgical treatment of diseases of the brain, spinal cord, and nerves

Neurology. Diagnosis and nonsurgical treatment of diseases of the brain, spinal cord, and nerves

Nuclear Medicine. Use of radioactive substances for diagnosis and treatment

Nuclear Radiology. Subspecialty of radiology that involves the use of radioactive materials in the diagnosis and treatment of disease

Obstetrics and Gynecology. Care of pregnant women and treatment of disorders of the female reproductive system and general medicine of the female

Occupational Medicine. Subspecialty of preventive medicine that deals with the special physical and psychological risks in the workplace

Oncology. Subspecialty of internal medicine concerned with the diagnosis and treatment of all types of cancer and other benign and malignant tumors

Ophthalmology. Diagnosis, monitoring, and medical/surgical treatment of vision problems and other disorders of the eye, including the prescription of glasses/contact lenses

Orthopedic Surgery (Orthopedics). Care of diseases of the muscles, and diseases, fractures, and deformities of the bones and joints

Otolaryngology (ENT). Medical and surgical care of patients with diseases and disorders that affect the ears, respiratory and upper alimentary systems, and related structures: in general, the head and neck

Otology. Subspecialty of otolaryngology that deals with the medical treatment of and surgery on the ear

Pathology. Diagnosis of conditions by examination of samples from organs, tissues, body fluids, and excrement

Physical Medicine and Rehabilitation (Physiatry). Diagnosis, evaluation, and treatment of patients with impairments and/or disabilities involving musculoskeletal, neurologic, cardiovascular, or other body systems

Plastic and Reconstructive Surgery. Surgery on abnormal structures of the body, caused by congenital defects, developmental abnormalities, trauma, infection, tumors, or disease, and generally performed to improve function but may also be done to approximate a normal appearance. At a minimum, five years of training are required in this specialty, with some programs lasting seven years. Hand surgery is a subspecialty of plastic surgery.

Preventive Medicine. Focuses on the health of individuals and the prevention of disease through immunization, good health practice, and concern with environmental and occupational factors

Public Health. Branch of medicine that deals with the protection and improvement of community health by organized community effort. It includes the monitoring and screening of populations to prevent the spread of communicable diseases. Many consider public health to be allied with, if not actually a subspecialty of, preventive medicine.

Pulmonary Diseases. Subspecialty of internal medicine concerned with diseases of the lungs and chest, including asthma, pneumonia, cancer, occupational diseases, bronchitis, emphysema, and other complex disorders

Radiology. Study and use of various types of radiation, including x-rays, in the diagnosis and treatment of disease

Rheumatology. Subspecialty of internal medicine that deals with diseases of the joints, muscles, and tendons, including arthritis

Surgical Critical Care (Traumatic Surgery). Subspecialty of surgery that deals with the treatment of the critically ill patient, such as the trauma victim and the postoperative patient, in the emergency department, intensive-care unit, trauma unit, burn unit, and other similar settings

Therapeutic Radiology (Radiation Oncology). Subspecialty of radiology that deals with the therapeutic applications of radiant energy, especially in the treatment of malignant tumors

Thoracic Surgery. Operative, perioperative, and critical care of patients with disease-causing conditions within the chest, including coronary-artery disease, cancers of the lung, esophagus, and chest wall, abnormalities of the great vessels and heart valves, and injuries to the airway and chest

Urology. Specialty that deals with the medical and surgical treatments of the genitourinary system

Vascular Surgery. Subspecialty of surgery that deals with medical disorders affecting the blood vessels, excluding those of the heart, lungs, and brain

SEE board certification; childbirth—choosing a practitioner.

PREGNANCY, DIAGNOSIS OF

Pregnancy may be diagnosed by home test kits or by blood or urine tests done at a practitioner's office or clinic. A positive pregnancy test should be followed by a medical examination to confirm the presence of the pregnancy.

SYMPTOMS OF PREGNANCY

The common symptoms of pregnancy are a missed period, nausea, and inexplicable fatigue. Other classic indicators are sore or enlarged breasts, headaches, and frequent urination.

PREGNANCY TESTING

Both blood and urine pregnancy tests work by testing for the presence of human chorionic gonadotropin (HCG). HCG is a hormone secreted by the fertilized egg as it passes through the fallopian tube into the uterus. It is found in the bloodstream as soon as six to eight days after fertilization and in the urine 17 to 28 days following fertilization.

Blood tests can detect pregnancy as early as seven days after ovulation and fertilization—before a missed period—in over 90 percent of pregnant women and are considered more accurate than urine tests. Blood tests identify HCG when levels are as low as one to five international units (IU) per liter in the bloodstream.

For this reason they are especially useful in detecting ectopic pregnancy (a condition in which the fertilized egg implants somewhere outside of the uterus), in which HCG levels are often too low to be detected by urine tests.

Higher-than-normal levels of HCG may indicate that there is a multiple pregnancy—twins, triplets, and so on. Certain types of rare tumors can also produce elevated HCG levels. Lower-than-normal levels of HCG may suggest ectopic pregnancy or impending miscarriage.

Urine tests can be done 17 to 20 days after fertilization. These tests take two or three minutes to complete.

UNEXPECTED PREGNANCY: KNOWING THE OPTIONS

There are many resources available for women who are uncertain about being pregnant. An objective counselor should discuss all options available, including continuing the pregnancy and raising a child, placing the child for adoption, and abortion options. Women should be aware that some "clinics," often called "crisis pregnancy centers," discourage the option of abortion and may not provide complete or objective information on the subject.

HOME PREGNANCY TESTS

Pregnancy may be diagnosed by home test kits that measure the levels of HCG in the urine. The instructions to perform the test must be precisely followed. To use the test, a woman collects a sample of her urine, then tests it with a special dipstick or other device. Some devices can simply be held in the urine stream. Generally, a change in color or other indicator shows whether or not the woman is pregnant.

Pregnancy tests can be purchased without a prescription in a drugstore or supermarket and are basically the same types of urine tests used by medical professionals. Some newer home tests can detect pregnancy just a few days after a missed period. While the home tests can be fairly accurate, positive results should be confirmed by a professionally administered test and a medical examination. Certain vitamins such as folic acid are needed for the growth of the fetus very early in pregnancy. Women intending to conceive should discuss the use of vitamins with her practitioner. Otherwise, a woman should visit her practitioner as soon as she realizes she is pregnant so that she may start vitamins early.

SEE abortion; adoption.

For more information on diagnosing pregnancy, contact:

Planned Parenthood Federation of America, Inc.
810 Seventh Avenue
New York, NY 10019
For the Planned Parenthood nearest you, call:
   800-230-PLAN
http://www.ppfa.org/ppfa

PREGNANCY, ECTOPIC

Ectopic pregnancy, or tubal pregnancy, occurs when a fertilized egg implants somewhere outside of the uterus, most often in one of the fallopian tubes, but occasionally on an ovary or in the abdominal cavity. If not treated, the growth of the embryo may rupture the fallopian tube, causing internal hemorrhage, infection, and possible death for the woman.

Ectopic pregnancies happen when the fertilized egg is stopped on its journey from the ovaries to the uterus via the fallopian tube. Scars in the tubes from infection, tubal surgery, endometriosis, and tubal abnormalities may block the passage of the egg. Ectopic pregnancy always results in the loss of the fetus and is now the leading cause of pregnancy-related death during the first trimester in this country.

According to the Centers for Disease Control and Prevention, 9 percent of all pregnancy related deaths were attributed to ectopic pregnancy in 1992. Ectopic pregnancies accounted for about 2 percent of all pregnancies; this rate is up 600 percent since 1970. Health experts attribute this rise to an increase in the incidence of sexually transmitted infections (which can scar the fallopian tubes) and induction of ovulation (an infertility treatment that involves the stimulation of ovaries with drugs to promote the release of eggs). Although pregnancy is rare after tubal sterilization, or while using an intrauterine device (IUD), there is an increased chance that such a pregnancy will be ectopic.

RISK

Ectopic pregnancy cannot be prevented, but there are some elements that predispose certain women to the condition. Risk factors include:

■ A history of pelvic inflammatory disease or endometriosis

■ An age of 30 years or more

■ Previous ectopic pregnancy

■ Abdominal surgery

■ Smoking

■ Prior fallopian tube surgery. Some 3 to 20 percent of women who have had fallopian tube surgery will have an ectopic pregnancy. However, the greater the success of the tubal surgery in fully restoring the normal function of the tubes, the lower the chance of an ectopic pregnancy.

■ Use of gamete intrafallopian transfer (GIFT), an infertility procedure that surgically places an egg fertilized outside the body into the fallopian tube. The egg generally implants in the uterus, but in rare cases may implant in the tube.

Although women cannot prevent or avoid an ectopic pregnancy, they should discuss the risk factors with their practitioner before they

ON THE HORIZON

A new alternative procedure is undergoing research. According to a 1995 study, the laparoscopic injection of highly concentrated glucose effectively treats early ectopic pregnancy in which the tube has not ruptured.

The glucose causes the embryo cells to burst, and within a few weeks, the blockage can be cleared easily. The procedure provides an alternative to tubal surgery, increasing the chances of keeping the fallopian tube and its reproductive capability intact.

become pregnant. A very thorough medical history in the prepregnancy planning stage should raise the red flags associated with increased risk.

SYMPTOMS

There may be no symptoms of an ectopic pregnancy during the first few weeks after conception; some women may not even know that they are pregnant. Often the condition goes undetected until the pregnancy ruptures, or breaks through, the walls of the fallopian tube.

Symptoms include:

■ Cramps and spotting early in the pregnancy

■ Vaginal bleeding

■ Severe lower abdominal pains on one side of the body

■ Nausea

■ Vomiting

■ Fainting spells

■ Dizziness

Pain can radiate along a nerve pathway to areas other than the site of the disorder. In ectopic pregnancies that cause bleeding in the abdomen, the pain often appears in the shoulder. Shoulder pain in women who are known to be, or who may be, pregnant can be a sign of a ruptured ectopic pregnancy.

DIAGNOSIS

Because symptoms vary and often do not appear until the pregnancy has progressed, ectopic pregnancy is difficult to diagnose. **Ultrasound,** a procedure that uses sound waves to create an image of the pelvic cavity, may be used to diagnose ectopic pregnancy. The change in the blood levels of the hormone human chorionic gonadotropin (HCG) may also be measured to aid diagnosis; lower than normal levels may suggest ectopic pregnancy. **Laparoscopy,** a procedure in which a thin viewing scope is inserted into the abdomen, may be used to allow practitioners to actually see the presence of an ectopic pregnancy. Earlier detection of ectopic pregnancy (through ultrasound studies or laparoscopic examination) has reduced rates of complications and death.

TREATMENT

Ectopic pregnancies must be diagnosed as soon as possible in order to prevent the fallopian tube from rupturing. Delicate microsurgery performed before the tube ruptures may save the tube if the pregnancy is diagnosed early. An ectopic pregnancy may be surgically removed or eased out of an end of a tube that has not yet ruptured. The drug methotrexate is now used to medically terminate an ectopic pregnancy.

If there is a normal second tube, a **salpingectomy** (removal of the fallopian tube) may be performed on the one containing the pregnancy. The tube may be removed through an opening in the abdomen (called an **open procedure**) or through a small incision near the navel, using a small viewing instrument called a **laparoscope.** The aim of the recently developed conservative surgeries is to preserve the tube and maintain fertility.

If the tube has ruptured, there may be severe hemorrhaging, making the woman's health a priority over saving the fallopian tube. In such cases, the tube is removed, sparing the adjacent ovary if possible. Antibiotics are also administered, since accumulated blood in the abdomen puts the woman at risk for peritonitis, an infection of the lining of the abdominal cavity, for which the mortality rate ranges between 12 and 57 percent (depending on the type of infection present). Improved antibiotics have lowered the mortality rate of peritonitis, but it still remains high.

Surgery to restore reproductive function after an ectopic pregnancy can be done with lasers or with an electrocautery device. Rates of pregnancy following laser surgery are slightly higher (53.3 percent) than the rates after electrocautery surgery, but the difference is not statistically significant.

FERTILITY AFTER ECTOPIC PREGNANCY

Depending upon the degree of scarring of the fallopian tubes and the functioning of the remaining tube (if one was removed), fertility may be impaired. Among women who want to get pregnant again after an ectopic pregnancy, success rates vary from 61 to 100 percent depending on the amount of damage to the tubes. Both the rate of fertilizations and the rate of pregnancies carried to term have been reported to be about 89 percent, with 10.9 percent of the pregnancies failing because of repeat ectopic pregnancy.

Scarring, which can interfere with the chances of future pregnancy, occurs by the eighth day after surgery in more than 50 percent of women operated on for ectopic pregnancy.

Scars can be repaired by laparoscopy and tend not to recur following such surgery.

In addition, the newer techniques for in vitro fertilization increase the chances of pregnancy in women who are missing fallopian tubes or who have scarring.

SEE laparoscopy; pregnancy—prenatal concerns.

PREGNANCY— PRECONCEPTION CONCERNS

A great deal of information about a pregnancy and the health of a future child can now be determined even before the pregnancy begins. Prepregnancy counseling is a series of examinations and evaluations that help to determine the effects a pregnancy will have upon a woman and whether or not there will be any health risks for a fetus. Such an evaluation, which looks at the health of the woman and the genetic and environmental risk factors, can minimize the risks of pregnancy before conception occurs. Women considering pregnancy may use the information while making the decision to have children and how best to reduce any risks.

GENETIC COUNSELING

Genetic counseling is professional advice concerning the possibility of transmitting a hereditary disorder to the child. A man or woman may be aware of potential problems found through blood tests, or they may be concerned about exposure they have had to environmental toxins. Women over the age of 35 have special concerns, such as higher rates of children with Down syndrome, as do women who have suffered repeated miscarriages.

The counseling involves researching the family history and personal medical histories of the parents. Age, habits, diet, hobbies, education, vocation, and nationality or ethnic background are included in addition to a review of family illnesses, abortions, and former partners. A detailed physical examination is performed, and specific laboratory tests may be done as well.

The counselor then tries to determine if there is a problem, and if so, whether it is genetic or caused by environmental factors. Any risks are considered by the woman and her partner. Those at risk of passing on genetic defects and who should seek counseling include:

■ Anyone who knows or suspects he or she has or carries a genetic disorder

■ Anyone concerned about exposure to medications, infections, chemicals, radiation, or other environmental factors that may be hazardous to pregnancy

■ Women over the age of 35

■ Those with a child or other relative with mental retardation or other delayed development

PREPREGNANCY COUNSELING

Before a woman tries to become pregnant, she and her partner should schedule a preconception office visit with an obstetrician/gynecologist. The preconception examination is the time when any concerns the woman has about her potential pregnancy should be addressed. The following subjects should be discussed:

■ Preexisting maternal medical conditions, particularly those that are chronic in nature, such as asthma, diabetes, epilepsy, high blood pressure, infections, chronic inflammatory bowel disease, and blood, neurological, or lung disorders

■ Medications the woman and her partner are currently taking (both prescription and non-prescription)

■ Previous pregnancy experiences, especially miscarriage, premature birth, ectopic pregnancy, delivery complications, and sensitivity to the Rh factor

■ Lifestyle factors of the woman and her partner such as smoking, alcohol consumption, illegal-drug use, and past sexual behaviors that may put the person at risk for HIV or other sexually transmitted infections

■ Concerns about the woman's age. The risk of miscarriage and birth defects increases with a woman's age. Teenage girls are at high risk of having low-birth weight or premature babies.

PREPREGNANCY SCREENING

Several diagnostic tests may be done before pregnancy to alert a woman to potential problems. A preconception screening should be done for **sexually transmitted infections,** such as syphilis, hepatitis, chlamydia, gonorrhea, and HIV/AIDS, especially if the woman may

GENETIC COUNSELING: QUESTIONS TO ASK

The goal of genetic counseling is to provide an accurate diagnosis of a known or suspected hereditary disorder and identify any exposure to dangerous substances. Look to the genetic counselor, who interprets the results of the examinations and laboratory tests, to answer these questions of yours:

■ Do I, my child, or another relative have a genetic disease?

■ What does being a carrier mean?

■ Is any member of my family a carrier of a genetic disease?

■ What are the chances that my future children or other members of my family will have a particular genetic problem?

■ What can be expected in the future for me or for a family member with a genetic disorder?

■ Where can good treatment and care for this disorder be obtained?

have been exposed to any infections through unprotected intercourse or IV drug use.

HIV testing and counseling for all women should be offered. Some 15 to 30 percent of babies born to women infected with HIV will have the virus and develop AIDS, and there is also a possibility that HIV can be passed to a baby through breast milk. Early medical care can help keep HIV-positive babies healthier.

Rubella, or **German measles,** screening is also necessary because this disease can lead to miscarriage, stillbirth, or serious birth defects. A woman planning to become pregnant should be vaccinated if she knows or suspects that she did not have the disease as a child. She should not attempt to conceive during the four months

GUIDELINES FOR WORK DURING PREGNANCY

The American Medical Association's Council on Scientific Affairs recommends that the following work activities be discontinued at these indicated weeks of pregnancy:

Job Function		Week of Gestation to Discontinue Activity
Secretarial and light clerical		40
Professional and managerial		40
Sitting with light tasks		40
Standing		
Prolonged (over 4 hours)		24
Intermittent:	More than 30 minutes per hour	32
	Less than 30 minutes per hour	40
Stooping and bending below knee level		
Repetitive:	More than 10 times per hour	20
	Less than 2 times per hour	40
Climbing vertical ladders and poles		
Repetitive:	4 times or more per 8-hour shift	28
Intermittent:	Less than 4 times per 8-hour shift	28
Climbing stairs		
Repetitive:	4 times or more per 8-hour shift	28
Intermittent:	Less than 4 times per 8-hour shift	28
Lifting		
Repetitive:	More than 50 pounds	20
	25 to 50 pounds	24
	Less than 25 pounds	40
Intermittent:	More than 50 pounds	30
	25 to 30 pounds	40
	Less than 25 pounds	40

✓ PRECONCEPTION CARE

A woman's health prior to pregnancy is extremely important to the future health of her child. In addition to getting good medical care, women who are planning to become pregnant should do the following:

■ Stop smoking. Women who smoke produce fewer eggs and are less likely to become pregnant than nonsmokers are. Smokers are also more likely to give birth to low-birth-weight babies, and sudden infant death syndrome risk is 10 times greater for their children than for those of nonsmokers. To stop smoking is the single greatest benefit a woman can give to both herself and her child.

■ Eat a well-balanced diet. You should eat a diet that includes foods high in nutri-ents but low in fat. Good food choices include whole grains for B vitamins and fiber; nonfat dairy products for calcium and riboflavin; and poultry, lean meats, and tuna packed in water or canola oil for iron and zinc. Ask your practitioner to recommend a multivitamin supplement.

■ Take folic acid. Have at least two half-cup servings a day of dark green and bright-colored vegetables. Other sources include lentils, garbanzo beans, spinach, black beans, and black-eyed peas. These vegetables are great sources of B vitamins, including folic acid. Several studies have shown that this important B vitamin (also known as folate) can reduce the risk of birth defects of the spine and brain by about 60

following vaccination and should use a reliable contraceptive.

Another screening test detects **hepatitis B** (or **HBV**), an infection that can be carried without overt symptoms. While few fetuses die from HBV infection, they may become chronic carriers of the infection after birth. There are preventive vaccines available, though there is no effective cure for the condition. Newborns whose mothers have HBV should be treated within 12 hours of birth to prevent infection.

PREPREGNANCY AND CONTRACEPTION

Experts recommend that a woman using oral contraceptives switch to a barrier method of contraception one month before trying to become pregnant. This will allow the body to return to its natural cycle. In addition, women using an intrauterine device (IUD) should have it removed. There is risk of miscarriage, infection, and premature birth if a woman becomes pregnant while an IUD is still in place.

Some contraceptives, such as the Pill, Norplant, or Depo-Provera, may affect the fetus if they are inadvertently used during pregnancy. A woman should discuss with her practitioner the risks associated with her chosen form of birth control and find out what to do in the event of a suspected pregnancy.

WORK-ENVIRONMENT SAFETY

The work environment of the woman may pose risks to the fetus. Women considering pregnancy should take precautions against being

percent. It is recommended by the United States Public Health Service that all women of reproductive age supplement their diets with 400 micrograms of folic acid by taking a multivitamin every day.

■ Reach a healthy weight. Women who are underweight have a higher risk of giving birth to premature, underweight babies, and those who are overweight have an increased chance of developing gestational diabetes, giving birth to an overgrown baby, and blood clots. A safe weight loss plan should be discussed with a practitioner. Dieting for weight loss during pregnancy is not recommended.

■ Reduce or eliminate alcohol and caffeine intake. Women who drink alcohol around the time of fertilization have a higher risk of having a child with fetal alcohol syndrome, a combination of birth defects.

■ Exercise. According to several studies, women who are in good cardiovascular health and exercise regularly before pregnancy give birth to healthier babies, have easier labors, and fewer back problems. They also get back to their prepregnancy weight more quickly. The American College of Obstetricians and Gynecologists recommends low-impact exercises such as walking or swimming for about 45 minutes at least three times a week for those looking to get into shape before pregnancy.

■ Drink eight glasses of water each day to help eliminate constipation.

exposed to occupational hazards such as chemicals, gases, radiation, and infectious diseases during pregnancy. Other risk factors include stress and excessive standing, lifting, climbing, and noise levels.

PREGNANCY IN WOMEN OVER AGE 35

Women over the age of 35 are at higher risk for complications during pregnancy, but mortality rates do not differ significantly from those giving birth under the age of 35. Women should consult with their practitioners about possible complications and monitor their pregnancies carefully for any potential problems.

Older women are more likely to have gestational diabetes, chronic high blood pressure, miscarriage, and toxemia. They are also likely to give birth to low-birth-weight, small-size babies. Women 35 and over also have more cesarean deliveries and give birth to more babies with Down syndrome. According to a 1995 report in *Obstetrics and Gynecology,* women over the age of 35 are:

■ Three times more likely to have chronic high blood pressure

■ Twice as likely to have uterine fibroid tumors

■ Five times more likely to go into labor prematurely

Fertility declines about 7 percent in women at age 30; by the age of 40, fertility declines by 50 percent. As fertility rates drop, the risk of miscarriage rises: women in their 20s have a 10 percent chance of miscarrying; those in their late 30s have an 18 percent chance; and women aged 45 have a 53 percent risk.

335

SEE birth defects; pregnancy—prenatal concerns.

For more information on genetic counseling, contact:

American Board of Medical Genetics
9650 Rockville Pike
Bethesda, MD 20814
301-571-1825
http://www.faseb.org/genetics

March of Dime Birth Defects Foundation
1275 Mamaroneck Ave.
White Plains, NY 10605
914-428-7100

For more information on prepregnancy counseling, contact:

American College of Obstetricians and Gynecologists
409 12th St., S.W.
Washington, DC 20024
202-638-5577
http://www.acog.com

Circle Solutions, Inc.
[formerly the Maternal and Child Health Clearinghouse]
2070 Chainbridge Rd., Suite 450
Vienna, VA 22182
703-821-8955

National Institute for Occupational Safety and Health
Department of Health and Human Resources
4676 Columbia Pkwy.
Cincinnati, OH 45226
800-356-4674
http://www.cdc.gov/niosh/homepage.html

PREGNANCY—
PRENATAL CONCERNS

The term "prenatal" describes the period of time during which the fetus develops in the uterus, prior to birth. Prenatal care is the medical care of a pregnant woman and fetus throughout pregnancy.

Pregnancy is divided into three trimesters. The first trimester of pregnancy consists of weeks one through 12. The second trimester covers weeks 13 through 26. The third trimester lasts from week 27 through week 40. A woman can find her own due date through simple arithmetic by taking the date of her last period, adding seven days, and then counting back three months.

THE FIRST TRIMESTER

During the first trimester, the woman's body goes through various changes in order to accommodate the growth and development of the fetus: the breasts become larger, the volume of blood circulating doubles, and the uterus enlarges to about three times its normal size.

The changes are more than just physical; pregnancy brings with it excitement, joy, amazement, and even fear and uncertainty. Adjusting to the idea of pregnancy is challenging, and it may take time. A woman and her partner must get used to the idea that they will become parents, and many people who felt they were prepared for parenthood may suddenly be frightened by the responsibility having a child brings. There may be worries about finances or how the pregnancy will affect a career or a relationship. A woman can discuss her emotions with a partner, friend, or practitioner to work through any concerns that keep her from enjoying her pregnancy.

During the first trimester, a woman should find an obstetrician or other birth practitioner for an examination. She may also want to make plans with her employer for maternity leave.

While many women have no difficulties during the first trimester, common problems that may occur include:

DEVELOPMENT OF THE FETUS

The pregnancy begins when the fertilized egg (or zygote), which has developed into a preembryo, implants in the lining of the uterus. At this point, it becomes known as an embryo and releases the hormone HCG (human chorionic gonadotropin) into the bloodstream. It is this hormone that is detected during a pregnancy test.

The cells of the embryo then begin to divide and develop into the fetus. By the end of four weeks after conception, the heart, head, nose, mouth, eyes, heart, lungs, brain, spinal column, and genitals are developing.

Limbs begin to develop during the sixth and seventh weeks. At the end of the eighth week, the fetus is about an inch long and weighs about one-thirtieth of an ounce. It is attached to the placenta (an organ that develops to nourish the fetus) by the umbilical cord. Also developing at this time are several internal organs, including the stomach and liver.

By 12 weeks, the fetus is three inches long. Fingernails and toenails of the fetus develop. Arms, hands, legs, toes, and feet are fully formed. Ultrasound (a diagnostic test that creates images using sound waves) can show head, hand, and leg movement. By the end of the first trimester, the fetus has developed into a recognizable human form and contains most of its organs and tissues.

Usually during the second trimester—weeks 13 through 26—the pregnancy becomes noticeable to others. At 16 weeks, the fetus weighs about four ounces. By the end of the second trimester, the fetus has grown to about 14 inches in length and weighs a little over two pounds. The movements of the fetus (quickening) are usually felt by the woman by the 20th week.

During the third trimester, the fetus grows from two pounds to about seven pounds as the uterus continues to enlarge. The fetus will complete its growth, in addition to the final development of its heart, circulatory system, and respiratory system. The soft bone plates of the head remain flexible to allow passage through the birth canal. Before a child's second birthday, the soft spots (called fontanelles) fuse together and harden.

THE FIRST PRENATAL VISIT

Your first prenatal visit will probably take longer than subsequent visits. First, your practitioner will ask you about your medical history. Here are some sample questions:

■ Have you ever been pregnant before? Have you ever had a miscarriage or an abortion?

■ When did you have your first period? Are your periods heavy? Light? Painful?

■ What illnesses have you had? What illnesses have your parents had? What illnesses have other members of your family had?

■ What kind of diet and lifestyle do you follow?

A physical examination will follow. Tests and measurements that should be performed include:

■ A pregnancy test

■ Height, weight, and blood pressure measurements

■ Eyes, ears, nose, throat, and teeth examinations

■ Heart, lungs, breasts, and abdominal examinations

■ An internal examination (pelvic examination) of the growth of your uterus and the amount of room in your pelvis for the baby

■ Examination for edema (fluid retention in tissues of the ankles, fingers, and legs)

■ A Pap test to screen for cervical cancer

■ A culture of the cervix to check for any sexually transmitted infections, such as gonorrhea

■ Blood tests to check for anemia and syphilis; to determine your blood type and Rh factor; and to see if you have had rubella (German measles) or hepatitis. In addition, the United States Public Health Service recommends voluntary HIV testing and counseling to all pregnant women.

■ A urine test to check for diabetes, kidney function, toxemia, or infection

The first prenatal visit is very important—not only for the necessary testing but also to establish good communication between you and the health-care provider. This is the time to ask your birth practitioner any questions you may have about your pregnancy or about your health in general. There's no such thing as a foolish question.

■ "Morning sickness." Nausea and, in extreme cases, vomiting occur in many pregnant women. Symptoms may last all day and into the evening, not just in the morning, and may be more severe at mealtimes. It is the most common complaint of women in early pregnancy and for many is the most uncomfortable. Symptoms usually cease at the end of the first trimester or the beginning of the second. Eating small, frequent meals and drinking water and juices throughout the day can help alleviate symptoms and prevent dehydration. Homemade ginger tea may also be useful in treating morning sickness.

In extreme cases, morning sickness can lead to weight loss and become severe enough to warrant hospitalization and/or intravenous feeding. Women should consult with their practitioners when experiencing morning sickness and weight loss.

■ Insomnia. Many women experience fatigue early in pregnancy as the body undergoes hormonal changes that can produce anxiety, resulting in difficulty sleeping. Fatigue can also be caused by stress, exhaustion, and depression. Over-the-counter sleep aids should be avoided, as they can harm the fetus. Standard drug-free remedies for sleeplessness, such as drinking a glass of warm milk, taking a warm bath, or having a massage, may help ease the insomnia. An increase in vitamin B_6 may help as well.

■ Bleeding or spotting. It not unusual to have some bleeding at the time of a missed period during the first trimester and occasional spotting throughout pregnancy. However, bleeding can also be a warning sign indicating a threatened miscarriage or ectopic pregnancy, especially when it occurs early in pregnancy. Pregnant women who experience any bleeding or spotting should consult their practitioners, who can determine whether it is minor or a symptom of serious problems.

■ Heartburn and constipation. Both heartburn and constipation are common during pregnancy. Heartburn most often occurs later in pregnancy but is also possible in the earlier stages. Constipation may be prevented by drinking eight glasses of water daily and increasing the amount of fiber in the diet. Women should consult their practitioners about treatments for either condition.

Some complications that may arise during the first trimester are:

■ Miscarriage. Also called spontaneous abortion, miscarriage occurs in 20 percent of pregnancies, and most often takes place between the sixth and 10th weeks. The most common causes of miscarriage are fetal abnormality, maternal hormonal imbalance, and anatomical defects of the uterus. Symptoms include slight bleeding or spotting, severe abdominal pain, severe cramps, and dizziness. Women experiencing any of these symptoms should consult their practitioners.

■ Ectopic, or tubal, pregnancy. An ectopic pregnancy occurs when the fertilized egg begins to develop outside the uterus, most often in a fallopian tube. This serious condition always results in the loss of the fetus and may result in death for the woman. Ectopic pregnancies happen in about 2 percent of all pregnancies. Warning signs include cramps and spotting early in pregnancy and, subsequently, more bleeding; shoulder pain; dizziness; and severe lower abdominal pain. If a woman has these symptoms, she should seek emergency care immediately.

THE SECOND TRIMESTER

The second trimester is often comfortable for the woman, as the discomforts felt in the first trimester have passed. Around this time, the growth of the pregnancy can be seen by others. Many women take on the "radiant glow" of pregnancy—caused not only by excitement but by an increased level of hormones that affects the skin. Women should become aware of the painless Braxton Hicks contractions, which may occur during this trimester and are often mistaken for the beginnings of labor.

Again, while many women have no difficulties, some common problems that occur during the second trimester are:

■ Edema, water retention that causes swelling of the feet and ankles

■ Nosebleeds and nasal congestion

■ Hemorrhoids and varicose veins

■ Leg cramps

■ Forgetfulness

■ Flatulence

■ Breast enlargement and discharge

■ Increased salivation and perspiration

Complications that may occur during the second trimester are:

■ Cervical incompetence. This is an abnormality of the cervix that prevents it from keeping the fetus securely within the uterus during pregnancy. Instead of remaining closed, the cervix dilates (widens). This condition may induce premature labor and may be the result of a malformation or a trauma to the cervix. Malformation has a higher incidence in DES daughters, women who were exposed in utero to the drug diethylstilbestrol.

With treatment, most women with this condition can carry their pregnancies to full term.

PRENATAL SELF-CARE

It is critical that you follow a healthful lifestyle while you are pregnant. Eating a nutritious diet and exercising regularly—in normal pregnancies if your practitioner approves—are vital to the health and well-being of both yourself and your fetus.

Here are some tips to help you get started on the right track:

■ Eat a well-balanced diet. Aim for a diet that includes foods high in nutrients but low in fat.

■ Make sure you get enough vitamins and minerals. Since it may be difficult to get these from foods alone, talk to your practitioner about prenatal vitamin and mineral supplements. The following list outlines the minimal vitamin and mineral needs of pregnant women, according to the National Research Council:

Protein (grams)	60
Vitamin A (micrograms)	800
Vitamin D (micrograms)	10
Vitamin E (milligrams)	10
Vitamin K (micrograms)	65
Vitamin C (milligrams)	70
Thiamin (milligrams)	1.5
Riboflavin (milligrams)	1.6
Niacin (milligrams)	17
Vitamin B_6 (milligrams)	2.2
Folic acid (micrograms)	400
Vitamin B_{12} (micrograms)	2.2
Calcium (milligrams)	1,200
Phosphorus (milligrams)	1,200
Magnesium (milligrams)	320
Iron (milligrams)	30
Zinc (milligrams)	15
Iodine (micrograms)	175
Selenium (micrograms)	65

Folic acid, a B vitamin (folate) found in broccoli, spinach, bok choy, and peppers, is important. Studies have shown this important B vitamin (also known as folate) can reduce the risk of birth defects of the spine and brain by about 60 percent.

■ Stop smoking. Smoking can cause birth defects and inhibit the fetus's growth. Women who smoke are more likely to give birth to low-birth-weight babies, and sudden infant death syndrome risk is 10 times greater for their children than for the children of nonsmokers.

■ Reach a healthy weight. Women who are underweight have a higher risk of giving birth to premature, underweight babies, and those who are overweight have an increased chance of developing gesta-

Practitioners may recommend bed rest or a **cerclage:** the surgical closing of the cervix with a suture. If not treated, cervical incompetence usually results in a miscarriage occurring most often in the second trimester.

■ Gestational hypertension. Temporary high blood pressure that develops in the woman after the 20th week of pregnancy is called gestational hypertension. Elevated blood pressure can be a sign of **preeclampsia,** a toxic condition occurring late in pregnancy. Gestational hypertension occurs more frequently in women aged 35 or over.

■ Preeclampsia (toxemia of pregnancy). Symptoms occur after week 20 and consist of high blood pressure, hand and facial swelling,

tional diabetes. Dieting for weight loss is not recommended during pregnancy.

■ Reduce or eliminate alcohol and caffeine intake. Alcohol can cause fetal alcohol syndrome, a combination of birth defects, while caffeine has been linked with an increased risk of miscarriage when consumed during pregnancy.

■ Increase fluid intake. It is recommended that women drink at least eight glasses of chemical-free water daily and increase the amount of fiber in their diets to help eliminate constipation.

■ Exercise. According to several studies, women who are in good cardiovascular health and who exercise regularly during pregnancy give birth to healthier babies and have easier labors and fewer back problems. They also get back to their prepregnancy weight more quickly.

The American College of Obstetricians and Gynecologists recommends low-impact exercises such as walking or swimming for about 45 minutes at least three times a week. Strenuous exercise and competitive games are discouraged, and the following guidelines should be adhered to:

■ Avoid deep, unsupported stretching.

■ Avoid bouncing, jerky, or twisting movements.

■ Avoid rapid changes in direction or speed.

■ Exercise on an exercise pad, not on bare wooden or carpeted flooring.

■ Do not exercise in hot, humid weather or when feverish.

■ Avoid hot tubs, steam rooms, or suanas, as these will increase body temperature and heart rate.

■ Do not exercise in high altitudes.

In addition, pregnant women should follow these recommendations when exercising:

■ Do not exceed a maternal heart rate of 140 beats per minute.

■ Do not exceed 15 minutes of strenuous activity.

■ Do not perform any exercise while lying on your back after the fourth month is completed.

■ Avoid exercises involving strong bearing-down.

■ Intake adequate calories to meet the extra energy required of pregnancy and exercise.

■ Do not exceed a maternal core temperature of 99.6°F.

and protein in the urine. These signs may develop over several days or quickly over 24 hours, and women with these symptoms should seek emergency care immediately, especially if the symptoms progress. Left untreated, the condition may become more severe, leading to eclampsia. **Eclampsia** is characterized by convulsions and sometimes coma. Preeclampsia occurs in about 5 percent of pregnancies, according to experts. Risk factors for preeclampsia include first pregnancy, an age of under 20 or over 40, and a history of high blood pressure, vascular disease, and kidney problems. Women at risk should consult with their practitioners about a more frequent testing schedule for blood pressure, urine sampling, and other diagnostic tests.

■ Gestational diabetes. A temporary form of diabetes called gestational diabetes may develop in normally nondiabetic women late in the second trimester or early in the third. Only 1 to 3 percent of cases of gestational diabetes put pregnancy at serious risk, according to experts.

■ Rh disease. The Rh factor, which can be detected through prenatal screening, is an antigen. It is a substance that stimulates an immune response in those without the factor, and is found in the red blood cells of most men and women who have blood described as Rh-positive. Those without the factor are known as Rh-negative.

Rh incompatibility occurs when the woman is Rh-negative and her fetus is Rh-positive (because the fetus may have inherited the partner's Rh-positive factor). If any of the fetus's Rh-positive blood cells enter the woman's bloodstream, the woman's body reacts to the Rh-positive blood cells by forming antibodies. During this first exposure, the fetus is rarely affected. However, during a subsequent pregnancy, the preexisting maternal antibodies will attack and destroy the fetus's blood cells. As early as four months into the subsequent pregnancy, such Rh incompatibility can result in fetal death by erythroblastosis, a type of anemia.

When both parents are Rh-negative, there is no threat of incompatibility. If the woman is Rh-negative and her partner is Rh-positive (or Rh status is not known), the woman's blood should be tested for Rh antibodies. If she has no antibodies against the Rh factor, she should have a preventive vaccine of Rh immunoglobulin at 28 weeks of pregnancy and again within 72 hours of delivery.

Treatment is necessary if antibodies appear at any point during the pregnancy. Fetuses found to be threatened by Rh incompatibility may be treated with a blood transfusion in which their blood supply is replaced with Rh-negative blood. The blood may be injected directly into the woman's abdomen or through the umbilical cord.

THE THIRD TRIMESTER

The third trimester of pregnancy lasts from week 27 through week 40. During this period, the shape of the abdomen changes a few weeks before the onset of labor as the fetus drops (usually headfirst) to or through the opening of the pelvis.

Complications that may occur during the third trimester include:

■ *Abruptio placentae* (or premature placental separation). The placenta partially or fully detaches from the uterine wall prior to the delivery of the baby. It is more likely to occur in women with high blood pressure or who use illicit drugs, such as cocaine. Warning signs are bleeding and cramping, which can be mild or severe.

■ *Placenta previa.* The placenta is abnormally low in the uterus, partially or fully covering the opening of the cervix. This happens when the fertilized egg becomes implanted in the lower half of the uterus rather than the upper half. *Placenta previa* occurs in one in 200 to 250 pregnancies. It can result in premature birth or stillbirth, depending on the severity; a cesarean delivery may be necessary in some cases. The signs of placenta previa are painless vaginal bleeding.

■ Preterm (premature) labor. When labor begins between weeks 20 and 37 of pregnancy, it is called preterm, or premature. Warning signs include contractions, backache, pelvic pressure, spotting, or bleeding. Some risk factors are in utero DES exposure, an abnormality in the uterus, and a history of premature delivery.

■ Premature rupture of membranes. Amniotic fluid leakage before the onset of labor indicates premature rupture of membranes. This condition may be followed by premature labor. If labor doesn't begin prematurely, bed rest and careful monitoring may be recommended. Whenever rupture of membranes occurs, the woman should immediately notify her practitioner. If this occurs prematurely, she should go directly to the hospital.

■ Postmaturity. When pregnancy extends past the point when the fetus is fully mature and able to survive outside of the womb (after 42 completed weeks), it is considered postmature. Practitioners may do testing, induce labor, or wait for labor to occur spontaneously, depending on the individual case and the number of days past the expected date of confinement.

SEE abortion; AIDS/HIV; birth defects; childbirth—choosing a practitioner; childbirth interventions; childbirth settings; miscarriage; pregnancy, ectopic; pregnancy—preconception concerns; pregnancy—prenatal testing.

For more information on prenatal care or concerns, contact:

Be Healthy
R.R. 1, Box 172
Glenview Rd.
Waitsfield, VT 05673
800-433-5523

Boston Women's Health Information Center
Davis Square
240A Elm St., 3rd Floor
Somerville, MA 02144
617-625-0271

Circle Solutions, Inc.
[formerly the Maternal and Child Health Clearinghouse]
2070 Chainbridge Rd., Suite 450
Vienna, VA 22182
703-821-8955

National Perinatal Association
3500 E. Fletcher Ave., Suite 209
Tampa, FL 33613
813-971-1008
npaonline@aol.com

Planned Parenthood Federation of America, Inc.
810 Seventh Avenue
New York, NY 10019
For the Planned Parenthood nearest you, call:
800-230-PLAN
http://www.ppfa.org/ppfa

PREGNANCY—
PRENATAL TESTING

Prenatal testing offers a woman the chance to evaluate the health of her pregnancy. The tests can be invaluable, detecting not only the gender and position of the fetus, but multiple pregnancies and some genetic and chromosomal abnormalities that may be present. This knowledge and accurate information allow proper counseling and preparation for the future parents.

With such information, the pregnancy can be monitored, and some problems can be promptly treated. Transfusions may be done to rectify an Rh incompatibility. Gene therapy procedures are being developed that may be used to correct chromosomal defects, such as those that cause cystic fibrosis. Prenatal testing that indicates a severe birth defect or a condition that threatens the life of the woman gives the woman the option of terminating the pregnancy.

There are roughly 250 disorders and diseases that can be diagnosed using prenatal testing, though many of them cannot be treated. Physicians also use the procedures to monitor certain complications as well as the growth and progress of the child. The primary prenatal tests are **alpha-fetoprotein screening, alpha plus screening, amniocentesis, chorionic villus sampling,** and **ultrasound.**

Tests for **structural disorders,** such as alpha-fetoprotein screening and ultrasound, can recognize abnormalities of the neural tube, the fetal structure that develops into the brain and spinal cord. Neural tube disorders include spina bifida, where the vertebrae fail to close and the spinal cord is exposed, and anencephaly, incomplete development of the brain.

Tests for **genetic and chromosomal disorders,** including alpha plus screening and chorionic villus sampling, can detect abnormalities such as Down syndrome, Rh disease, hemophilia, and Tay-Sachs disease. Some tests, such as amniocentesis, can detect both structural and genetic disorders.

The testing procedures are usually recommended in high-risk pregnancies. Though there is potential for birth defects in any pregnancy, the following factors in the woman increase the chances of problems and may prompt testing:

■ An age of more than 35

■ A family history of a genetically inherited disease or defect

■ Previous pregnancies with complications

■ Chronic disease, such as diabetes, epilepsy, or high blood pressure

■ Exposure to teratogens—drugs, medications, and other environmental factors known to possibly cause birth defects

ALPHA-FETOPROTEIN SCREENING

Alpha-fetoprotein screening is done at 15 to 20 weeks of pregnancy to detect levels of alpha-fetoprotein (AFP) in the woman's bloodstream. AFP is a chemical present in the neural tube of the fetus, the structure that develops into the brain and spinal cord. If the neural tube is abnormal, the AFP escapes and may result in higher levels of AFP in the woman's blood. Though genetic abnormalities cannot be detected with this screening, a low level of AFP has been associated in some cases with Down syndrome.

The screening is done with a simple maternal blood test. There is a 20 percent chance the test will miss a neural tube defect. In addition, only one out of 25 abnormal screens indicates an actual neural tube defect. AFP levels vary naturally according to the number of fetuses and their gestational ages. When there is a multiple pregnancy, or when the dates of pregnancy are inaccurate, the AFP readings may seem too high and cause misleading results.

A second AFP screening is usually done to verify the initial results. If the results are abnormal, the next step is an examination that verifies the gestational age of the fetus and determines if there is a multiple pregnancy. Once this is verified, an ultrasound can be done to visualize most neural tube defects. An amniocentesis should be offered as the definitive test for neural tube defects. If any structural abnormalities are found, a chromosomal analysis should be done.

ALPHA PLUS OR TRIPLE SCREENING

The alpha plus or triple screening examination measures the alpha-fetoprotein, estriol, and human chorionic gonadotropin levels of the woman with a simple blood test. That information, along with the woman's age, weight, pregnancy dates, and results from a diabetes test, is analyzed by a computer which estimates the risk of Down syndrome and other genetic abnormalities.

Alpha plus may be used to help to decide whether amniocentesis is necessary. If the results show a risk of birth defects equivalent to or higher than that of a 35-year-old woman, then amniocentesis may be recommended. According to a 1993 article in the *Medical Post,* alpha plus is expected to diagnose 70 percent of Down syndrome cases and 70 percent of neural tube defects.

AMNIOCENTESIS

Amniocentesis is a procedure in which a needle is inserted through the woman's abdomen into the uterus and amniotic sac, the fluid-filled membrane that houses the fetus. Using ultrasound to guide the needle, a small amount of amniotic fluid is withdrawn for analysis. The test is usually done between 15 and 20 weeks of pregnancy. Local anesthesia can be used. Results of the test are available in 10 to 14 days.

The gender of the fetus, as well as many birth defects, including neural tube disorders and Down syndrome, can be detected using amniocentesis. The procedure is also used to monitor the fetal condition when a fetus has been affected by Rh disease in an Rh-negative woman.

Amniocentesis can cause minor complications, such as cramping, spotting, and the leakage of fluid into the vagina. There is also the risk of serious problems, such as infection, spontaneous abortion (miscarriage), maternal hemorrhage, and fetal injury if the needle strikes the fetus. Experts say the risk of such serious complications is about one in 200.

Because the test is not done until week 15 of the pregnancy, and results can take 10 to 14 days, women who consider terminating the pregnancy based on amniocentesis results may face a second-trimester abortion.

CHORIONIC VILLUS SAMPLING (CVS)

Considered by some to be an alternative to amniocentesis, chorionic villus sampling involves collecting a small sample of chorionic villi, the fingerlike projections of the amniotic sac that later develop into the placenta. The American College of Obstetricians and Gynecologists (ACOG) recommends that CVS be performed between nine and 12 weeks of pregnancy.

There are two types of CVS, both performed with the guidance of ultrasound imaging equipment. In transcervical CVS, a thin tube is passed into the vagina and through the cervix to obtain the sample. With transabdominal CVS, a needle is inserted through the abdomen to obtain chorionic villus tissue.

Chorionic villus sampling can detect genetic disorders, such as Down syndrome, but not neural tube disorders. Results of the sampling are available within three to four days. It can be done earlier in pregnancy than amniocentesis.

The risks of CVS include cramping, spotting, and the leakage of fluid into the vagina. More serious complications are uterine infection, spontaneous abortion (miscarriage), maternal hemorrhage, and fetal injury. Studies show that the rate of miscarriage after CVS is .6 percent higher than after amniocentesis. (This means that for every 200 procedures of CVS performed, one more miscarriage will occur than with the same number of amniocentesis procedures.) CVS before nine weeks of pregnancy has also been linked to fetal limb deformities, thought to be caused by the trauma of the procedure during a crucial developmental period.

ULTRASOUND

With this technique, sound waves are "bounced" off the bones and tissues of the fetus to construct pictures, called sonograms, that show its shape and position. The ultrasound is done by passing a scanner, called a transducer, back and forth over the abdomen. A computer is used to translate the echoes into an image on a television monitor.

Routine ultrasound for women with low-risk pregnancies is performed after 16 weeks to see how the fetus is developing. It can reveal the number, gender, and gestational age of the fetus (or fetuses) as well as any major structural defects. The test cannot detect genetic or chromosomal disorders, such as Down syndrome. Ultrasound is also used during amniocentesis and chorionic villus sampling to provide an image of the needle as it is guided into the amniotic sac.

While ultrasound is considered a routine prenatal test for women with low-risk pregnancies, studies have shown that it does not have any real benefit for the fetus. However, the test may lay to rest a woman's fears about the health of the fetus or give her the option to choose abortion in the event of defects.

In high-risk pregnancies, ultrasound is recommended for many situations. It is used to detect ectopic pregnancies and can be employed after a threatened miscarriage to tell whether the fetus is still alive. It can be used to assess the fetus, monitor growth, and examine the placenta. There are no known risks that accompany ultrasound.

A variation of the test is *vaginal ultrasound,* in which a probe is inserted into the vagina to scan the uterus. Vaginal ultrasound is usually used for complications of pregnancy that occur in the first three months.

SEE abortion; birth defects; pregnancy—prenatal concerns.

PREMENSTRUAL SYNDROME

About 20 to 50 percent of all women of childbearing age suffer from some degree of premenstrual syndrome (PMS). PMS, also known as premenstrual tension or congestive dysmenorrhea, is the monthly occurrence of one or more symptoms during the week before or the first few days of menstruation.

PMS occurs in teenage girls, but it is more common in women over 30, especially those approaching menopause. In 10 percent of those women who have it, PMS causes severe symptoms that can interrupt work or other daily activities.

SYMPTOMS

There are at least 150 symptoms of PMS, both physical and psychological, with varying occurrences and intensity. Symptoms can be loosely classified into four groups:

■ Breast tenderness and/or enlargement. Prior to menstruation, breast tissue prepares for a possible pregnancy following ovulation. This can make breasts enlarged and sore.

■ Fluid retention and abdominal bloating. Higher levels of estrogen in the body inhibit the normal flushing of water from the body, so less water taken in during this time is eliminated. The water gradually accumulates in cells and body tissues and may cause weight gain. Fluid retention may also cause fingers and ankles to swell.

■ Appetite changes and carbohydrate craving

■ Premenstrual tension. This includes depression (from mild mood swings to manic despair), tiredness, irritability, increased anger, anxiety, and frustration.

Other symptoms of PMS are: backaches, nightmares, insomnia, constipation, sweating, breathing difficulties, shakiness, urinary difficulties, and a heightened sensitivity to noises, odors, and touch. PMS also intensifies certain ailments, such as asthma, migraine headaches, vaginal yeast infections, and rheumatoid arthritis.

Some women do report *positive* premenstrual changes, including increased creativity, energy, and sexual interest.

CAUSES OF PREMENSTRUAL SYNDROME

The precise cause of premenstrual syndrome is still unknown. Many scientists believe it is a disorder of the reproductive endocrine system that occurs when progesterone levels peak to prepare for a potential pregnancy, sometime during the week prior to menstruation. Another possible cause involves a brain chemical called serotonin, a substance that calms and gives a feeling of well-being. Some studies have linked low levels of serotonin, associated with ovulation, to depression. Some experts also feel PMS may be inherited by a woman from her mother.

TREATING PMS

At one time, PMS was considered an imaginary or psychological illness, and some practitioners still see it that way. Although it is far from being understood, most practitioners now regard PMS as

✓ TO HELP PREVENT OR ALLEVIATE PMS

■ Keep a chart. Before you can treat PMS, you must determine that you have it. To diagnose PMS, keep a monthly record of physical and emotional changes. If the symptoms are present every month for at least three months, if they occur premenstrually and do not start before ovulation, and if they disappear completely for a minimum of seven days after menstruation, you are likely to have PMS.

■ Eat a high-complex-carbohydrate, low-fat diet. Carbohydrates increase brain serotonin levels, reducing mood swings. In addition, a low-salt diet reduces bloating. Eating "mini-meals" (six a day) will maintain the mood-enhancing effect of carbohydrate consumption, which lasts two to three hours after eating. Avoid simple sugars, as found in candy, table sugar, and honey. This may be difficult because many women desire sweets premenstrually.

■ Exercise. Aerobic activity can minimize and even eliminate many PMS symptoms. By raising your body temperature, you can help regulate the production of the hormones estrogen and progesterone in your body. For best results, aerobic exercise should raise your heart rate above 120 beats per minute for 20 to 30 minutes, three to four times weekly.

■ Reduce caffeine and alcohol intake. Caffeine increases irritability, anxiety, and mood swings and may increase breast tenderness in some women. Alcohol, which may affect some premenstrual women more quickly, can also make you more emotional.

■ Try herbal remedies. Evening primrose oil, catnip, vitex (agnus castus), mugwort, spearmint, and valerian are among those remedies thought to be effective. Consult an herbal therapist before beginning treatment.

■ Relax. All PMS symptoms are aggravated by stress. Relaxation and meditation exercises, including yoga and massage, can ease PMS symptoms.

a temporary hormonal disorder that can be treated with self-help techniques. For a severe case, there are several options available from a practitioner. Oral contraceptives may be used to lessen the symptoms in some women. Diuretics, medications that help eliminate water from the body, can be prescribed to relieve bloating. Treatments also include vitamins and minerals (including B_6, magnesium, and omega-6 fatty acids), tranquilizers, and progestin. Prozac, an antidepressant, is currently being used to treat PMS. Possibilities should be discussed with a practitioner.

SEE menstrual cycle and ovulation; migraine headache.

For more information on PMS, contact:

PMS Access
P.O. Box 259641
Madison, WI 53725
800-558-7046
608-257-8682
http://womenshealth.com

RADIATION THERAPY

Radiation therapy uses high-energy rays or radioactive materials to destroy the reproductive material, called DNA, of cancerous cells and inhibit their ability to grow and multiply. In radiation therapy, high-energy x-rays or radioactive cobalt (a radioactive material) produces ionizing radiation that is used to destroy the DNA of cancerous cells. Radioactive minerals, such as phosphorus, gold, iodine, and radium, are also used. Radiation may be used to treat most forms of cancer. Almost half of all cancer patients undergo radiation therapy, alone or in combination with another treatment.

Administered internally or externally by an expert known as a radiation oncologist, radiation therapy may be used to help shrink a tumor to make its surgical removal easier. It may also be used after surgery to destroy remaining cells, or in place of surgery when a tumor cannot be removed. It is also used as a palliative therapy to treat the symptoms of incurable cancer. Radiation therapy is often used in conjunction with chemotherapy to destroy cancerous cells, especially in the treatment of breast cancer.

EXTERNAL RADIATION TREATMENT

The most common form of radiation therapy, external radiation, is administered through a high-powered x-ray machine known as a **linear accelerator.** The machine creates an invisible beam of electrons that is directed to the site of the cancer. Radiation therapy is a local therapy and should affect only the cells that are in the treated area.

It may be administered through a hospital's outpatient service or clinic. The dosage and length of radiation therapy depend on the type of cancer being treated and its stage. The average dosage is about two to four minutes of radiation for five consecutive days each week over a period of two to eight weeks.

INTERNAL RADIATION TREATMENT

Internal radiation is administered through radioactive implants placed inside the body, usually inside a body cavity (such as the vagina) or within a tumor. Internal radiation is administered in the hospital. Implants are usually left in place for a number of days, and the treatment may be repeated several times over the course of two weeks depending on the type of cancer and its stage.

SIDE EFFECTS OF RADIATION

Side effects of radiation therapy include:
- Loss of appetite
- Nausea and vomiting
- Fatigue
- Sunburnlike reddening and blistering of the skin. Fair-skinned individuals are affected by this more than those with darker skin.

Other side effects vary greatly according to where the radiation is administered. For example, patients who are treated in the upper chest

MENOPAUSE CAUSED BY RADIATION THERAPY

Women who undergo radiation therapy in the pelvic area may experience medically induced menopause, a condition in which the ovaries stop functioning either temporarily or permanently. A woman may experience a sudden onset of menopausal symptoms, such as hot flashes, vaginal dryness, ceased periods, depression, and mood swings, or she may develop these symptoms more gradually, depending on the type of treatment administered and its dosage.

In rare situations, a surgical procedure called **oophoropexy** may be done to actu-ally move the ovaries away from the treatment area and the effects of the radiation. When the treatment is completed, the ovaries are moved back into place. This procedure is not beneficial if the radiation is combined with chemotherapy because the chemotherapy will adversely affect the ovaries regardless of where they are located.

It is important to discuss the effects of treatment and the possible menopausal symptoms that may occur with a gynecologic oncologist, a specialist in treating cancer of the female reproductive organs.

---

or throat area experience an extremely dry, sore throat, and patients with lung cancer may develop a very dry cough or sputum. Antiemetics (antinausea drugs) may be used to reduce nausea and vomiting, and skin creams may be used to soothe burned skin.

RISKS OF RADIATION

Exposure to radiation always injures some normal tissue and is not without its risks, though they are very difficult to determine with certainty. The Food and Drug Administration, through its Center for Devices and Radiological Health, attempts to set standards for exposure to radiation equipment.

Radiation exposure is measured in "rem," a unit that describes the biological effects on a person from a dose of radiation. One rem equals 1,000 millirems (mrem). The average person is exposed to background (naturally occurring) radiation of roughly 300 mrem per year, with 200 mrem from environmental radon alone.

The amount of radiation a person receives from medical sources is dependent on a number of factors: the type of equipment, strength of radiation field generated, duration and exposure, and amount of shielding used. Doses of more than 100 rem when received by large portions of the body will cause **acute radiation syndrome,** and symptoms such as nausea and vomiting begin to appear. As the doses reach even higher levels, serious problems, such as infection, fever, hemorrhage, loss of hair, diarrhea, and loss of body fluids, may occur, as well as injury or death to the skin, mucous membranes, and bone marrow.

SEE cancer; chemotherapy; specific cancers.

For more information on radiation therapy, contact:

American Cancer Society
1599 Clifton Rd., N.E.
Atlanta, GA 30329
800-ACS-2345
404-320-3333
http:\\www.cancer.org

**American Society for Therapeutic Radiology
and Oncology**
American College for Radiology
1891 Preston White Dr.
Reston, VA 22091
703-648-8900
http:\\www.acr.org

ChemoCare
231 North Ave., W.
Westfield, NJ 07090-1482
800-55-CANCER
908-233-1103 (New Jersey)
   Offers support for those undergoing
   radiation and chemotherapy treatments.

Radiation Research Society
2021 Spring Rd., Suite 600
Oak Park, IL 60521
708-571-2881
http:\\www.cjp.com\radres\

REPETITIVE MOTION INJURIES

A number of musculoskeletal disorders are grouped under the heading "repetitive motion injuries" (RMIs), or "repetitive strain injuries." These disorders include **carpal tunnel syndrome, tendinitis, tenosynovitis,** and **"tennis elbow."** They generally occur as a result of activities in which the fingers and wrists are moving and bending, or being held in an awkward position, for long periods of time. This can cause inflammation of the tissue surrounding the bones, putting painful pressure on nerves. There may also be pain in the head and neck.

RMIs are more common among women than men, possibly because women are more likely to have jobs, such as typing or using a cash register or calculator, that require small, repetitive movements. A recent study from the U.S. National Institute of Occupational Safety and Health (NIOSH) reported that one in five employees who used a video display terminal suffered repetitive strain injuries.

CARPAL TUNNEL SYNDROME

Some 35 percent of those with jobs requiring repetitive movements get carpal tunnel syndrome, and 30 percent of those with carpal tunnel get it in both hands at the same time. It occurs when the tissues covering the tendons in the fingers become inflamed, putting pressure on the main nerve in the wrist. Carpal tunnel may also occur during and after pregnancy and while breast-feeding. At these times, high hormone levels lead to edema (water retention and swelling), which can put more pressure on the nerves. Weight gain and arthritis may also contribute.

351

✓ TO PREVENT REPETITIVE MOTION INJURIES

■ Be sure you are sitting in a comfortable position. A computer keyboard, ideally, should be 26 to 28 inches from the floor (the average desk is 30 to 32 inches from the floor). You should sit 14 to 24 inches from the computer screen. The screen should be positioned so that the top of the screen is 10 degrees below eye level. The middle of the screen should be 20 degrees below eye level.

■ Take frequent breaks from your computer, cash register, or workstation if your job puts you at risk for injuries. The Washington State Department of Labor and Industries prevents video display terminal workers from typing for more than an hour at a time and for more than five hours a day. Try switching to a different, non-repetitive task for a change.

■ If your job puts you at risk for repetitive motion injuries, discuss your options with your supervisor. Find out if you can get a new desk or computer, or discuss redesigning tools or workstations so that they won't strain your wrists and arms. Make arrangements to trade jobs for a few hours a day with a coworker who has a different kind of job.

Symptoms of carpal tunnel include pain in the wrists and arms, a burning sensation, the feeling of "pins and needles," and numbness. Treatment consists of nonsteroidal anti-inflammatory drugs (NSAIDs), such as ibuprofen, and a wrist splint to rest the joint. Weight loss and diuretics (medications that help the body rid itself of water) may help the condition. Treatment of arthritis may also help.

In severe cases, surgery may be necessary. The procedure cuts the ligament of the wrist to relieve pressure on the nerve. While at one time this procedure required six to eight weeks of recovery, now the stitches may be removed in as little as $1^1/_2$ weeks.

OTHER FORMS OF RMI

Tennis elbow, which occurs most often in tennis players, is the result of constant rotary motions of the forearm as the hand and wrist remain in the same position. The movements inflame the tendons on the outside of the elbow because of the constant irritation of the twisting and rotating, and cause pain near the elbow joint. This condition may be treated by putting the forearm in a splint so that it may rest or by applying moist heat. **Tendinitis** is the inflammation of tissue that attaches the muscles to the bone. **Tenosynovitis** is inflammation of the membranes that line the joints of the body. Both may be treated with NSAIDs and rest. Massage therapy may be a useful treatment.

For more information on repetitive motion injuries, contact:

U.S. National Institute of Occupational Safety and Health
Department of Health and Human Resources
4676 Columbia Pkwy.
Cincinnati, OH 45226
800-356-4674
http://www.cdc.gov/niosh/homepage.html

REPRODUCTIVE SYSTEM AND SEX ORGANS OF THE WOMAN

EXTERNAL SEX ORGANS

The external sex organs are contained in an area known as the **vulva.** The **outer lips** (labia majora) and the **inner lips** (labia minora) form soft folds that protect the opening of the **urethra,** the passage through which urine leaves the body, and the opening of the vagina. The urethra is not a sex organ, though it is located in the vulva.

The lips also protect the **clitoris,** a highly sensitive organ about the size of a pea, which is located just above the opening of the urethra. The clitoris, which has specialized nerve endings, swells during sexual arousal and is a source of sexual pleasure when stimulated.

Also located in the vulva are the **Bartholin's glands,** located on each side of the vaginal opening, and the **Skene's glands,** which are on each side of the opening to the urethra. The glands secrete fluids that provide lubrication during sexual excitement.

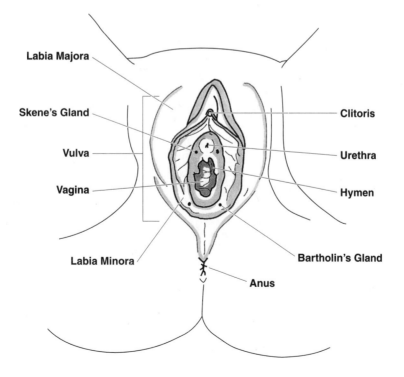

Labia Majora

Skene's Gland

Vulva

Vagina

Labia Minora

Clitoris

Urethra

Hymen

Bartholin's Gland

Anus

INTERNAL REPRODUCTIVE ORGANS

The internal reproductive organs of the woman are the vagina, the cervix, the uterus (commonly known as the womb), the fallopian tubes, and the ovaries. These organs are supported by the pelvic girdle, a structure of bones and muscles shaped like a basin.

VAGINA

The **vagina** is a passage four to five inches long between the vulva and the cervix, the opening of the uterus. The opening of the vagina is located behind the urethra and in front of the **anus,** the opening through which stool passes from the body.

During vaginal intercourse, the vagina receives the penis. It is also the path by which the menstrual flow leaves the body, and it serves as the birth canal. The vagina is lined by a smooth surface that contains many mucous glands and is supported by muscle and fibro-elastic tissue that can accommodate and respond to sexual and reproductive needs.

The **hymen** is a stretchable membrane, about $1/8$ inch thick, that stretches across the opening of the vagina. The opening of the hymen varies in size, and the hymen may be "torn" by the entry of the penis into the vagina during the first sexual intercourse, causing slight bleeding. The presence or absence of bleeding is not a sign of virginity because of the great anatomical variations and since it may be stretched by exercise or use of tampons before first intercourse takes place. In addition, some women are born without an intact hymen.

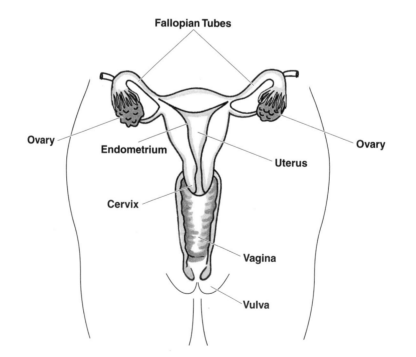

Fallopian Tubes

Ovary

Endometrium

Ovary

Uterus

Cervix

Vagina

Vulva

CERVIX

The cervix is the part of the uterus that projects into the vagina. The cervix contains glands that aid conception by providing mucus. The mucus is greater in volume, thinner, and more favorable to sperm just prior to and at ovulation so that the man's sperm can easily swim toward the egg in the fallopian tube. The secretions of the cervix also act to block many infectious agents from causing uterine infections.

UTERUS

The uterus is a hollow, muscular organ suspended by ligaments in the pelvic girdle. Its triangular interior, lined by the **endometrium,** can hold about a teaspoonful of liquid. Roughly the shape of a small pear, the uterus is about three inches long and weighs about two ounces. After conception, the fertilized egg attaches to the wall of the uterus, where it can develop into an embryo and then a fetus. The muscles of the uterus contract during labor, while the cervix opens, allowing for the delivery of the fetus.

The endometrium thickens each month with a network of intricate blood vessels and tissues. This growth is stimulated by the hormones estrogen and, after ovulation, progesterone, which are released from the ovaries.

If a fertilized egg (known as a **zygote, blastocyst,** or **preembryo**) does not implant in the uterus, the endometrium breaks down. The resulting blood and tissues flow through the cervix and vagina and out of the body. Known as **menses, menstruation,** or the **menstrual period,** the flow lasts from three to seven days. Only about three to four tablespoons of the flow are blood; the rest is fluid and tissue.

Pregnancy begins when a preembryo attaches to the endometrium. It is from the endometrium that the growing embryo, which develops into the fetus, will receive food until the **placenta,** an organ that develops from the outer layer of the fertilized egg, forms to nourish it.

During pregnancy, the capacity of the uterus increases by 500 times, and its muscles become much stronger. It grows in size and weight so that it can sustain the labors of birth.

FALLOPIAN TUBES

There are two fallopian tubes, one on each side of the uterus. Each tube extends from the top of the uterus and ends near one of the ovaries. These two $3\frac{1}{2}$-inch, spaghetti-thin tubes are supported by a curtain of tissues containing blood vessels. The tubes receive the eggs that are released by the ovary at the time of ovulation. Contractions of the fallopian tubes and the movements of small, hairlike structures (cilia) within the tubes propel the egg toward the uterus. The fallopian tubes also provide a place for fertilization of the egg to take place.

OVARIES

The two almond-shaped ovaries hang by ligaments to each side of the uterus and to the walls on either side of the pelvis. They are about $1\frac{1}{4}$ inches long and, together, weigh about one-quarter ounce. The ovaries produce the female hormone estrogen as well as progesterone and a small amount of testosterone. They also house and nourish thousands of eggs, or ovum. A woman is born with all of the eggs she will ever have, about 500,000; however, only about 400 mature eggs are produced that are capable of being fertilized.

At puberty, which usually happens around the age of 12 years, a series of hormone and growth changes occurs which helps the body of a girl to develop into the body of a woman. The pelvis widens, the hips become rounded, the breasts become fuller, and pubic hair begins to grow. These changes prepare the body for childbirth.

During the first few days of the menstrual cycle, the pituitary gland secretes FSH (follicle-stimulating hormone), a hormone that stimulates several of the dormant egg cells in the ovary. One of the eggs (or perhaps more than one) is selected for ovulation during the cycle and pushes to the surface over the next two weeks. It appears as a fluid-filled follicle the size of a marble protruding from the surface of the ovary. The follicle secretes estrogen. At midcycle, the pituitary gland then secretes another hormone (LH, or luteinizing hormone) that causes the follicle around the egg to burst, and the ripe egg is picked up by the fallopian tube for transport to the uterus. If sperm are present, the egg is fertilized at this time, usually while it is in the fallopian tube. In the second half of the cycle, the ruptured follicle develops into a corpus luteum and secretes progesterone.

Between the ages of 45 and 55—the average age is 50—a woman's ovaries stop releasing eggs, her hormone production decreases, and her menstrual periods end. The end of the last period is called **menopause.** Menopause can occur at once or gradually, and affects women to varying degrees both physically and emotionally. The gradual period of change leading into menopause is called **perimenopause** or the **climacteric.**

BREASTS

While the breasts are not part of the reproductive system per se, they are closely related to the reproductive and sexual processes. The breasts contain a complex system of glands and ducts that produce milk for the newborn after pregnancy and may provide sexual plea-sure when stimulated.

During childhood, the breast tissue remains dormant; around the age of 12, hormones cause fat deposits to develop in the breasts, and they begin to swell. The nipples grow, and the areola, the halo around the nipple, takes on a heavier pigmentation. Breast development may be uneven and varies from person to person.

Each breast contains about 17 independent milk-producing units filled with microscopic alveoli that produce droplets of milk. The milk filters into branching ducts and finally into the main stem that ends at the nipple.

During pregnancy, the breasts receive hormonal stimulation from the placenta, causing the weight and size of the breasts to approximately double. When the baby is born, milk production begins. For the first few days, the fluid is yellowish and watery. This fluid, called colostrum, contains lymphocytes (disease-fighting white blood cells) and immunoglobulins (antibodies) that pass on the mother's immunities to the baby and protect it from disease. Usually on the fifth day, milk begins to flow to provide nourishment for the baby.

The breasts take glucose from the mother's blood and change it into lactose with the help of enzymes. Also brought to the baby through the breasts are minerals, especially calcium, which helps develop bone, and vitamins essential for health. Nursing provides most babies with all the necessary nourishment they need until approximately six months of age.

During menopause, as the body's production of estrogen decreases, the breasts lose some—but not all—of their fat deposits. The glandular structure of the breasts also begins to disappear, causing the breasts to lose their fullness and become smaller.

SEE breast-feeding; endocrine system; menstrual cycle and ovulation.

SAFER SEX

Enjoying sex is a normal, natural part of life. Everyone is sexual—women and men, young or old, straight or gay, married or single. However, there are risks involved in having sex, risks that include sexually transmitted infections (STIs). In fact, one out of every four people becomes infected at some time during life. **Safer sex** refers to anything done to reduce the risk of infection. By practicing safer sex, women and their partners can reduce the risk of contracting dangerous STIs while continuing to enjoy sex.

Safer sex is important to women because they are at higher risk than men for getting an STI. This is because the vagina is more easily infected than the penis and the anus. A woman's chance of being infected by a man with HIV (the virus that causes AIDS) is twice as great as a man's chance of being infected by a woman with HIV.

Women generally have fewer symptoms than men and are less likely to know if they are infected; damage may be done to the body even before symptoms develop. Sexually transmitted

NOT ALL STIS ARE TRANSMITTED THE SAME WAY

If you have **unprotected vaginal** or **anal intercourse,** you are at high risk for:
- Trichomoniasis
- Bacterial vaginosis
- Gonorrhea
- Chlamydia
- Syphilis
- Chancroid
- Human papilloma virus (HPV). Some strains of the virus cause genital warts; others are associated with cervical cancer.
- Herpes simplex virus (HSV), which can cause genital herpes
- Hepatitis B virus (HBV)
- Cytomegalovirus (CMV)
- Pubic lice
- Scabies
- Human immunodeficiency virus (HIV), which can cause AIDS

If you have **oral sex,** you are at high risk for:
- Gonorrhea
- Syphilis
- Chancroid
- Herpes simplex virus
- Hepatitis B virus
- Cytomegalovirus

If you have **sex play without sexual intercourse,** you are at high risk for:
- Herpes simplex virus
- Cytomegalovirus
- Pubic lice
- Scabies

In addition, there are many other diseases, including the flu and mononucleosis, that are also sexually transmitted.

Remember also that there is a vaccine for hepatitis B, one of the most dangerous STIs.

infections may increase the risk of ectopic pregnancy, cause sterility and birth defects, and lead to major illness and death. Some STIs cannot be cured and stay in the body a lifetime.

Partners interested in safer sex can explore different ways to turn each other on and may discover new sexual excitements. By communicating desires, and being clear about how and where they like to be touched, partners can help one another increase their sexual pleasure. Many partners find that exploring safer sex can make sex more satisfying. It can:

- Improve partner communication
- Increase intimacy
- Prolong sex play
- Enhance orgasm
- Broaden the scope of sexual pleasure
- Relieve anxiety
- Strengthen relationships

WHEN IS SEX SAFE?

If neither partner has ever had sex with anyone else, or if neither partner was ever infected with a sexually transmitted disease, there is no risk of STIs. Most people have only one partner—at a time. However, most people have several partners during a lifetime and may carry infections from one partner to another. Partners who pass on STIs may not have known they were infected or may have hoped they wouldn't infect their partners. Or they may be less than honest about their sexual history and activity.

The risk of being infected with an STI is greater when drugs and alcohol are being used. Such drugs can lower inhibitions and make it more likely that unsafe activity will take place. Feelings of embarrassment, insecurity, anger, and the desire to be swept away may also contribute to risky sexual activity because partners

are less likely to talk about practicing safer sex.

If a woman and her partner have decided to have sex with only each other, they may give up safer sex after being tested to be sure neither person is infected. Some infections, like HIV, may take years to develop symptoms. A health-care practitioner can diagnose these infections.

REDUCING THE RISKS

The most important ways for a woman to practice safer sex and reduce her risk are to:

- Keep a partner's bodily fluids—blood, semen, and preejaculate (the few drops of semen that may be present before ejaculation)—out of her own vagina, anus, and mouth.
- Avoid contact with any sores caused by STIs.

A woman should avoid sex if she has any sores caused by an STI and should keep her own bodily fluids out of her partner's body.

SAFER SEX AND SATISFACTION

There are many ways to have safer, satisfying sex. Unprotected vaginal and anal intercourse have the highest risks for the most dangerous STIs. Lower risk sex play includes:

- Masturbation and mutual masturbation
- Mutual pleasuring or "outercourse"—sex play without penetration
- Erotic massage and body rubbing
- Oral sex
- Deep kissing
- Vaginal intercourse with a condom or vaginal pouch
- Anal intercourse with a condom or vaginal pouch

CONDOMS
AND SAFER SEX

Condoms are the best protection for enjoying sexual intercourse. They can help make sex last longer, and they can help prevent premature ejaculation.

Latex condoms offer good protection against:

- Vaginitis caused by infections like trichomoniasis and bacterial vaginosis
- Pelvic inflammatory disease
- Gonorrhea
- Chlamydia
- Syphilis
- Chancroid
- Human immunodeficiency virus/AIDS

Latex condoms offer some protection against:

- Genital warts
- Herpes
- Hepatitis B virus

Vaginal pouches offer some protection against STIs as well. They allow women to take responsibility for protection against STIs, and they can be worn whether or not a man remains erect. Women should remember that most forms of birth control, such as the Pill, Norplant, Depo-Provera, diaphragms, cervical caps, and IUDs, do not protect against STIs. Spermicides offer some protection against chlamydia, gonorrhea, and trichomoniasis. They cannot be relied on to protect against viruses like HIV, herpes simplex, and human papilloma.

SEE AIDS/HIV; contraception; sexually transmitted infections.

For more information on safer sex, contact:

Planned Parenthood Federation of America, Inc.
810 Seventh Avenue
New York, NY 10019
For the Planned Parenthood nearest you, call:
    800-230-PLAN
http://www.ppfa.org/ppfa

SECOND OPINION

A second opinion is advice or thoughts from another practitioner on a diagnosis of a condition, method of treatment, or the necessity of treatment. Second opinions about suggested medical procedures are often very valuable because they help clarify the options in health care that are available. It is important for a woman to realize that she has a right to seek as many opinions as she wishes.

SEEKING A SECOND OPINION

Seeking a second opinion is common practice. A woman's practitioner may initiate the second opinion by referring the woman to another practitioner or specialist. Or the woman herself may decide to seek another practitioner's opinion on the diagnosis, treatment, and cost of treatment for the condition that concerns her. Many medical

✔ WHERE TO FIND A SECOND OPINION

A good place to begin the search for a physician who will render a second opinion is the *Official ABMS Directory of Board Certified Medical Specialists* in your local library's reference section. In addition, many local hospitals and medical societies sponsor referral or second opinion services, though their resources may be limited to doctors with facility privileges or society memberships.

Also check with your employer's benefits department or ask your insurance company to provide you with a list of physicians it uses for its second opinion program. A Medicare beneficiary may contact the local Social Security Administration office for a directory of doctors who participate in the Medicare second opinion program.

If you belong to a managed-care plan, your choice of specialists who provide second opinions may be limited. Some plans limit your choice to specialists who have contracts with the plan. Others may permit you to select the specialist of your choice; however, it may cost you an additional deductible if you go outside the plan. Always check with the plan administrator if you have any questions concerning the protocol for requesting a second opinion.

---

insurers have made second opinions mandatory before they will agree to pay for a procedure. The search for a second opinion should not be limited to procedures that involve surgery. Many types of therapy performed in a hospital are risky or invasive even though they do not involve surgery.

WHY A SECOND OPINION?

Second opinions are valuable because they can help women explore their options in health care and make informed choices. Not all practitioners agree on medical problems, how to diagnose them, and how to treat them, and clarifying options through a second opinion is important, especially if a trip to the hospital is being considered. Another view on the medical problem could help to avoid unnecessary treatment and complications. Every woman should consider finding a practitioner independently for a fair and original second opinion.

SEE medical rights; practitioners, how to choose.

SEXUAL ASSAULT

Sexual assault is any attack, verbal or physical, with sexual connotations that is inflicted on another person. There are no firm statistics on how often sexual assault occurs because so many incidents remain unreported. The National Women's Survey estimates that 683,000 rapes occur each year; however, the Department of Justice Bureau of Justice Statistics estimates only 130,000 incidents of rape each year. The National Organization for Women reports that half of all workingwomen experience some form of sexual harassment. Overwhelmingly, women and children are the victims of sexual assault, though it happens to men as well.

Rape, incest, and sexual harassment are some forms of sexual assault. Any form of sexual assault is a crime of violence, power, and control. It is not a sexual crime. It can happen any time of the day, anywhere, and to any person regardless of age, gender, race, ethnicity, disability, sexuality, or social class.

Survivors of sexual assault may feel:
- Anxiety or confusion
- Emotional shock
- Fear
- Depression
- Low self-esteem
- Shame or guilt

Victims may also experience nightmares, insomnia, sexual intimacy problems, and flashbacks. Those who have been assaulted may turn to alcohol or drugs. Victims of incest or childhood sexual assault may become victims of other abuse during their adult years. Counseling is often recommended for victims of assault.

RAPE

Rape is a violent crime that causes both physical and emotional anguish for the victim. The violation of rape is humiliating and traumatizing. It is possible that no other crime does as much damage to a woman's sense of self and well-being.

The legal definition of rape varies from state to state. In most locations, rape is considered vaginal penetration of a woman without her consent. The definition has been expanded to include oral and anal contact as well. Most important, rape is committed against another person *without that person's consent.* It is important to remember that rape is never provoked by the victim and is never the victim's fault.

A woman always has the right to say no to intercourse and have her wishes honored. It does not matter if she does not fight back or if there is no evidence of a struggle, such as bruises. Almost all rape victims experience such fear and confusion that they cannot physically fight their attacker.

ACQUAINTANCE RAPE

In 75 percent of all rapes, the victim knew her attacker as a friend or date. This is known as date rape or acquaintance rape. Most date rapes are linked to the use of alcohol and in part to a societal belief instilled in men showing that when a woman says no, she really means yes. It is common on college campuses and is of

THE PLANNED PARENTHOOD WOMEN'S HEALTH ENCYCLOPEDIA

✔ WHAT TO DO IF YOU ARE RAPED

Have someone you trust help you through the following process:

■ Contact your local rape crisis center immediately (listed in the phone book) and ask them for the best procedure for medical care, support, and police procedures. Many centers will send a representative to meet you at the emergency room to act on your behalf.

■ Get to the emergency room immediately. Don't shower, change clothes, or urinate. Don't disturb the place where the assault took place. These precautions help to preserve evidence.

■ Talk to emergency room personnel or your crisis counselor about emergency contraception, especially if you are at midcycle and aren't using another form of con-

traception. Also ask to be tested for any sexually transmitted infections, since many have no symptoms.

■ Report the crime to the police as soon as possible. Some areas allow anonymous reporting. The police may be able to arrest the rapist and preserve needed evidence, and you don't need to decide right away if you wish to prosecute. A prompt report also works in the victim's favor in the courtroom, if legal action is taken.

■ Be sure to get postrape counseling. Recovery from rape may take months— even years—and support is a necessary part of the healing. Your local hospital can put you in touch with a local domestic abuse and rape crisis center where you can find counseling and support.

---

increasing concern to workingwomen, who often travel and dine with colleagues.

Knowing the attacker is not presumed consent, even when on a date—or in the context of marriage. The influence of drugs and alcohol does not imply consent to having sex, although it often makes women vulnerable to sexual assault. If a man spends money on a date with a woman, he is not entitled to sex at the end of the night. Nor does a relationship or prior relationship with the attacker—even if he is the victim's husband or partner—imply consent. A woman also has the right to change her mind after consenting to sex.

To help prevent date rape, a woman should make her wishes and desires perfectly clear to

the man. Most colleges now recommend that men ask women for their consent at each step of a sexual relationship. Women are encouraged to be aggressive rather than compliant. Women are also advised to stay in control and not give in to the influence of alcohol or drugs.

INCEST

Incest is any sexual contact between family members who are not marital partners. It happens most often between brothers and sisters and is also common between fathers and daughters (father-daughter incest is considered criminal). As with rape, many incidents of incest are never reported. In some cases, children report their experiences but are not believed.

Depression, anxiety, isolation, low self-esteem, chronic pain, stress disorders, substance abuse, personality disorders, irritable bowel syndrome, and fear of sexual intimacy are common effects of intergenerational, nonconsensual incest. (Consensual sex play between same generational children who are related is common and may not have the damaging effects of nonconsensual incestuous relationships.) Usually, the damage is not caused by the sex act itself, but by emotional responses that may develop over the years. Counseling with a therapist or through a support group should be considered by anyone whose well-being has been jeopardized by past or continuing incestuous relationships. Counseling can also help people free themselves of incestuous relationships.

SEXUAL HARASSMENT

Sexual harassment is any unwelcome sexual advance (ranging from verbal innuendo and jokes to physical advances and rape) that is a condition of employment or education, or that makes the environment uncomfortable or hostile. It may include lewd comments, visual undressing, a pat on the behind, or touching of the breasts. While the perpetrators may feel they are being flattering, harassment can cause victims to feel violated, insulted, and inferior.

According to the law, harassment occurs when the victim must submit to sexual conduct to get a job, a promotion, admission to a school, or any related benefits. Harassment also occurs when the conduct creates a hostile workplace or educational environment that interferes with the victim's performance or participation.

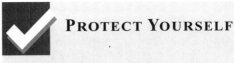

PROTECT YOURSELF

There are measures you can take to help reduce your risk of becoming a victim of rape and violent sexual assault. They include:

■ Lock the doors of your home and your car, even when you are inside.

■ Leave lights on inside and outside the house.

■ Have your house and car keys ready when going from your house to your car or your car to your house.

■ Don't list your full name in the phone book or on the mailbox if you live alone.

■ Don't walk alone, if possible. Walk at a steady pace with confidence. Stick to well-lighted, open areas. If you feel uncomfortable on the sidewalk of a lonely road, walk in the street.

■ Carry a whistle or pepper spray. If you are threatened, scream and run, if you think it will help.

■ Don't accept rides from people that you don't know well.

■ Be aware of your surroundings; look around and behind you.

■ Think about what you would do in the event of an attack. Prepare to resist your attacker.

■ Avoid getting drunk or high.

■ Don't open your door to strangers. Ask repair people, police, and utilitymen to show proper identification by slipping it under the door.

ENDING SEXUAL HARASSMENT

Women who are victims of sexual harassment should:

■ Avoid the harassers. If possible, don't work with them or go to school with them.

■ Tell the harasser how you feel. Be specific, telling him how you feel about what was said or done, and that you want him to stop.

■ Don't keep it to yourself. If the advances are happening in the workplace or at school, tell the person you are going to tell his boss. If the harasser is your boss, go over his head. Many corporations have policies on sexual harassment that can be followed.

■ Keep records of the incidents. They may be useful in stating your case.

■ If necessary, take legal action. Sexual harassment is becoming more recognized by society as a crime. Often, going public with an accusation brings other women forward who were victims.

■ Don't take the blame. Victims of sexual harassment are often thought to have provoked the advances by dressing a certain way or staying late at the office. However, harassment is more likely a tool of power and control than of sex.

SEE contraception, emergency; depression; domestic violence.

For more information on rape, contact:

National Coalition Against Sexual Assault
P.O. Box 21378
Washington, DC 20009

National Victim Center
2111 Wilson Blvd., Suite 300
Arlington, VA 22201
800-877-3355 (referrals)
703-276-2880 (office)
http://www.nvc.org

Rape Crisis Center Hotline
202-333-7273
Provides access to the Sexual Assault and
Child Sexual Abuse National Directory of
Victim Survivor Services and Prevention,
which gives referrals to local organizations.

For more information on sexual harassment, contact:

Nine-to-Five Hotline
National Association of Working Women
1430 W. Peachtree St., Suite 610
Atlanta, GA 30309
800-522-0925
404-876-1604

SEXUAL DYSFUNCTION

Sexual dysfunctions are a group of disorders that frequently or always prevent a person from enjoying sexual intercourse or experiencing orgasm. These dysfunctions affect both men and women and affect nearly everyone at some point in life.

The most common sexual dysfunction among men and women is a decreased sexual desire, or **libido.** There is no "normal" level for sex drive, which varies over the life span in each person, and from person to person. A decreased libido can be the result of illness, a history of sexual abuse, or medications. Fatigue and anxiety, caused by caring for a newborn child or by a heavy workload, can also lower the sex drive. Pregnancy, menopause, and oral contraceptives can all decrease or increase libido, depending on the person. Women who have had their ovaries surgically removed and suffer a loss of testosterone may have a drastic change in libido after surgery. If a decreased libido interferes with sexual satisfaction, a woman and her partner should discuss the problem with a practitioner, who may decide to refer them to a sex therapist.

SEXUAL DYSFUNCTIONS AMONG MEN

The most common sexual dysfunction among men is **premature ejaculation.** Any ejaculation that happens before it is desired—usually before the partner is fully aroused or satisfied—is premature. Premature ejaculation is often caused by two circumstances: overeagerness and performance anxiety, both psychologically based causes. A condom may be worn to lessen sensation and prolong ejaculation. The man may also practice the "squeeze technique," in which the tip of the penis, just below the glans, is squeezed gently just before orgasm to cause the loss of the desire to ejaculate.

The second most common sexual dysfunction among men is **impotence,** which can be psychologically or physically based. All men are impotent at some time in their lives, perhaps due to fatigue, drug and alcohol use, anxiety, or other temporary condition. Chronic impotence is usually organic, caused by diabetes, obesity, alcohol, circulatory problems, some nervous disorders, and some prescribed drugs. It can also be caused by an injury to the penis, congenital conditions, and certain surgical procedures.

Impotence should be discussed with a practitioner to rule out physical causes. A sex therapist or counselor may be able to help solve psychological impotence with therapy. Increased age can lead to an increase in organic diseases that can increase impotence. If impotence occurs later in life, it is important to consult a practitioner, as its cause may well be symptomatic of an illness. Delayed ejaculation can develop usually as a result of medication or drug side effects (alcohol, heroin, tricyclic medication, and many others). Painful ejaculation can occur because of sexually transmitted infections or various drug side effects. If impotence is permanent and physical, a flexible implant or an inflatable device may be inserted into the penis to simulate an erection.

SEXUAL DYSFUNCTIONS AMONG WOMEN

The sexual dysfunctions women usually experience are **anorgasmia** (the inability to experience orgasm), **dyspareunia** (pain during sexual

FINDING HELP

Everyone experiences some form of sexual dysfunction in his or her life. It is often caused by guilt, anxiety, fatigue, and substance abuse, and it usually disappears when issues are addressed. If it persists, see your practitioner for a medical examination and a review of possible causes.

Your practitioner might suggest a sex therapist. This professional, trained to treat individuals and partners, reviews the partners' sexual history and provides an explanation of reproductive anatomy. The therapist will also assign exercises for the couple to practice at home designed to increase communication, lessen anxiety, and increase understanding of individual sexual pleasures.

A reputable sex therapist can be found by contacting the American Association of Sex Educators, Counselors, and Therapists. Remember that a professional therapist will never engage in sexual activity with clients, or encourage practices such as observed sex, group sex, partner switching, or other questionable situations.

intercourse), and **frigidity** (inability to enjoy a loving, sexual experience).

Painful intercourse and anorgasmia can be caused by any number of conditions, including a lack of knowledge concerning personal sexual response, an inattentive partner, feelings of guilt about sex, memories of traumatic events such as rape or incest, and physical disorders of the female reproductive system. Anorgasmia is experienced by 30 to 60 percent of all women at some time. Primary anorgasmia (never having an orgasm) usually has different causes than secondary anorgasmia (being currently unable to have an orgasm). Secondary anorgasmia is often related to environmental or partner factors.

The cause of frigidity is just as elusive: hormonal fluctuation can produce mood swings that affect the libido. A woman's own internal chemistry can also affect her libido, or a woman may be experiencing personal "turnoffs." In 90 percent of women with frigidity, treatment is effective. A gynecologist should be consulted if there is any pain during sexual intercourse, or frigidity.

Some women experience a rare condition called **vaginismus.** This is an involuntary tensing of the vaginal muscles that prevents penetration of any sort. It is usually caused by fear or anxiety. A woman, with the help of a practitioner, can learn to gradually relax those muscles, perhaps with the use of a set of dilators or her own fingers.

SEE sexual response.

For more information on sexual therapy, contact:

**American Association of Sex Educators,
    Counselors, and Therapists**
P.O. Box 238
Mount Vernon, IA 52314-0238

SEXUAL ORIENTATION

Sexual orientation refers to the gender for which a person has sexual desire. Sexual desire between men and women is called heterosexuality. Heterosexual women and men are often called straight. Sexual desire between people of the same gender is called homosexuality. Homosexual women are often called lesbian, and both homosexual men and women are often referred to as gay. Bisexuality is the sexual desire for people of both genders. Asexuality is the absence of sexual desire. While many definitions of heterosexuality, homosexuality, and bisexuality include sexual activity, not everyone acts upon their sexual desires. Some people may consider themselves to have no particular sexual orientation.

LESBIANISM

Lesbians are homosexual women who desire other women for sex partners. Some women realize their lesbianism early in their lives; others discover it much later, sometimes after years of heterosexual marriage.

Homophobia, the irrational fear and hatred of homosexuality that is present in society, often keeps lesbians from "coming out" and being open with friends, family, and coworkers about their sexual orientation. Some women who reveal their lesbianism must face insults and embarrassment, and many lose their jobs, family members, or even custody of their children.

While being homosexual within a heterosexist society is stressful, lesbian individuals and communities enjoy a great deal of pride and excitement. More and more, informal and for-mal organizations of lesbians are forming to provide each other with support and to celebrate the satisfaction they receive from their lifestyle. Many lesbians ignore the pressure to conform to other social ideals about womanhood.

LESBIAN HEALTH

Physically, lesbians are no different from straight women and should generally receive the same health care. However, differences in sexual behaviors affect the incidence of certain gynecological problems and result in distinctive health-care needs. For example:

■ If women have exclusively lesbian relationships, they need no birth control. They will not need obstetric care unless they decide to conceive a child by donor insemination or sexual intercourse.

■ Syphilis and gonorrhea are rarely seen among lesbians, since these diseases are not easily transmitted from one woman to another.

■ Genital herpes and genital warts can be sexually transmitted from woman to woman. Lesbians who have symptoms of these STIs, which are spread easily, should seek treatment and avoid intimate contact, including kissing and touching, until the lesions are completely healed.

■ Yeast infections, trichomonas, and bacterial vaginosis are all vaginal infections that can be transmitted from woman to woman during sexual activity.

■ Bladder infections are less common among lesbians than straight women, though they do occur.

■ Instances of sexually transmitted infections may increase if lesbians have several sex partners or relations with bisexual women.

■ Transmittal of HIV is rare from woman to woman but is possible. Sexually active lesbians, like all sexually active people, should become informed about safer sex.

■ Although lesbians are no more predisposed to alcoholism than straight women, alcoholism appears to be a hazard of the stress of being a lesbian within a homophobic culture. Because bars are one of the few meeting places for homosexuals, alcoholic behavior is encouraged further. Some researchers estimate that more than 30 percent of lesbians suffer from alcoholism (compared with an estimated 5 to 10 percent of the general population). Many chapters of Alcoholics Anonymous and Al-Anon now have lesbian meetings, making it easier for these women to seek help.

HEALTH CARE FOR LESBIANS

Since lesbians have fewer infections and no need for birth control, they generally visit their health-care practitioners less often and, consequently, receive less routine health care than heterosexual women. As a result, they may develop more gynecological problems than straight women because they avoid regular checkups. Routine screening tests are imperative for early detection of breast, cervical, and ovarian cancers, and lesbians should have pelvic exams, Pap tests, and breast exams at regular intervals to ensure that any problems are found as soon as possible. The large proportion of lesbians who choose not to bear children may be at higher risk for breast cancer, endometriosis, and fibroids.

Lesbians may also avoid having annual gynecological exams because they experience—or are afraid they may experience—heterosexist, prejudicial, or otherwise insensitive treatment from some health-care practitioners. Lesbians who want to have children often encounter prejudice from medical professionals who refuse to inseminate gay women. Rather than risking their health, they should seek out practitioners who are accepting. While some women may decide not to disclose their sexual orientation to their practitioners, health-care professionals generally provide better care when they know a patient's complete background and sexual history.

Treatment complications may also occur when a lesbian seeks therapy for common mental health conditions like depression if a misguided and misinformed therapist attempts to "cure" her sexual orientation or sees it as the root of all her problems. Lesbians should check with friends, women's centers, or national or local gay resource centers for referrals of therapists accepting of and knowledgeable about lesbianism.

The best way to find out if a health professional is comfortable with homosexuality is to simply ask, either during an initial interview or over the phone before making an appointment. Many lesbians prefer therapists who are "out" lesbians or gay men. National resource groups and lesbian and gay community centers may be able to provide referrals.

EMOTIONAL WELL-BEING

The experiences of lesbians in society may place them at increased risk for some mental health problems and may protect them from other psychological problems.

The daily stress of living within a society that does not accept and often does not even recognize a lesbian's way of life can affect her emotional health. Many lesbians live a life of secrecy, hiding their sexual preferences from family and coworkers. Those who announce their sexual orientation, or "come out," often suffer prejudice, abuse, and loneliness.

Seeking support from a lesbian culture and community is vital in maintaining self-esteem and emotional well-being. However, lesbians and gay men have different cultures, and there is not one "gay" culture, which may make it difficult for lesbians to find friends and potential partners. Lesbian women can help themselves and others by starting lesbian interest and support groups in their areas and participating in those already in existence.

For more information on lesbian and gay concerns, contact:

Gay and Lesbian Advocates and Defenders
P.O. Box 218
Boston, MA 02112
617-426-1350

Lesbian Resource Center
1808 Bellevue Ave., Suite 204
Seattle, WA 98122
206-322-3953

National Gay and Lesbian Task Force
2320 17th St., N.W.
Washington, DC 20009
202-332-6483
http://www.ngltf.org

Office of Lesbian and Gay Concerns
Unitarian Universalist Association
25 Beacon St.
Boston, MA 02108
617-742-2100 ext. 470

P-FLAG (Parents, Families and Friends of Lesbians and Gays)
1101 14th St., N.W., Suite 1030
Washington, DC 20005
202-638- 4200
http://www.pflag.org

SEXUAL RESPONSE

In 1966 sex researchers William Masters and Virginia Johnson identified four cycles of the human sexual response cycle. These specific stages are **desire, excitement/plateau, orgasm, and resolution.** They can be reached through a variety of sexual activities, including vaginal, anal, and oral intercourse, and masturbation.

The response cycle can be triggered by a particular situation, an attractive person, personal fantasy, or images in a magazine or on the television. Sexual arousal can also be suppressed. Many other priorities, such as work or study, can cause people to ignore sexual stimulation. Religious beliefs may have a profound effect on the suppression of sexual response. The fear of pregnancy, AIDS, or a past traumatic experience often causes people to suppress their desires.

DESIRE

The desire stage is also known as the arousal stage. During this stage, the heart beats faster, blood pressure increases, and the blood flow to the sex organs increases. A woman's clitoris and vaginal tissues swell and become lubricated, and a man's penis becomes erect. There is also an increase in muscle tension, the skin becomes flushed, and the nipples become erect. During this stage, a woman and her partner may use fore-play, such as kissing and petting, to increase sexual stimulation and reach the excitement/plateau stage. Masturbation, sex toys, lubrications, and erotica may be used during the desire stage.

EXCITEMENT/PLATEAU

During the second stage, the excitement/plateau stage, sexual excitement is heightened. A woman's clitoris and a man's penis become engorged and sensitive as the blood flow to the genitals of both men and women increases. The pulse, breathing rate, muscle tension, and blood pressure also increase significantly.

ORGASM

The third stage is the orgasm, also called the climax. Orgasm is a series of powerful and rapid contractions of many different muscles, including the uterine and vaginal muscles, the pubic muscles, and the anal sphincter. The contractions occur in both women and men at .8-second intervals. Orgasm is accompanied by feelings of great physical pleasure during which the muscular tension that had built up in the second stage is finally released.

For a woman, the orgasm generally lasts 13 to 51 seconds, while for a man it lasts 10 to 30 seconds. In women, the contractions are centered in the pelvic muscles, though they are felt throughout the body. In men, the contractions are concentrated in the genitals—though they are also felt throughout the body—and are followed by ejaculation, the releasing of semen through the tip of the penis.

Most women can reach orgasm through stimulation of the clitoris, which produces contractions centered in the vaginal entrance, called a **vulvar orgasm.** Vaginal stimulation produces a **uterine orgasm,** centered in the uterus. About 30 percent of women can also reach orgasm through stimulation of the **Grafenberg spot,** or **G-spot,** located on the front wall of the vagina, about an inch into the vaginal canal. The spot swells when stimulated, and produces a strong feeling of sexual pleasure. Such stimulation leads to a uterine orgasm. Many experts, however, dispute the existence of the G-spot. Vulvar orgasms tend to be shorter, more intense, and more likely to be multiple than uterine orgasms.

RESOLUTION

The final stage is resolution. This is when the body gradually returns to normal. The muscles relax, the breathing and heart rate decrease, and the blood flows away from the genitals. At this point, most men experience a period of time, known as a refractory period, during which they cannot be aroused again and experience another orgasm. Women, however, are able to be aroused and experience additional orgasms. Some women may have multiple orgasms, without refractory periods, if the stimulation continues.

SATISFYING SEXUAL EXPERIENCES

Women were once considered to be passive partners who took no pleasure in sex. Today, a woman's equal right to sexual pleasure is generally recognized. Sex is no longer what men do to women. Both partners may be committed to pleasing one another, and both may experiment with passive and aggressive roles.

A woman today is also more free to understand and experience her body. Discussions about sex are more common, and a woman is encouraged to explore her own body through masturbation to discover what will bring her to orgasm. In fact, many women who find it difficult to reach orgasm learn to pleasure themselves and reach climax using masturbation. A woman and her partner are able to make sex satisfying by talking about their own preferences, fantasies, and desires.

Years ago, sex manuals praised the virtues of simultaneous orgasms, when both partners reach climax at the same time. Today, however, it is recognized that it is not necessary in order to have a satisfying sexual experience—in fact, the pressure to achieve simultaneous orgasm may lead to sexual dysfunction. Recent surveys show that fewer than 24 percent of the men they surveyed, and only 14 percent of the women, believe that a simultaneous orgasm is a must for gratifying sex.

Women who came of age during the sexual revolution are more likely to insist on having orgasms when they are ready and are less apt to be accommodating to the man's need. These women are more likely to reach orgasm through oral sex or the use of a vibrator.

SEE sexual dysfunction.

SEXUALLY TRANSMITTED INFECTIONS

Sexually transmitted infections (STIs), also called sexually transmitted diseases (STDs), are spread through sexual contact, including vaginal, anal, and oral intercourse. Some can be spread through touching and kissing. There are more than 30 STIs, including chlamydia, genital herpes, human papilloma virus (HPV), genital warts, hepatitis B, gonorrhea, syphilis, trichomoniasis, bacterial vaginosis, and the human immunodeficiency virus (HIV) that can cause AIDS.

One out of four Americans will contract an STI during his or her lifetime. Approximately 12 million new STI cases are diagnosed each year in the United States. Many STIs have no symptoms until serious and permanent damage has occurred.

PREGNANCY AND STIS

Some STIs can be passed from a woman to her developing fetus during pregnancy or to her child during birth. Some STIs can result in the death of the fetus in the womb. Others can cause serious birth defects, developmental disabilities, and other health problems for newborn infants—problems that can last a lifetime or even cause death. Pregnant women and women who want to become pregnant should consider being tested for STIs.

Following are descriptions of STIs, common symptoms, and means of transmission, as well as diagnosis and treatment. Each section also discusses ways to protect against the spread of STIs.

BACTERIAL VAGINOSIS (BV)

BV is an inflammation of the vagina—vaginitis—that is caused by a change in the normal balance of vaginal bacteria. The change is characterized by an increased number of anaerobic bacteria with a decreased number of normal lactobacilli, healthy bacteria. Hundreds of thousands of women in the United States develop BV every year. It is not usually sexually transmitted, but sexual intercourse may intensify BV by altering the bacterial balance.

Common symptoms:

■ Heavy and unusual vaginal discharge that is often grayish and frothy and may have a fishy odor, especially after intercourse

■ Irritations of the vagina (often because of another infection)

Diagnosis: Microscopic examination of vaginal discharge

Treatment: One partner—sometimes both—is treated successfully with antibiotics.

Protection: Condoms offer very good protection against BV.

CHANCROID

Chancroid is an especially dangerous sexually transmitted bacterium because the sores it causes increase the chances of getting HIV. Once very common, reported cases of chancroid have fallen to fewer than 1,500 per year in the United States. This may be due to increased condom use among American men.

Common symptoms:

■ First, a small boil or ulcer—called a bubo—appears, usually on the genitals. It doesn't heal like a common pimple. Later, the bubo becomes an open sore. There may be pus and pain.

■ Women may have no sores, but they may have painful urination or bowel movements, painful intercourse, rectal bleeding, or vaginal discharge.

Untreated chancroid can infect and swell the glands located in the groin. Men are more commonly infected than women. Symptoms usually appear within a week of infection.

How chancroid is spread: Vaginal, anal, and oral intercourse

Diagnosis: Chancroid ulcers can be confused with herpes, syphilis, and other conditions. Microscopic examination of the discharge from the bubo may be necessary.

DON'T LET EMBARRASSMENT BECOME A HEALTH RISK

Many people find it very difficult to talk about their sexual health. Some even find it shameful. But discomfort and shame can get in the way of common sense. They can keep people from taking good care of themselves and their partners. Choose a practitioner with whom you can be comfortable while discussing these issues. Keep yourself healthy by speaking frankly and openly with your health-care provider about your sex life and your sexual health concerns. Some practitioners don't ask—so take charge and speak up.

Treatment: Both partners can be treated successfully with oral antibiotics.

Protection: Condoms offer very good protection against chancroid.

CHLAMYDIA

Chlamydia is a bacterium. It can cause sterility in women and men. In women, it infects the cervix and can spread to the urethra, fallopian tubes, and ovaries. It can cause bladder infections and serious pelvic inflammatory disease (PID), ectopic pregnancy, and sterility. In men, it infects the urethra and may spread to the testicles. Chlamydia can also lead to arthritis. In infants, chlamydia can cause pneumonia, eye infections, and blindness. It is the most common and most invisible STI in America. Four million American men and women become infected every year.

Common symptoms:

■ Discharge from the penis or vagina

■ Pain or burning while urinating; more-than-usual urination

■ Excessive vaginal bleeding, abdominal pain, nausea, fever

■ Painful intercourse

■ Inflammation of the rectum

■ Inflammation of the cervix

Seventy-five percent of women and 25 percent of men with chlamydia have no symptoms. Many women discover they have chlamydia only because their partners are found to have the disease—or they discover they had it in the past when they are treated for infertility. If symptoms do appear, they appear in seven to 21 days. A urinary tract infection in a male partner may be a sign to a woman that she has chlamydia.

How chlamydia is spread:

■ Vaginal and anal intercourse

■ From the birth canal to the fetus

■ Rarely, from the hand to the eye

Diagnosis: Chlamydia can be confused with gonorrhea and other conditions. Microscopic examination of tissue samples or a urine test is necessary for correct diagnosis.

Treatment: Both partners can be treated successfully with antibiotics.

Protection: Condoms offer very good protection against chlamydia.

CYTOMEGALOVIRUS (CMV)

CMV is a virus that is transmitted through many bodily fluids. It is also sexually transmitted. It is the most common infection in America that is spread from a woman to the developing fetus—10 to 20 percent of infants born to women with CMV get it. Every year, CMV causes permanent disability, including hearing loss and mental retardation, for 4,000 to 7,000 babies. CMV is also very dangerous for people with weakened immune systems. It can cause blindness and mental disorders. CMV remains in the body for life.

Common symptoms:

■ Swollen glands, fatigue, fever, and general weakness. CMV causes 8 percent of the cases of mononucleosis.

■ Irritations of the digestive tract, nausea, diarrhea

■ Loss of vision

There are usually no symptoms with the first infection. But reinfection with CMV, or infection with other STIs such as HIV and hepatitis B, may reactivate the virus and cause illness.

How CMV is spread: In saliva, semen, blood, cervical and vaginal secretions, urine, and breast milk by:

■ Close personal contact

■ Vaginal, anal, and oral intercourse

■ Blood transfusion and sharing IV drug equipment

■ Pregnancy, childbirth, and breast-feeding

Between 40 and 80 percent of Americans get CMV through contact with other children by the time they reach puberty. Adults, however, usually get CMV through sexual activity.

Women who want to become pregnant and who may have the virus should consider testing for CMV.

Diagnosis: Blood test

Treatment: There is no cure. Symptoms may be managed with a variety of intravenous drugs. No treatment is effective during pregnancy.

Protection: Condoms can provide protection against CMV during vaginal, anal, and oral intercourse, but kissing and other intimate touching can spread the virus.

GENITAL WARTS

See "Human Papilloma Virus."

GONORRHEA

Gonorrhea is a bacterium that can cause sterility, arthritis, heart problems, and disorders of the central nervous system. In women, gonorrhea can cause pelvic inflammatory disease (PID), which can result in ectopic pregnancy or sterility. During pregnancy, gonorrhea infections can cause premature labor and stillbirth. To prevent serious eye infections that are caused by gonorrhea in newborn babies, drops of silver nitrate or antibiotic are routinely put into the eyes of infants immediately after delivery. More than 1 million cases of gonorrhea are reported every year in the United States.

Common symptoms:

■ For women: frequent, often burning urination; pelvic pain; a green or yellow-green discharge from the vagina; swelling or tenderness of the vulva; and arthritic pain

■ For men: a puslike discharge from the urethra or pain during urination

Eighty percent of the women and 10 percent of the men with gonorrhea show no symptoms. If they appear, they appear in women within 10 days. It takes from one to 14 days for symptoms to appear in men.

How gonorrhea is spread: Vaginal, anal, and oral intercourse

Diagnosis: Microscopic examination of urethral or vaginal discharges. Cultures may be taken from the cervix, throat, urethra, or rectum.

Treatment: Both partners can be successfully treated with oral antibiotics. Often people with gonorrhea also have chlamydia. They must be treated for both infections at the same time.

Protection: Condoms offer very good protection against gonorrhea.

HEPATITIS B VIRUS (HBV)

Although 90 to 95 percent of adults with HBV recover completely, the virus can cause severe liver disease and death. Unless they are treated within an hour of birth, 90 percent of the infants born to women with HBV will carry the virus. Pregnant women who may have been exposed to HBV should consider being tested before giving birth so that their babies can be vaccinated at birth or treated if they become ill. Like other viruses, HBV remains in the body for life.

HBV is the only STI that is preventable with vaccination. But about 200,000 Americans get HBV every year because they have not been vaccinated. There are now about 1.5 million people with HBV in the United States.

Common symptoms:

■ Extreme fatigue, headache, fever, hives

■ Nausea, vomiting, lack of appetite, tenderness in the lower abdomen

■ Later symptoms: dark urine, clay-colored stool, yellowing of the skin and white of the eye (jaundice)

HBV may show no symptoms during its most contagious phases. If symptoms do appear, they appear within four weeks.

How HBV is spread: In semen, saliva, blood, and urine by:

■ Intimate and sexual contact, from kissing to vaginal, anal, and oral intercourse

■ Use of unclean needles to inject drugs

■ Accidental sticking with contaminated needles in the course of health care. Usually the infection is passed from an infected patient to a health-care worker.

Hepatitis B is very contagious.

Diagnosis: Blood test

Treatment: None. In most cases, the infection clears within four to eight weeks. Some people, however, remain contagious for the rest of their lives.

Protection: Condoms offer some protection against HBV during vaginal, anal, and oral intercourse, but the virus can be passed through kissing and other intimate touching. Infants, children, and adults who do not have HBV can be protected from infection with an HBV vaccine. Everyone should be vaccinated against HBV.

HERPES

There are two forms of genital herpes—herpes simplex virus-1 and herpes simplex virus-2. Herpes-1 is most often associated with cold sores and fever blisters, while herpes-2 usually affects the genitals. Both forms of herpes have similar symptoms and may be sexually transmitted. During pregnancy, herpes may cause miscarriage or stillbirth. If active herpes infections are present during childbirth, newborn infants may suffer serious health damage, including developmental disabilities and, rarely, death. Congenital herpes infection occurs more commonly during a primary herpes infection and is less common during recurrent herpes outbreaks. More than 30 million Americans have genital herpes. A half million new cases are diagnosed every year. The herpes simplex virus (HSV) remains in the body for life.

Common symptoms:

■ A recurring rash with clusters of blistery sores appearing on the vagina, cervix, penis, mouth, anus, buttocks, or elsewhere on the body

■ Pain and discomfort around the infected area, itching, burning sensations during urination, swollen glands in the groin, fever, headache, and a general run-down feeling

Symptoms usually appear from two to 20 days after infection—but it may be years before the primary outbreak occurs.

Recurrences are sometimes related to emotional, physical, or health stresses. During recurrences it is important to observe strict rules of day-to-day hygiene. Wash hands frequently and do not touch the sores. If the sores are touched inadvertently, wash hands immediately. Be particularly careful when handling contact lenses and touching the eyes.

How HSV is spread:

■ Touching, sexual intimacy (including kissing)

■ Vaginal, anal, and oral intercourse

HSV may be passed from one partner to another, or from one part of the body to another, whenever contact is made with an active herpes virus.

HSV is most contagious from the time the sores are present until they are completely healed and the scabs have fallen off. Unfortunately, recent studies show that some people may be contagious when they have no symptoms. Mucous membranes of the mouth, anus, vagina, penis, and the eyes are especially susceptible to infection.

Diagnosis: HSV can be confused with syphilis, chancroid, and other STIs. Examination of the sores and laboratory culturing of fluid samples taken from the sores are important. Definitive diagnosis by lab culture may not be possible if the sores are dried or scabbed. This means a visit to the practitioner early in the outbreak is important.

Treatment: No cure. Symptoms can be relieved and the number of recurrences reduced with a drug called acyclovir.

Protection: Partners should refrain from sexual intimacy from the time they know the blisters are going to recur until after the scabs have completely fallen off the healed sores. Condoms offer some protection when the virus is not active.

HUMAN IMMUNODEFICIENCY VIRUS (HIV)

HIV infections weaken the body's ability to fight disease and can cause acquired immune deficiency syndrome (AIDS)—the last stage of HIV infection. HIV is the most dangerous STI, and it affects people of all ages. It is now the leading cause of death for American women and men between 25 and 44 years old. It is believed that more than 1 million Americans have HIV. Like other viruses, HIV remains in the body for life.

Common symptoms:

■ Constant or rapid, unexplained weight loss, diarrhea, lack of appetite

■ Fatigue

■ Persistent fevers, night sweats, dry cough

■ Light-headedness, headaches, mental disorders

■ Thick, whitish coating of yeast on the tongue or mouth (thrush)

■ Severe or recurring vaginal yeast infections

■ Chronic pelvic inflammatory disease

■ Purplish growths on the skin

There may be no symptoms for 10 years or more. About 5 percent of those with HIV may not develop symptoms.

How HIV is spread: In blood, semen, vaginal fluids, and breast milk by:

■ Anal, vaginal, and oral intercourse

■ Sharing contaminated needles for injecting IV drugs

■ Transfusion of contaminated blood products

■ To the fetus during childbirth

■ To the child during breast-feeding

Diagnosis: There are blood tests to detect HIV antibodies. Diagnosis of AIDS is based on the presence of one or more of a variety of conditions and "opportunistic" infections related to an HIV infection.

Treatment: No cure or vaccine. Many AIDS-related conditions—such as pneumonias, cancers, and a variety of infections that take advantage of weakened immune systems—can be managed to some extent with a variety of treatments. However, AIDS is fatal, and at this time, no one has recovered.

Protection: Condoms offer very good protection against HIV.

HUMAN PAPILLOMA VIRUS

There are 60 different human papilloma viruses (HPVs). They cause a variety of warts and other conditions and may remain in the system for life. A few HPVs cause genital warts, but most genital HPV infections are not visible and have no symptoms. Some of these are associated with cancer of the cervix, vulva, or penis. Every year, about 1 million Americans are infected with genital HPVs—40 million women and men are now infected.

Common symptoms:

■ Warts on the genitals, in the urethra, in the anus, and rarely in the throat

■ Genital warts are soft to the touch, may look like miniature cauliflower florets, and often itch.

■ Untreated genital warts can occasionally grow to block the openings of the vagina, anus, or throat and become quite uncomfortable.

It usually takes from two to three weeks after infection for warts to develop. In women, genital warts grow more rapidly during pregnancy or when other vaginal infections are present.

How genital HPVs are spread:

■ Vaginal and anal intercourse

■ Very rarely, genital warts spread to the fetus during childbirth.

Diagnosis:

■ Microscopic examination of tissue sample

■ Clinical evaluation of warts during a physical or gynecologic exam

■ Special magnifiers called colposcopes can detect genital HPVs that cannot be seen with the naked eye during pelvic exams.

■ Pap tests may reveal precancerous conditions caused by genital HPVs. Early treatment prevents cancer of the cervix.

Treatment: HPV often recurs, and genital warts can be treated in a number of ways. They can be removed by carefully applying, and often reapplying, a prescription medication, podofilox, to the wart. Practitioners offer other treatments, including standard surgery, laser surgery (vaporizing the wart with a beam of high-powered light, cryosurgery (freezing the wart with liquid nitrogen), and application of podophyllin or acid.

Protection: Condoms may offer some protection against genital HPVs, but the viruses may "shed" beyond the area protected by a condom.

MOLLUSCUM CONTAGIOSUM

Hundreds of thousands of cases of the virus molluscum contagiosum, a disease of the skin and mucous membranes, are diagnosed every year.

Common symptoms: Small, round, pinkish white, waxy-looking, dimpled growths in the genital area or on the thighs. Symptoms usually appear between two and 12 weeks after infection, but they may not appear for years. If not treated, molluscum may cause dermatitis and infection to develop in the area of the polyp.

How molluscum contagiosum is spread: Vaginal, anal, and oral intercourse as well as other intimate contact.

Diagnosis: Microscopic examination of tissue taken from the sore

Treatment: Growths may be removed with chemicals, electrical current, or freezing.

Protection: Condoms may offer some protection against molluscum contagiosum, but the virus may "shed" beyond the area protected by the condom. Molluscum is often not sexually transmitted.

PELVIC INFLAMMATORY DISEASE (PID)

PID is a condition that harms a woman's reproductive system. PID occurs throughout the pelvic area, in the fallopian tubes, the uterus, the lining of the uterus, and in the ovaries. Treated or untreated, PID can lead to sterility, ectopic pregnancy, and chronic pain. The more episodes of PID a woman has, the greater are her chances of becoming sterile. PID is not always the result of an STI—but in many cases it is. The STIs that most commonly cause PID are gonorrhea and chlamydia. More than a million new cases of PID are diagnosed every year in the United States. It is believed that millions of others go undiscovered.

Common symptoms:
- Fever, chills
- Nausea, vomiting
- Pain during intercourse
- Pain in the lower abdomen
- Spotting and pain between menstrual periods or during urination
- Unusually long or painful periods, and unusual vaginal discharge

Treatment: Antibiotics, bed rest, and sexual abstinence. Surgery may be required to remove abscesses or scar tissue or to repair or remove reproductive organs.

Diagnosis:
- Pelvic exam
- Microscopic examination of vaginal and cervical secretions
- Laparoscopy. An optical instrument is inserted through a small cut in the abdomen to look at the reproductive organs.

Symptoms can be confused with those of appendicitis and other infections. Diagnosis can be difficult if patients are too embarrassed to admit sexual activity.

Protection: Condoms offer very good protection against the STIs commonly associated with PID.

PUBIC LICE

Every year, millions of people treat themselves for pubic lice, also called crabs or cooties.

Common symptoms:
- Intense itching in the genitals or anus
- Mild fever
- Feeling run-down
- Irritability

Itching usually begins five days after infestation begins. Some people don't itch and don't know they are infested.

How pubic lice are spread:
- Contact with infected bedding, clothing, and toilet seats
- Intimate and sexual contact

Self-diagnosis: Seen with the naked eye or with a magnifying glass, pubic lice look like tiny crabs. They are pale gray but darken in color when swollen with blood. They attach themselves and their eggs to pubic hair, underarm hair, eyelashes, and eyebrows. Their eggs are white and are deposited in small clumps near the hair roots.

Treatment: Follow the directions on the package insert of an over-the-counter medication. Some of the brands available are Kwell, A-200, and RID. Repeated head-to-toe applications may be necessary. Pregnant women and infants must use products especially designed for them, like Eurax. Everyone who may have been exposed to pubic lice should be treated at the same time. All bedding, towels, and clothing that may have been exposed should be thoroughly washed or dry-cleaned.

Protection: Limit the number of intimate and sexual contacts.

SCABIES

The scabies mite burrows under the skin. It can hardly be seen with the naked eye. It belongs to the same family of insects as the spider. It is not always sexually transmitted. Schoolchildren often pass it to one another.

Common symptoms:
- Intense itching, usually at night
- Small bumps or rashes that appear in dirty-looking, small curling lines, especially on the penis, between the fingers, on buttocks, breasts, wrists, thighs, and around the navel

Often symptoms are not visible. It may take several weeks for them to develop.

How scabies is spread:
- Close personal contact
- Bedding and clothing

Diagnosis: Although people can diagnose themselves, diagnosis is often difficult. Microscopic examination of a skin scraping or biopsy by a practitioner may be necessary.

Treatment: Follow the directions on the package insert of an over-the-counter medication such as Kwell or Scabene. Repeated neck-to-toe applications may be necessary. Everyone who may have been exposed to scabies should be treated at the same time. All bedding, towels, and clothing that may have been exposed should be thoroughly washed or dry-cleaned.

Protection: Limit the number of intimate and sexual contacts.

SYPHILIS

Untreated, the syphilis bacterium, called a spirochete, can remain in the body for life and lead to disfigurement, mental disorder, or death. The number of reported cases of syphilis in the United States has dropped below 120,000. This may be due to increased condom use among American men.

Common symptoms:
Syphilis has several phases that may overlap one another. They do not always follow in the same sequence. Symptoms vary with each phase, but there are no symptoms most of the time.

- Primary Phase: Sores, called chancres, often appear from three weeks to 90 days after infection. They last three to six weeks. They appear on the genitals, in the vagina, on the cervix, lips, mouth, or anus. Swollen glands may also occur during the primary phase.

- Secondary Phase: Other symptoms often appear from three to six weeks after the sores appear. They may come and go for up to two years. They include body rashes that last from two to six weeks, often located on the palms of the hands and the soles of the feet. There are many other symptoms, including mild fever, fatigue, sore throat, hair loss, weight loss, swollen glands, headache, and muscle pains.

- Latent Phase: No symptoms. Latent phases occur between other phases or can overlap them.

- Late Phase: One-third of untreated people with syphilis experience serious damage of the nervous system, heart, brain, or other organs, and death may result.

How syphilis is spread:
- Vaginal, anal, and oral intercourse
- Kissing
- To the fetus during pregnancy

Syphilis is especially contagious when sores are present early in the disease—the liquid that oozes from them is very infectious. People are usually not contagious during the latent phases of the first four years of syphilis infections. Untreated syphilis remains latent for many years or a lifetime, but can be spread from a pregnant woman to her fetus.

The effect of syphilis on a fetus is very serious. If untreated, the risks of stillbirth or serious birth defects are high. Birth defects include damage to the heart and brain as well as blindness. It is very important for pregnant women to consider testing for syphilis early and, sometimes, throughout their pregnancies. Pregnant women with syphilis can be treated to prevent damage to the fetus.

Diagnosis:
■ Microscopic examination of fluid from sores
■ Blood tests
■ Examination of spinal fluid

Treatment: Antibiotics are successful for both partners—but damages caused by the disease cannot be undone.

Protection: Condoms offer very good protection during vaginal, anal, and oral intercourse.

TRICHOMONIASIS

"Trich," a bacterium, is a common cause of vaginitis. Up to 3 million Americans develop trichomoniasis every year.

Common symptoms:
■ Frothy, often musty-smelling discharge
■ Itching in and around the vagina
■ Blood spotting in the discharge
■ Swelling in the groin
■ Urge to urinate more often than usual

Only rarely do men have symptoms. Sometimes women have no symptoms. It takes from three to 28 days for symptoms to develop.

How trichomoniasis is spread: Vaginal intercourse

Diagnosis: Microscopic examination of vaginal discharge

Treatment: Antibiotics are successful for both partners.

Protection: Condoms offer very good protection against trich.

SEE AIDS/HIV; contraception; gynecologic examination; pelvic inflammatory disease; pregnancy—preconception concerns; safer sex; vaginitis.

For more information about STIs, contact:

American Social Health Association
P.O. Box 13827
Research Triangle Park, NC 27709
919-361-8400
National STD Hotline
800-227-8922
http://sunsite.unc.edu/asha

Herpes Resource Center
P.O. Box 13827
Research Triangle Park, NC 27709
919-361-8488
National Herpes Hotline
919-361-8488

National Institute of Allergy and Infectious Diseases
National Institutes of Health
Bldg. 31, Room 7A50
9000 Rockville Pike
Bethesda, MD 20892-2520
301-496-5717
niaidoc@niaid.nih.gov

Planned Parenthood Federation of America, Inc.
810 Seventh Avenue
New York, NY 10019
For the Planned Parenthood nearest you, call:
800-230-PLAN
http://www.ppfa.org/ppfa

SKIN

The skin is the most visible and largest organ in the body. It protects the body from the sun, bacteria, and infection. The skin regulates body temperature, stores fat and water, senses the environment, excretes sweat, and aids in the body's synthesis of vitamin D.

Proper skin care does not need to be complicated or expensive. In fact, most experts recommend washing skin daily with a mild cleanser, then gently patting it dry. To help prevent skin cancer, a daily foundation of sunscreen is also recommended for the face, which is exposed to the sun more often than most other parts of the body.

COMPONENTS OF THE SKIN

The skin is composed of the epidermis, dermis, and subcutaneous tissue. The **epidermis,** the outermost layer of the skin, is composed of flat squamous cells, round basal cells, and a stratum corneum (a nonliving keratinous layer). Also found in the epidermis are keratinocytes (producers of keratin), melanocytes (producers of melanin), and Langerhans' cells (linked with immune system surveillance). The epidermis not only regulates water loss (through openings called pores), produces melanin and keratin, and serves as the barrier between the environment and the internal organs but also is the site of new skin cell production.

The **dermis,** made up of an upper section called the papillary dermis and a lower section called the reticular dermis, contains reticuloendothelial cells, fibrous connective tissue, follicles, blood and lymph vessels, sweat and sebaceous (oil) glands, sensory nerves, and muscle. The **subcutaneous tissue** is mainly composed of fat, which protects against injury and insulates the body. It is also a reserve of calories.

COMMON DISORDERS OF THE SKIN

The occurrence of major problems of the skin has been attributed to cell and follicle dysfunction, parasites, hormonal changes, various allergens and irritants, infection, heredity, and excessive sunlight exposure. Common skin disorders and afflictions include acne, rosacea, psoriasis, dermatitis, bacterial infections, and skin cancer.

Acne, a skin disorder resulting in an eruption of pimples on the skin, commonly affects—but is not limited to—teenagers because changing levels of hormone activity cause the sebaceous glands to produce an excess of oil (sebum). Sebum, skin cells, and bacteria collect and build up in the follicles of the skin and cause pimples to form. The sebum ruptures the follicle walls allowing whiteheads (a closed pore), blackheads (an open pore), and pimples to appear on the skin's surface. Sebaceous cysts appear when the sebum does not rupture the skin and instead, a lump forms under the skin.

The treatment of acne usually involves the application of some kind of topical antibacterial product, such as benzoyl peroxide or tretinoin (Retin-A). Antibiotics may be used, in both topical and oral form, to combat the infection. These include oral and topical tetracycline, erythromycin, and topical clindamycin. Other treatment methods are the use of Accutane (oral isotretinoin), cortisone injections, hormone therapy (to regulate the hormones that trigger the overproduction of oil), and ultraviolet-light therapy. In the case of cystic acne, minor surgery and dermabrasion (use of a rough surface to slough away imperfections) may be implemented to remove sebaceous cysts.

Rosacea is a skin condition that results in redness and inflammation of the face, primarily affecting the nose and cheeks. As rosacea progresses, the skin flushes and exhibits tiny pimples (papules and pustules) and dilated blood vessels (telangiectasia). This skin condition appears to be aggravated by many factors that increase blood flow to the head. These include strenuous exercise, increased temperature, emotional stress, hot foods, and alcohol. Avoidance of these factors may diminish the frequency of outbreaks of rosacea.

Rosacea may escalate into a condition known as rhinophyma. **Rhinophyma** is characterized by a bulbous nose and red lines and bumps on the skin's surface. The treatment of rosacea involves the use of topical steroid applications and both topical and oral antibacterial products. Rhinophyma may be treated with laser or scalpel surgery and dermabrasion.

Psoriasis is characterized by a scaling of the skin caused by the overproduction of skin cells. The scales may have a silverish appearance and can be removed by softening and scrubbing them. The thickening, pitting, or crumbling of fingernails may be a result of psoriasis. It is not dangerous or contagious and may be triggered by stress, illness, or cold temperatures. Common treatments of psoriasis include the use of topical steroid preparations or coal tar preparations, ultraviolet-light therapy, drugs such as anthralin and methotrexate, and PUVA therapy (the use of psoralen and ultraviolet light).

Dermatitis and **eczema** are general terms used to describe any inflammation of the skin. One type of dermatitis, **atopic eczema,** results from an allergic reaction to various allergens ranging from wool to detergent. The itching, blistering, and crusting rash that results from atopic dermatitis can be treated with oral antibiotics, ultraviolet-light therapy, and topical corticosteroids. Avoiding the allergen, stress, and extreme temperatures also aids in treating atopic dermatitis.

Allergic contact dermatitis results from exposure to any allergen to which the body is sensitive. Allergens could include the sun, dyes, cosmetics, plants (poison ivy, oak, sumac), clothing, metal compounds, and ingredients in certain medications. Contact dermatitis results in inflamed, red, itchy skin and blisters. Treatment consists of the identification and the removal of the offending allergen. The use of topical corticosteroid cream may also be helpful before the blistering phase of allergic contact dermatitis appears.

Seborrheic dermatitis is a condition where the skin is red and inflamed and causes yellowish, greasy scales to appear on the scalp (dandruff), face, and other areas of the body. The itching and general discomfort of seborrheic dermatitis can be treated with hydrocortisone creams (for facial seborrheic dermatitis) and shampoos for the scalp containing zinc pyrithione, selenium sulfide, sulfur and salicylic acid, or tar.

AGING

During middle age and after menopause, women's skin becomes thinner and loses some of its flexibility and elasticity. The change is due to the slowdown of cell renewal and decreased production by the oil and sweat glands. Often

HAIR

Encased in follicles beneath the skin are hair roots. Hair covers most of the body and consists of dead skin cells filled with the protein keratin. The main function of hair is to help the body retain heat by diminishing the loss of body warmth. The average head can contain more than 100,000 hairs.

Thinning Hair

There are a variety of reasons for thinning scalp hair, a condition known as **alopecia.** It is not uncommon for women to undergo short periods of hair thinning especially when they are under stress. Normally, scalp hairs are all in different phases of growth. When many hairs are in one particular phase of growth in which they break easily, it may appear as if clumps of hair are falling out. This situation is often seen in women who have just delivered. It may also be a result of a hormone change, fever, anti-cancer drugs or chemotherapy, or a thyroid disorder. Some women experience thinning hair due to an androgenic disorder, a problem caused by irregular levels of testosterone and other androgens in the system.

Most postmenopausal women experience thinning scalp and pubic hair, due to increased levels of androgen (the male hormone produced by the adrenal glands) and lower estrogen levels.

If none of the above changes apply—and if more significant biological imbalances are absent—anemia could be causing your hair loss. Consult your practitioner. Anemia can be detected with a simple blood test. The presence of an underactive thyroid gland (which creates the condition hypothyroidism), of which hair loss is often a symptom, should also be explored by your practitioner.

Excessive Hair Growth

A gradual increase in facial and body hair growth, called **hirsutism,** is a common condition in women. Linked usually to hormone changes, hirsutism may begin at any time in life. While a sudden, significant increase in body hair may indicate another serious disorder (such as an adrenal or ovarian disorder), hair growth does not need to be treated unless it bothers you personally. Hormonal therapy can often alleviate the condition, or hair can be removed through electrolysis.

the result is dry skin and increased definition of wrinkles. There also may be a change in pigmentation, another result of slower cell renewal, as well as the cumulative effect of exposure to sunlight. Avoiding excessively dry environments (with the use of a humidifier), overbathing, and overuse of soap, combined with regular use of skin moisturizers and oils, will help make drying skin look smoother and feel better.

Currently, researchers are experimenting with substances that speed up skin cell renewal, such as low concentrations of vitamin A acid. One such product, tretinoin, marketed as Retin-A, has long been prescribed for acne and has been found to smooth out fine wrinkles, improve skin texture, and give a rosy glow to sun-damaged skin. However, these improvements appear only after regular use over a period of six weeks or longer. In addition, as the product promotes the rebuilding of the outer layer, it causes the skin to noticeably peel and makes the treated skin extremely sensitive to sun. When the drug is discontinued, its benefits (and side effects) appear to gradually stop.

Some experts recommend hormone replacement therapy, which contains estrogen, as a means of restoring the skin's flexibility and elasticity. However, there is no scientific evidence that estrogen supplements are effective in treating wrinkles and other signs of aging.

SEE aging; cancer, skin.

For more information on skin, contact:

American Hair Loss Council
P.O. Box 809313
Chicago, IL 60606-9313
800-274-8717

American Society for Dermatological Surgery
930 N. Meacham Rd.
Schaumburg, IL 60173
800-441-2737

Skin Cancer Foundation
245 Fifth Avenue
New York, NY 10016
212-725-5176

SMOKING

At a time when the smoking rate of the general population is decreasing, the smoking rate for women is increasing. Although 1.5 million people in the United States quit smoking each year, some 50 million adults continue to smoke in spite of repeated warnings of severe health consequences, such as lung cancer, emphysema, chronic bronchitis, and coronary heart disease. In fact, lung cancer related to smoking currently causes more deaths in women than breast cancer does.

More women are smoking now than ever before. In 1993 it was reported that 22.5 percent of American women smoked, and if the current trend continues, women will soon smoke at higher rates than men. The increase in the number of women smokers has been attributed to advertisements that portray smoking as both glamorous and a weight control measure.

Since 1977, the rate of high school senior women who smoke has surpassed that of high school men. Of all high school seniors, 25 percent had their first cigarette by the sixth grade, 50 percent by the eighth grade, and 75 percent by the ninth grade. Statistics continue to show that 19 percent of high school women smoke on a daily basis.

ADDICTIVE PROPERTIES OF SMOKING

Not only is smoking dangerous to one's health, it is also addictive. Smoking becomes addictive for two reasons: the habit-forming ritual of placing a cigarette in the mouth, lighting it, and inhaling at regular intervals, and the addictive properties of **nicotine,** a drug that is only found in the tobacco leaf. People can develop an addiction to nicotine just as easily as they can develop an addiction to cocaine and heroin. In 1988 the Surgeon General's Office reported that one "hit" of nicotine reaches the brain in seven seconds, while a "hit" of heroin injected into the bloodstream takes 14 seconds to reach the brain. The frequent "hits" of nicotine experienced with smoking make it one of the hardest addictions to break.

RISKS

The continued use of tobacco by women has resulted in the stark reality that more women now die from lung cancer than breast cancer. Pregnant women who continue to smoke have an increased risk of miscarriage, stillbirth, premature birth, and complications of pregnancy. They also expose their unborn children to possible birth defects and other effects of smoking.

Cigarette smoking can also cause or contribute to emphysema (lung disease characterized by breathlessness), chronic bronchitis (inflammation of air passages in the lungs), and coronary heart disease. Women over 35 years of age who smoke are more than 10.5 times as likely to die from emphysema or chronic bronchitis than are nonsmoking women. Smokers are more than twice as likely to suffer from a heart attack than nonsmokers are, and are more likely to die suddenly (within an hour) from a heart attack than a nonsmoker is.

Smoking has been reported to contribute to an earlier menopause and an increase in osteoporosis (breakdown of bone density). Studies have also shown that urinary estrogen levels are lower in premenopausal smokers. Women who smoke are also at a risk of forming blood clots. Use of estrogen (in the form of oral contraceptives) while smoking may put women at extremely high risk for heart disease and stroke due to blood clots. Therefore, women who smoke should not use the Pill.

LUNG CANCER

Cigarette smoking is responsible for 87 percent of all lung cancers, making it the number one cause of lung cancer, expected to claim some 157,000 lives annually.

Although the incidence rate of lung cancer in men is on the decline, it is rising in women. In fact, lung cancer is now the leading cause of all cancer deaths among women, surpassing that of breast cancer. It is estimated that more than 70,000 women will die from lung cancer annually. According to the U.S. Department of Health and Human Services, there has been a 400 percent increase of lung cancer in women over the last three decades.

SPECIAL CONSIDERATIONS FOR PREGNANT WOMEN

Smoking can be particularly dangerous to a woman and her unborn child if she smokes while she is pregnant. A report by the Office of Smoking and Health, U.S. Department of Health and Human Services, revealed that 20 percent of all women smoke during pregnancy.

If a woman smokes during pregnancy, there is a greater chance that she will have a miscarriage, give birth prematurely, or have a low-

WHAT YOU CAN DO TO QUIT SMOKING

■ Depend on family, friends, and colleagues for support. Quitting smoking is tough, and the more people you have for support, the better.

■ Set a date to quit smoking. Put it in writing and tell others who will hold you to it. Celebrate the anniversary of the date on a weekly, monthly, or yearly basis.

■ Join a stop-smoking program. To find one, contact the local chapter of the American Cancer Society, Smokenders, or the American Lung Association.

■ Exercise. Not only does exercise help you keep your mind off smoking, it can help you get your body into shape and keep off those extra pounds that many quitters fear.

■ Make a list of reasons to quit. The list may include your health, the health of your family and coworkers, the desire to become pregnant, the money you will save by not smoking, or the fact that you will be more welcome in restaurants or more comfortable in a nonsmoking airplane or theater.

■ Know the effects that quitting will have on your body. According to the American Cancer Society:

—Within 20 minutes of quitting, the blood pressure and pulse drop to normal.

—Within 24 hours of quitting, the risk of heart attack drops.

—Within 48 hours of quitting, the nerve endings begin to grow again, enhancing the senses of smell and taste.

—Within two to three weeks of quitting, circulation improves and lung function increases by 30 percent.

—Within nine months of quitting, coughing, congestion, and shortness of breath recede, the cilia in your lungs are growing back, and your ability to fight infection increases.

—Within five to 10 years of quitting, your risk of lung cancer is down, and your death rate is almost that of a nonsmoker. Some precancerous cells are replaced by healthy cells.

■ Stay healthy. Try to get enough rest and eat a balanced diet.

■ If you slip and do smoke, stop to think what made you smoke. Stress, anxiety, or a situation in which you habitually smoked (such as during a coffee break) can trigger the urge. Make an effort to avoid that situation in the future.

■ When the urge arises, try the four D's: **Delay** lighting a cigarette; take a **Deep** breath; **Drink** water; then, **Do** something else to keep your mind off smoking.

---

birth-weight baby. Both premature births and low birth weights can lead to other complications and longer hospital stays for the newborn. In fact, smoking during pregnancy is responsible for 14 percent of all premature births and 10 percent of all infant deaths.

Smoking during pregnancy allows nicotine and carbon monoxide to enter the fetus through the placental wall. These chemicals interfere with the fetus's ability to receive the correct amount of nutrients and oxygen needed for normal development. They may affect the child after birth as well. Smoking during pregnancy can result in a child who is more susceptible to colds and lung problems. The child may also be mentally slower than children of nonsmokers, and he or she will run an increased risk of also smoking.

The only way for a pregnant women to prevent cigarettes from affecting the fetus during pregnancy is to quit smoking. Cutting back or switching to a low-tar brand will not eliminate all of the risks for the fetus. The best time for a woman to quit smoking is before she becomes pregnant. If she does this, the fetus can grow and develop as if the woman never smoked.

Smoking during lactation, or breast-feeding, exposes the baby to the same nicotine that the mother inhales. Even if a mother is not breast-feeding her child, she should refrain from smoking around the baby. A baby's lungs are more susceptible to the effects of secondhand smoke than an adult's lungs. Continual exposure to secondhand cigarette smoke can contribute to bronchitis, pneumonia, colds, coughs, and middle-ear infections for the child.

SECONDHAND SMOKE

People who choose not to smoke are still at risk from the smoke released into the air by smokers. Inhaling another person's smoke is called passive smoking or secondhand smoking. In the 1986 Surgeon General's Report, passive smoking was listed as a cause of lung cancer and other smoke-related diseases. The risk of lung cancer is 30 percent higher for nonsmoking wives of smokers than it is for nonsmoking wives of nonsmokers. It is believed that secondhand smoke causes 37,000 heart disease deaths and 13,000 cancer deaths per year.

QUITTING THE HABIT

Many people who attempt to quit smoking experience withdrawal symptoms, which is a normal reaction when any addictive substance is no longer put into the body. The worst symptoms—drowsiness, headaches, and fatigue—usually occur within the first few days of quitting. Other withdrawal symptoms are difficulty concentrating, anxiety, a constant craving, irritability, restlessness, and digestive problems. Symptoms vary drastically from person to person. Some women suffer from many of the withdrawal symptoms, while others may only have one or two. Withdrawal symptoms last only about two weeks. The addiction to the habit of smoking may take many months or years to conquer completely.

It is never too late to quit smoking, and the benefits to the body cannot be overstated. Once a person stops smoking, the body begins to reverse the harmful effects of smoking. The cilia, or hair in the lungs, which are damaged or impaired by smoking, begin to function normally. Some people may have a more frequent and productive cough in the first few weeks after quitting as the lungs begin to work more effectively. The vasoconstricting effects of smoking on the arteries is eliminated, as is the increased risk of hypertension, coronary heart disease, and stroke. After 15 years of not smoking, an ex-smoker's health returns to nearly the same level as that of a nonsmoker.

Use of the nicotine patch, a prescription patch that slowly releases nicotine into the bloodstream, can help ease the withdrawal symptoms but is not a cure-all. It is important to follow a practitioner's instructions while using the patch and to remember not to smoke a cigarette during its use—the combination of the two can cause an overload of nicotine, accelerating heart rates and drastically raising blood pressure. Nicotine gum, also a prescription containing nicotine, has the same effect as the patch. The patch and nicotine gum have few side effects.

SEE addiction; cancer, lung.

For information on smoking, or for help with breaking the smoking habit, contact:

Action on Smoking and Health
2013 H St., N.W.
Washington, DC 20006
202-659-4310
http://ash.org

American Cancer Society
1599 Clifton Rd., N.E.
Atlanta, GA 30329-4251
800-227-2345
404-320-3333
http://www.cancer.org

American Heart Association
7320 Greenville Ave.
Dallas, TX 75231
800-AHA-USA-1
214-373-6300
http://www.amhrt.org

American Lung Association
1740 Broadway
New York, NY 10019
800-LUNG-USA
212-315-8700
http://www.lungusa.org

International Network of Women Against Tobacco
American Public Health Association
1015 15th St., N.W.
Washington, DC 20005-2605
202-789-5622

National Cancer Institute
Office of Cancer Communications
9000 Rockville Pike, Room 10A16
Bethesda, MD 20892
800- 4-CANCER
http://www.icic.nci.nih.gov/

Office on Smoking and Health Hotline
Centers for Disease Control and Prevention
4770 Buford Highway, N.E., Mailstop K-50
Atlanta, GA 30341-3724
800-CDC-1311 (recorded message)
770- 488-5705 (live person)
http://www.cdc.gov/

Smokenders
4455 E. Camelback Rd., Suite D150
Phoenix, AZ 85018
602-840-7414
smokenders@aol

STRESS

There are many causes of stress that are unique to women. Menstruation, infertility, pregnancy, and menopause are physical sources of stress. Women become single parents more often than men do, and face poverty, domestic violence, incest, and sexual assault more frequently. In addition, women often juggle careers and motherhood, facing social pressures that require them to fulfill both full-time roles.

Later in life, women are often called upon to become full-time caregivers for a child, partner, or elderly parent with an infirmity, a situation that can cause considerable stress. The National Family Caregivers Association reports that three-fourths of all caregivers are women. In addition, because women on average live longer than men, they are more likely to become widowed. The death of a partner may bring with it not only the stress of grief but also financial worries.

FIGHT OR FLIGHT

The feeling of stress actually refers to the physical response the body mounts to a perceived threat, whether the threat is real or imagined, physical or psychological. When the nervous system senses danger, it prepares for the "fight or flight" response by releasing into the bloodstream adrenaline and other stress-triggered hormones.

Adrenaline causes the heart to beat faster, the mouth to become dry, the level of blood pressure to rise, and the muscles to tighten and ready for action. In addition, sugar is released into the system by the liver to provide extra energy, and the digestive and immune systems slow down so that blood can be diverted to other parts of the body.

Stress often has a positive effect. Stressors such as planning a wedding, pursuing a new romantic interest, being pregnant, or tackling a challenging project at work can stimulate activity and create a feeling of exhilaration. However, when stress becomes long-term or out of control, the repeated physical responses have a negative effect on the body.

SYMPTOMS OF STRESS

Negative stress can cause a number of physical and mental health problems. Stress has long been associated with heart disease and often is a factor in chronic lower back pain and types of depression and anxiety disorders. When stress leads to insomnia, loss of sleep, the body's ability to fight off infection and disease is diminished.

Symptoms of stress include:
- Headache
- Sudden mood swings
- Elevated blood pressure
- Insomnia
- Lack of concentration
- Fatigue
- Amenorrhea (loss of periods)
- Vaginismus (a condition in which the opening of the vagina involuntarily constricts and cannot be easily relaxed)
- Painful intercourse
- Decreased interest in sex
- Lack of orgasm
- Excessive smoking or drinking
- Eating disorders, such as anorexia nervosa and bulimia

TREATING STRESS

While the symptoms of stress may be treated as they appear, it is necessary to deal with the origins of stress through such things as relaxation techniques and lifestyle changes. For some, treatment may mean removing the cause of stress, possibly by changing jobs or seeking help with family responsibilities. Psychotherapy, a type of counseling that helps individuals overcome the problems that trigger anxiety, may help those who are unable to handle emotionally stressful situations.

A family of tranquilizers known as benzodiazepines—which includes Valium, Librium, and Xanax—may be prescribed to treat severe anxiety or sleeplessness, or it may be combined with other drugs for the treatment of stress-related ulcers. Such drugs are addictive and should only be used for a short period of time under a physician's supervision. Benzodiazepines are usually used with psychotherapy.

Many alternative therapies may be used to treat stress. Meditation, yoga, and Chinese medicine are often used to help slow the mind and

HOW STRESSFUL EVENTS AFFECT YOUR LIFE

To rate how much stress you are experiencing in your life, add up the numbers listed for life events you have undergone within the last year. If you score more than 200, you have a 50 percent chance of becoming seriously ill from stress; a score of 300 or more raises your chance of illness to 80 percent.

Life Event	Score
1. Death of a spouse	100
2. Divorce	73
3. Marital separation	65
4. Jail term	63
5. Death of a close family member	63
6. Personal injury or illness	53
7. Marriage	50
8. Being fired	47
9. Marital reconciliation	45
10. Retirement	45
11. Change in health of a family member	44
12. Pregnancy	40
13. Sexual difficulties	39
14. Having a baby	39
15. Business readjustment	39
16. Change in financial state	38
17. Death of a close friend	37
18. Change to a different line of work	36
19. Change in number of arguments with spouse	35
20. Mortgage large in relation to income	31
21. Foreclosure of mortgage or loan	30
22. Change in responsibilities at work	29
23. Son or daughter leaving home	29
24. Trouble with in-laws	29
25. Outstanding personal achievement	28
26. Spouse begins or stops work	26
27. Begin or end school	26
28. Change in living conditions	25
29. Change in personal habits	24
30. Trouble with boss	23
31. Change in work hours or conditions	20
32. Change in residence	20
33. Change in schools	20
34. Change in church activities	19
35. Change in recreation	19
36. Change in social activities	18
37. Small mortgage in relation to income	17
38. Change in sleeping habits	16
39. Change in number of family get-togethers	15
40. Change in eating habits	13
41. Vacation	13
42. Christmas	12
43. Minor violations of the law	11

Source: Reprinted with permission from *Psychosomatic Research,* vol. 11, Holmes and Rahe, "Social Readjustment Rating Scale," 1967. Pergamon Press Ltd., Oxford, England.

the body, prompting relaxation. Alternative therapies may also speed the healing of any stress-related illness. Mind/body therapies, such as hypnotherapy, may be used to help the individual deal with emotions that lead to stress. Herbal remedies such as chamomile, valerian, ginkgo, linden flower, and passionflower are all reputed to have calmative qualities.

PREVENTING STRESS

To help prevent stress and relieve stressful situations:

■ Exercise. Any sustained physical exercise will reduce stress by using up extra adrenaline while increasing your sense of control and distracting you from your worries. Exercise also helps you feel good physically. Walking, aerobics, swimming, and jogging are a few stress-relieving exercises that can be done without a partner.

■ Be sure to get enough sleep.

■ Maintain a balanced diet. Proper nutrition can help prevent the effects of stress and may help fight off stress-related illnesses.

■ Practice moderation in all things. By cutting down on alcohol, cigarettes, late-night hours, overtime, and excess commitments, you can cut down on stress and its negative effects.

■ Find a quick trick that calms you. Some find relaxation in counting backward from 100 to 1, in taking deep breaths, or in closing their eyes.

■ Experiment with meditation, an ancient technique similar to self-hypnosis that relaxes the mind and body. The idea is to give the mind a chance to relax by taking a break from sight, sound, information, and demanding thoughts.

■ Share your feelings. A long-running Johns Hopkins University study begun in 1946 has shown that people who don't reach out to others in times of stress suffer a greater incidence of cancer and suicide.

■ Try to eliminate or modify stressors in your life. Though it may be difficult to change your occupation or your family life, working fewer hours, calling on a relative for help, or giving up extra activities may be what is needed to ease stress.

■ Experiment with massage, yoga, or other alternative therapies to relieve stress. Such remedies will aid relaxation as well as healing.

■ Consider getting a pet you can relate to. Pets can be relaxing and help reduce stress. However, if the needs of a pet are too much for you to handle, it may actually add to stress.

SEE depression.

For more information on stress, contact:

American Institute of Stress
124 Park Ave.
Yonkers, NY 10703
914-963-1200
stressl24@aol.com

National Family Caregivers Association
9621 E. Bexhill Dr.
Kensington, MD 20895-3104
301-942-6430
caregiving@aol.com

National Mental Health Association
1021 Prince St.
Alexandria, VA 22314-2971
703-684-7722
http://www.worldcorp.com/dc-online/nmha

Women's Programs Office
American Psychological Association
750 First St., N.E.
Washington, DC 20002-4242
202-336-6044
pubinterest@apa.org

STROKE

Stroke is the third leading cause of death and the major cause of disability among American adults. According to the American Heart Association (AHA), stroke strikes an estimated 500,000 Americans each year and kills about 150,000. Although the incidence of stroke is about 19 percent higher for men, approximately 1.5 million women are alive today who have been affected by it. Stroke accounts for approximately one-third of all causes of paralysis in women between the ages of 17 and 44.

A stroke, also called a cerebrovascular accident (CVA), apoplexy, or cerebral infarction, is an injury to the nervous system that occurs when blood vessels fail to deliver an adequate amount of blood to the brain. A stroke may result in death, or damage to the brain, which may cause physical paralysis, weakness, communication difficulties, and many other neurological problems. The effects may be permanent, depending on the portion of the brain affected, the severity of the stroke, and the victim's response to rehabilitation.

While more people are surviving strokes now than ever before (the death rate declined more than 50 percent between 1960 and 1990), the majority of long-term survivors still experience major changes in their lifestyles. The AHA estimates that 15 percent require institutional care; one-third depend on someone else to care for their basic activities of daily living; and more than half report a decrease in their social life.

TYPES OF STROKE

There are two principal types of stroke: ischemic and hemorrhagic.

An **ischemic stroke** is usually caused by a blockage in a blood vessel. Blood clots and low blood flow caused by a narrowing of the arteries both result in an inadequate supply of blood to the brain that can result in ischemic stroke.

The type of ischemic stroke depends on where the blockage originates. In **cerebral thrombosis,** the most common type of stroke, the blockage originates in an artery that supplies blood to the brain. In **cerebral embolism,** a clot or other foreign material originating elsewhere in the body is carried through the bloodstream and lodges in an artery leading to the brain. This traveling matter, know as an embolus, often forms in the heart.

Ischemic strokes may also vary in duration and effects. A **transient ischemic attack (TIA),** or ministroke, is caused by a temporary blockage of the blood flow to the brain. The blood flow in a TIA quickly returns to normal, and all symptoms disappear within 24 hours. More than one-third of the people who have had a TIA ultimately have a stroke. **Reversible ischemic neurological deficit (RIND)** occurs when the strokelike symptoms last longer than 24 hours but leave only minor deficits. **Partially reversible ischemic neurological deficit (PRIND)** occurs when the symptoms last more than three days and produce minor dysfunction.

The second type of stroke, **hemorrhagic stroke,** is usually the result of the rupture of a blood vessel, caused by a head injury, the rupture of an aneurysm (a bulge in the wall of a blood vessel), or the leakage or rupture of a congenitally weak or malformed blood vessel.

Hemorrhagic stroke type is determined by location. In **cerebral hemorrhage,** the ruptured or leaking artery is actually located in the brain tissue. It accounts for about 10 percent of all strokes. In **subarachnoid hemorrhage,** the bleeding is on the surface of the brain between brain and skull. It accounts for about 7 percent of all strokes.

SIGNS OF STROKE

The warning signs of a stroke are:

- Sudden weakness, numbness, tingling or other unusual sensations, or paralysis in the face, arm, or leg, particularly on one side of the body
- Sudden dimness or blurring of vision, particularly in one eye
- An inability to speak or understand spoken language, called aphasia
- An inability to recall the word for an item, or disconnected speech, called anomia
- Sudden, severe headache
- Unexplained dizziness, unsteadiness, or falls
- Sudden unconsciousness

Anyone experiencing any of these symptoms may be having a stroke and should seek medical attention immediately.

RISK

The risk factors of stroke include:

- Age. Nearly three-quarters of all strokes occur in people 65 or older.
- Race. African Americans are about 60 percent more likely to have a stroke than whites are.
- Smoking
- Sickle-cell anemia. One in 14 people with sickle-cell anemia eventually has a stroke.
- Diabetes. One-fifth of stroke sufferers are diabetic.

- Tendency toward migraine headaches. Studies show a link between migraines and strokes in women under 45, particularly if they have a history of both migraines and smoking.
- A history of transient ischemic attacks (TIAs), or ministrokes. TIAs are strong predictors of stroke and should be considered a warning sign.
- Hypertension. Because hypertension (high blood pressure) may result in decreased blood flow to the brain and weakened blood vessel walls, it is a strong risk factor for stroke.
- A history of heart disease and atherosclerosis (hardening of the arteries).
- Use of some illegal drugs, such as cocaine
- Obesity and sedentary lifestyle. These factors do not place a person at risk for stroke, but rather predispose a person to the development of other risk factors of stroke, such as heart disease.
- Oral contraceptives. High-dose oral contraceptives have been associated with an increased risk for stroke. Studies show that the more commonly used low-dose oral contraceptives rarely increase the risk of stroke. However, they should not be used by women having other risk factors, including heavy smoking, physical inactivity, and stress. Women over the age of 25 who smoke and take high-dose oral contraceptives are 22 times more likely to have a stroke than those who do neither.

TREATMENT

Immediate treatment following a stroke involves monitoring vital signs and stabilizing the individual. In ischemic stroke, the first step is to improve blood and oxygen flow to the brain. This may be done by administering anticoagulants (such as heparin) or platelet inhibitors (such as aspirin), drugs that thin the blood and dissolve and prevent clots. Surgery may be done to open the artery and improve blood and oxygen flow. A hyperbaric chamber, which uses oxygen under pressure, may reduce brain damage.

For hemorrhagic stroke, treatment includes drugs to lower the blood pressure, slowing the flow of blood. Injection of a special substance into the leaking artery may plug the leak. Surgery may also be necessary to close ruptured blood vessels. A procedure known as evacuation may also be performed to relieve the pressure of the blood building up within the skull.

Treatment for stroke also includes preventive measures such as treating and controlling the risk factors of stroke, such as heart disease, TIAs, diabetes, and hypertension.

REHABILITATION

Rehabilitation therapy often starts soon after the medical emergency is over. Individuals may have difficulty getting around, doing day-to-day tasks (such as grooming and preparing meals), and communicating. Many also become depressed or develop another psychological disability. As a result, a rehabilitation program often involves several types of care and may include speech therapy, physical therapy, and psychological and occupational therapy (therapy that helps teach basic, everyday skills).

A stroke victim should be evaluated to determine which therapies are needed in what combination to provide maximum effects. The assessment should be based on the severity of the disorder, the mental state of the patient, and the environment (such as a supportive network of friends and family). Rehabilitation can take place in a hospital, a nursing facility, at an outpatient clinic, or at home. Those who need intensive (three hours a day or more) rehabilitation programs are usually treated at a hospital. If mobility and daily functioning are not a problem, the care can take place at home.

The extent of the recovery is usually established by the end of six to nine months, but some patients continue to show steady improvement over a long time. A network of supporters, whether friends, family, or members of a support group, is an important factor in the rehabilitation process, which may continue long after formal therapy has been discontinued. Mechanical assists such as wheelchairs, braces, extenders, and computers can go far in improving the quality of life of one who has had a stroke.

SEE blood pressure; cholesterol; heart disease.

For more information on stroke, contact:

AHA Stroke Connection
[formerly the Courage Stroke Network]
American Heart Association
7272 Greenville Ave.
Dallas, TX 75231
800-AHA-USA1
214-373-6300
http://www.amhrt.org

National Stroke Association
96 Inverness Dr., E., Suite I
Englewood, CO 80112-5112
800-STROKES
http://www.stroke.org

Stroke Clubs International
805 12th St.
Galveston, TX 77550
409-762-1022

TOXIC SHOCK SYNDROME

Toxic shock syndrome (TSS) is a rare illness that is believed to be caused by bacteria in the bloodstream. It has been estimated that each year six to 17 of every 100,000 menstruating women and girls will get toxic shock syndrome. TSS may also occur in individuals infected with the group A streptococcus bacteria, which produce toxins as they rapidly reproduce.

TSS begins with flulike symptoms suddenly, usually during menstruation. Symptoms of TSS include:

■ High fever (101°F or higher)

■ A sudden sunburnlike rash that spreads over the body

■ Vomiting

■ Peeling of the skin, especially on the hands and feet

■ Fainting

■ Dizziness

■ Diarrhea

■ Drop in blood pressure

Though it is not known how the bacteria enter the bloodstream, toxic shock syndrome has been linked to extended tampon use. When placed in the vagina, tampons, especially the high absorbency variety, seem to provide an ideal place for the bacteria to thrive. In 80 percent of TSS cases, the women had used high-absorbency tampons. In a few rare cases, use of the contraceptive sponge and the diaphragm has triggered TSS by retaining infected fluids in the vagina.

TSS can lead quickly to shock, kidney failure, and death. If the symptoms of toxic shock syndrome appear, a woman should remove the tampon, diaphragm, or any other object from the vagina and seek emergency medical care immediately. A treatment of antibiotics and intravenous fluids will be used to kill the bacteria and replace lost liquids.

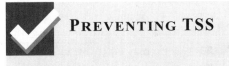

PREVENTING TSS

To avoid toxic shock syndrome:

■ Use sanitary pads instead of tampons.

■ Use a less absorbent type of tampon made for a regular or light flow and be sure to change them regularly, about every four hours. Never leave absorbent objects in the vagina for long periods of time.

SEE menstrual cycle and ovulation.

URINARY TRACT INFECTIONS

Urinary tract infections (UTIs) include infections of the bladder, the ureters (the tubes that lead from the kidneys to the bladder), and the urethra (the tube that carries urine from the bladder to the outside of the body). Infections of the bladder are also called cystitis. UTIs are most often caused by bacteria that have spread from the rectum to the vagina and then to the urethra and bladder, but may also be caused by bacteria from sexually transmitted infections. UTIs, which may resemble vaginal infections but are not the same, can cause the tissues of the urinary tract to become swollen and sensitive. They affect women much more often than men because the woman's urethra is shorter than a man's (about one inch to his six), and bacteria may enter through it more easily. A woman's urethra is also closer to the anus than is a man's.

Almost all women will have a urinary tract infection at some point in their lives. The typical UTI disappears in about a week; however, 20 percent of women experience infections that recur periodically. Women are more likely to have a UTI during pregnancy or menopause, and women with diabetes are also prone to these infections.

Although painful, UTIs are seldom serious health threats. The symptoms include:

■ Burning pain during urination

■ The urge to urinate when the bladder is nearly empty

■ A frequent urge to urinate, especially during the night

■ Involuntary loss of urine
■ Lower abdominal or back pain
■ Blood or pus in the urine
■ Fever

CAUSES OF UTIs

Under normal conditions, there are bacteria present in the digestive tract, and certain kinds of activity may promote their presence in the urinary tract. Sexual intercourse, especially in the conventional position with the man on top of the woman, can drive bacteria present on the vulva into the urethra. This condition, because it is brought on by frequent intercourse, is sometimes called honeymoon cystitis. UTIs are also brought on by the irritation of intercourse, especially when the penis is inserted before the vagina is fully lubricated. Anal intercourse or digital play around the anus, followed by continued sexual activity without washing, may also cause UTIs.

Diaphragms are associated with the development of UTIs in some women. Bubble baths, swimming pools with treated water, and some contraceptive foams can also trigger symptoms of urinary tract infections in those with allergic reactions. Certain types of clothing, such as non-absorbent, sweat-retaining clothing, can increase transmission of bacteria from the anus to the vagina and urethra and promote infection.

UTIs often occur in pregnant women because the pressure of the fetus may prevent the bladder from emptying completely, giving the bacteria a place to grow. It is also thought that increased levels of estrogen in the body during pregnancy help bacteria to grow. A pregnant woman with the symptoms of a UTI should see her practitioner because untreated infections may lead to premature labor.

Women in menopause are also prone to urinary tract infections. This is thought to be because in some women the bladder and urethra become more fragile and because the hormonal changes can alter the normal balance of bacteria in the system. Older women who have a cystocele (a bladder that has dropped into the vaginal canal) or who suffer a loss of bladder control may also have UTIs because all of the urine may not be emptied from the bladder during urination.

DIAGNOSIS

Urinary tract infections are usually bacterial in origin. Therefore, diagnosis involves testing a urine sample, taken from midstream during urination to avoid contamination, for the presence of infection. There is a chance that the test will not detect an early infection if the urine is not concentrated enough. Home tests for urinary tract infections are available over-the-counter but are neither very sensitive nor reliable. A practitioner should be consulted for confirmation of the diagnosis and treatment.

TREATMENT

Sulfonamides (sulfa drugs) and antibiotics are used to treat urinary tract infections. Phenazopyridine hydrochloride (Pyridium), a drug that turns the urine orange, may be prescribed to

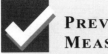

PREVENTIVE MEASURES

To prevent urinary tract infections or discourage them from returning:

■ Drink eight or more glasses of fluid a day. Avoid soft drinks, which promote the growth of bacteria.

■ Drink unsweetened cranberry juice, which contains acids that inhibit the growth of bacteria. According to a 1994 study in the *Journal of the American Medical Association,* women who drank 10 ounces of cranberry juice a day were 58 percent less likely to have a UTI.

■ Urinate immediately before and after sexual intercourse. This helps keep the tract clean and flush out any bacteria.

■ Urinate often, and go to the bathroom as soon as you feel the urge to urinate. This prevents bacteria from building up in the bladder. Pour water over the labia and pat dry.

■ Change your sexual position if it is a trigger for UTIs.

■ Keep the pubic area clean and dry. Wear cotton underpants, panty hose with a cotton crotch, and avoid tight jeans to allow the area to breathe. Tampons and sanitary napkins should be changed frequently.

■ Use condoms or vaginal pouches during vaginal intercourse to prevent sexually transmitted infections.

■ After a bowel movement, wipe from front to back to avoid spreading bacteria to the urethra. Rinsing or washing the area is very effective if you suffer from frequent UTIs.

relieve inflammation and pain. A woman should also drink at least eight glasses of water a day to flush the bacteria out of the system. Unsweetened cranberry juice, which contains benzoic acid, increases the levels of acid in the urinary tract so that bacteria cannot flourish and the infection disappears more quickly—no other juices have this benefit. Cranberry juice may also enhance the effects of drugs. It can also be purchased in capsule form. Some herbal remedies are also thought to relax the urinary tract and expel bacteria. A follow-up urine test should be done after treatment to be sure the bacteria are gone.

SEE sexually transmitted infections; vaginitis.

For more information on UTIs, contact:

Planned Parenthood Federation of America, Inc.
810 Seventh Avenue
New York, NY 10019
For the Planned Parenthood nearest you, call:
   800-230-PLAN
http://www.ppfa.org/ppfa

UTERINE PROLAPSE

A prolapsed uterus, a uterus that partially descends into the vagina, is due to the weakening of the pelvic floor muscles. The condition is often the result of childbirth (difficult labor, a large baby, or many pregnancies), obesity, constipation, or fibroid tumors or other pelvic tumors. A prolapsed uterus tends to worsen after menopause and usually occurs after age 60. It is usually diagnosed during a pelvic examination.

SYMPTOMS

While a woman may not experience symptoms with a uterine prolapse, there may be:

- A sensation of heaviness or pressure in the vagina
- Urinary incontinence (the involuntary leaking of urine)
- Backache
- Painful or difficult intercourse
- Constipation

In severe cases, the uterus may protrude out of the vagina, causing irritation to the cervix, the narrow opening of the uterus. Uterine prolapse may cause difficulty walking.

TREATMENT

In mild cases, treatment may involve taking replacement hormones, which may help to thicken the vaginal walls and strengthen pelvic muscles. For overweight women, losing weight can relieve pressure on the organs. Kegel exercises, designed to tighten the muscles around the vagina and rectum, may also be practiced. (For more information on Kegel exercises, see "Strengthening the Pelvic Floor" on p. 228.)

For more severe cases, the use of a **pessary** may help relieve the symptoms. A pessary is a device, similar in design to a diaphragm, that helps hold the uterus in place. Pessaries come in many shapes and sizes, so it is up to the woman and her practitioner to determine the most appropriate type based on the woman's body and lifestyle. Only one type, the ring pessary, can be worn during sex. These devices need to be removed and cleaned frequently, usually by the patient, to avoid irritation and infection. For these reasons, some women find pessaries too inconvenient to use for long, and most practitioners offer them only as a temporary solution to younger women and as the only option for women too old or unfit for surgery.

Uterine resuspension involves surgically repositioning the uterus and other organs that have dropped, shortening the stretched ligaments and reinforcing the muscles around the vagina and rectum. Many physicians do not endorse this type of surgery, since overcorrection may make sex difficult. There is also the chance that the uterus will fall again. Studies report that the uterus descends again in 10 to 20 percent of cases after uterine resuspension, although usually not as far as the first time.

In severe cases, a **hysterectomy,** removal of the uterus, will solve the problem of prolapse. Many practitioners offer this surgery as the primary option, although its use is controversial because there are less invasive alternatives.

Once the uterus is removed, other organs can shift, unless the surgeon also tightens up sagging ligaments and muscles and repositions other organs. Other side effects, such as urinary disorders, decreased sexual function, and bladder and bowel problems may accompany hysterectomy. A woman considering a hysterectomy should seek a second opinion.

PREVENTING UTERINE PROLAPSE

To help prevent uterine prolapse:

■ Practice Kegel exercises.

■ Avoid constipation. Drink eight glasses of water a day and eat a high-fiber diet. Constipation, which promotes prolonged "bearing-down" efforts, is a symptom, and also a contributing factor, of uterine prolapse.

■ Maintain a healthy weight. Extra pounds put extra pressure on the uterus and other internal organs.

■ Exercise. Being active helps to maintain your weight and also strengthens the muscles that help keep organs in the right place.

■ Try alternative methods. Acupuncture and yoga are two therapies that may help you to avoid prolapse.

■ Give birth in a squatting, or other upright, position. A vertical birth position eases the pressure put on the vagina, allows gravity to assist in the birth, and requires less use of interventions such as forceps. However, experts say that cesarean section and episiotomy do not prevent prolapse.

■ Don't smoke. A smoker's cough may aggravate prolapse.

SEE hysterectomy; incontinence, urinary.

VAGINITIS

Vaginitis, or inflammation of the vagina, can result from a vaginal infection or exposure to a sexually transmitted infection. The walls of the vagina become irritated and infected by bacteria, yeast (most often candida), parasites, or viruses, all of which cause vaginal discharge, itching, irritation, and discomfort. Vaginitis may also cause vaginal bleeding, pain in the lower abdomen, and pain during sexual intercourse. Some 75 percent of all women will have at least one vaginal infection in their lifetime, and 22 million will have repeat infections.

Because vaginitis has many different causes, a woman should see her medical practitioner for an accurate diagnosis if she experiences any symptoms. The symptoms of vaginitis may sometimes closely resemble those of a urinary tract infection. To determine the cause of an infection, a pelvic exam is done in conjunction with a microscopic examination of the discharge. Abnormal Pap test results may also be a sign of vaginitis.

YEAST INFECTIONS

Yeast infections, caused by a yeast called candida, are the most common form of vaginitis. Known as candidiasis, or moniliasis, this infection occurs when the normal balance of healthy bacteria in the vagina changes, creating an environment in which the candida can easily grow. Antibiotics may trigger yeast infections because they prompt the growth of yeast. Menopausal women not taking hormone replacement therapy are more likely to contract this form of vaginitis because without natural hormones, the vaginal lining is thinner and more prone to infection.

The major symptoms of yeast infections include:

■ Thick, cottage-cheese-like vaginal discharge

■ A yeasty odor

■ Itching or irritation of the vagina and the vulva

A woman should have her practitioner verify the presence of a yeast infection before beginning treatment. Treatment usually involves antifungal creams, ointments, or suppositories, and oral medications have recently become available. Eating plain yogurt containing the live acidophilus culture, or taking tablets with the culture, may also ease symptoms. Some women find applying the yogurt directly to the vagina, or inserting a tampon soaked in plain yogurt, soothing.

Over-the-counter yeast creams, such as Monistat and Gyne-Lotrimin, may be used to treat a recurring yeast infection that has already been diagnosed by a medical practitioner in the past. However, if the symptoms do not subside in a week, the woman should return to her practitioner.

TRICHOMONIASIS

Trichomoniasis, or "trich," is the most common sexually transmitted infection that causes vaginitis. It is caused by a parasite, a trichomona, which can be identified by microscopic examination of vaginal fluids. Trichomonas can also invade and cause infection in the urinary tract. However, it does not invade the uterus and fallopian tubes and will not affect fertility.

Symptoms include:

■ Frothy yellow or greenish vaginal discharge

■ A disagreeable odor

■ Itching, soreness, and inflammation of the vulva and inside the vagina

■ Blood in vaginal discharge

■ Burning during urination

■ Frequent urge to urinate

■ Swelling in the lower abdomen

The most effective treatment for trichomoniasis is the antibiotic metronidazole (Flagyl), which may have side effects, including nausea, diarrhea, a metallic taste in the mouth, and headache. It should not be taken during the first three months of pregnancy or while breast-feeding, if possible. Alcohol must be avoided while taking metronidazole because it can cause headache, difficulty breathing, nausea, vomiting, dizziness, confusion and sudden collapse. Other treatments include antibiotic suppositories or the application of antibacterial creams and gels. Some herbal remedies may be effective as well.

Because trichomoniasis is sexually transmitted, both partners should be treated simultaneously to eradicate the organisms. Men often do not have symptoms. Men's symptoms, if they occur, include burning during urination and pus or watery discharge from the penis. To prevent reinfection, partners should use condoms or vaginal pouches during treatment.

YEAST INFECTIONS AND DIET

Some women who experience recurring yeast infections have found that an antiyeast diet/drug regimen can relieve symptoms and prevent future infections. The link between yeast infections and diet is controversial. If she has any doubts, woman should not treat herself for a yeast infection unless a diagnosis has been made by a practitioner.

A growing number of experts believe that foods high in sugar may fuel the growth of candida in the body and that other foods, such as yogurt containing live cultures and garlic, can inhibit the growth of the organism.

The following recommendations are offered for preventing yeast infections through diet:

■ Eat more vegetables.

■ Avoid simple sugars and simple carbohydrates, such as candy, cake, and ice cream.

■ Cut back or eliminate fruit, especially dried fruit, from your diet.

■ Have a daily cup of yogurt containing live *Lactobacillus acidophilus* or take tablets or capsules containing the culture. These can help inhibit the growth of candida in the digestive tract and vagina.

■ Take antibiotics only if absolutely necessary.

■ Take natural antifungal medicines, such as caprylic acid, citrus seed extracts, or garlic products. These can be found in most health food stores.

■ Limit or avoid foods containing yeasts, molds, or ferments, such as cheese and bread, if you are allergic.

BACTERIAL VAGINOSIS (BV)

Infections may also be caused by bacteria, including *Gardnerella vaginalis* and group B streptococcus infection, which usually originate in the bowel and migrate to the vagina. The group B strep infection may affect a pregnant woman and the fetus by causing complications in the pregnancy. Bacterial vaginosis was once known as nonspecific vaginitis, before its causes were identified.

Symptoms of BV include:

- An off-colored, grayish vaginal discharge
- An unpleasant, fishy odor
- Irritation of the vagina and vulva
- Frequent urination or urinary urgency
- Irritation during intercourse

Bacterial vaginosis is usually diagnosed through microscopic examination of the discharge, and treatment varies with the diagnosis. Current treatment usually involves the use of antibiotic vaginal creams containing clindamycin (Cleocin) or metronidazole (MetroGel).

Bacterial vaginosis can be sexually transmitted. Circumcised men are less likely to pass BV to their partners because the surface of the penis is dry and inhospitable to bacteria. However, uncircumcised men may pick up and pass on the bacteria more easily because the foreskin provides an environment for growth. In men, there may be no symptoms. Men are generally not treated unless a woman has a repeat episode after treatment. Some studies show that treating the man does not decrease recurrences.

OTHER CAUSES OF VAGINITIS

In addition to bacterial causes of vaginitis, inflammation of the vagina can be triggered by mechanical or chemical factors. Vaginal ulcera-

PREVENTING VAGINITIS

The vagina, which is moist and warm, is an ideal breeding ground for bacteria. By making the environment less conducive to bacteria, you can reduce your risk of vaginitis.

To prevent all forms of vaginitis:

- Practice safer sex. Use a condom or vaginal pouch during intercourse.
- Wear breathable underwear, panty hose with a cotton crotch, or loose-fitting pants.
- Do not share towels. Trichomoniasis, for example, can survive at room temperature for several hours and can be transmitted by a moist towel or washcloth.
- Do not sit around in a wet bathing suit.
- Always wipe away from the vagina after bowel movements and urination. Pour water over the labia and pat dry to avoid leaving urine in the area.
- Avoid scented soaps and detergents. Do not use vaginal sprays on the vulva. Do not leave soap or shampoo residue between the vulvar lips after bathing.
- During treatment for vaginitis, use a condom or vaginal pouch to stop the spread of the bacteria.

tions, which can be brought on by herpes or gonorrhea, can become infected and cause inflammation. Microscopic tissue tears within the vagina may also become infected and trigger vaginitis. Atrophic vaginitis can occur after menopause because of lack of estrogen. Women with atrophic vaginitis complain of vaginal dryness and painful intercourse.

Irritation may occur with the use of vaginal sprays and deodorant soaps, shampoos, spermicides, and douches that can cause reactions in some women. Bubble baths can also trigger vaginitis. Generally, when use of these products stops, the vaginitis subsides. Vaginitis may also be caused by the presence of a foreign body in the vagina, such as a forgotten tampon or diaphragm. In this case, the irritation and inflammation end when the object is removed, and the woman is treated with antibiotics to prevent infection from occurring.

SEE sexually transmitted infections; urinary tract infections.

For more information, contact:

Planned Parenthood Federation of America, Inc.
810 Seventh Avenue
New York, NY 10019
For the Planned Parenthood nearest you, call:
   800-230-PLAN
http://www.ppfa.org/ppfa

VARICOSE VEINS

Varicose veins are swollen veins that usually occur in the legs. Varicose (meaning "enlarged" in Latin) veins are common in older women and sometimes develop in women who are pregnant. Hemorrhoids, which are varicose veins located in the anus, are common in pregnant women. Women are five times more likely than men to get varicose veins, though men are more likely to have hemorrhoids.

The veins in the legs, which keep blood moving to the heart, work against gravity with the help of small valves that keep blood from flowing backward. Varicose veins occur when one of the valves fails, allowing blood to collect in one spot. The vein swells, and shows through the skin as a purple or blue-tinged area.

Varicose veins tend to run in a family, and those of German and Irish descent, Ashkenazi Jews, and Middle Europeans are more likely to develop them. In addition, higher hormone levels, such as those found in pregnant women, are thought to dilate veins and possibly cause valve failure.

SYMPTOMS

Although unsightly, most varicose veins do not cause problems, unless they become infected or clots develop in them. However, the following symptoms may occur:
- Muscle cramps
- Swollen ankles and legs

■ Dry skin or ulcerated patches on the legs (caused by a deficiency of blood)

■ A feeling of fatigue and soreness in the calves of the legs

In rare instances, varicose veins may cause **phlebitis,** inflammation of the vein. This is usually associated with a blood clot. The clots cause pain in the legs but rarely travel to the heart or the lungs.

TREATMENT

Varicose veins do not disappear, and they may worsen over the years. If there is no pain or other problem, cosmetic creams are available to help hide the veins. A woman prone to varicose veins may wear elastic stockings to promote circulation in the legs and prevent present veins

SPIDER VEINS

Spider veins are small, thin, purple capillaries on the thighs that become visible. They commonly develop in women 30 to 50 years old and also in pregnant women. Though they are much smaller and more delicate than varicose veins, spider veins develop for the same reasons, sometimes as a result of varicose veins. Thet are also stimulated by female hormones, especially estrogen.

There is no health risk involved with spider veins, and any treatment is purely cosmetic. They may be treated with **scleropathy** or through **electrodesiccation,** a procedure that applies an electric current to the capillary to close it off. The small veins may also be closed with an injection of collagen.

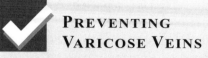

PREVENTING VARICOSE VEINS

To prevent varicose veins:

■ Avoid standing or sitting for long periods of time. If you must stand or sit, move around or change position often.

■ Don't sit with your legs crossed.

■ Elevate your feet at times throughout the day, preferably by lying flat. This encourages blood to flow back toward the heart.

■ Wear elastic support hose to keep blood from pooling near the feet.

■ Don't wear tight girdles, garters, shoes, or socks. These may interfere with circulation.

■ Stay in shape. The muscles used during exercise help move blood up from the legs. Extra weight also puts a strain on the veins in the legs.

■ Elevate the foot of the bed several inches to decrease pressure on veins while you sleep.

■ Make sure you are sitting in a comfortable position. To promote circulation, the ideal chair should pitch downward at three degrees and have a "waterfall" edge. This keeps pressure off the thighs.

■ Don't smoke. Smoking has been linked to the development of varicose veins.

from worsening and new varicose veins from appearing.

There are several medical solutions for varicose veins. In each one, the vein is closed off or removed, forcing the blood to flow through other veins. With **scleropathy,** an irritating solution that causes inflammation is injected into the vein, causing it to close together. **Laser treatment** uses a highly focused beam of light to inflame the walls of the vein and close it off. These procedures are usually done on superficial veins and may be done by a plastic surgeon during an in-office procedure.

A procedure performed for more severe varicose veins, usually done by a vascular surgeon, is **ligation and stripping** of the veins. In this surgery, the **saphenous vein,** the main vein that runs from the pelvic region to the foot—there is one in each leg—is cut and removed, usually with an instrument that turns it inside out as it is pulled out. Then visible varicose veins are removed as well. As a result of the procedure, the veins deep within the leg take over the job of returning the blood to the heart. However, deep veins can become overloaded, a more serious problem.

Another procedure, **plication,** is the wrapping of a nearby muscle around the varicose vein to cause a slight constriction. When the person walks, the muscle acts as a valve, forcing the blood toward the heart. Because the cosmetic results of the surgery depend upon how much exercise the person gets, this procedure is not usually used.

Hemorrhoids, varicose veins in the anus, cause pain and bleeding during bowel movements and are caused by pressure resulting from constipation, obesity, pregnancy, and prolonged coughing. They are treated with a high-fiber diet to relieve constipation. Sitz baths and topical creams may also soothe symptoms. If problems continue, the hemorrhoids may be removed using cryosurgery, which destroys the hemorrhoid through freezing. They may also be removed surgically or through laser treatments. In both cases, the recovery period may be painful and the hemorrhoids may recur.

SEE cryosurgery.

WEIGHT REDUCTION

W eight reduction, the process of losing excess body fat, is an issue with which many women struggle. According to the National Center for Health Statistics, 27 percent of women of all ages are overweight, a condition that can cause health risks.

Women who are obese—meaning they weigh 20 percent more than their optimal weight—have an increased risk of diabetes, heart disease, urinary incontinence, and several other chronic conditions. Varicose veins, infertility, high blood pressure, and cancers of the gallbladder, ovaries, uterus, and pancreas are also more common in obese women. However, obese women do have the benefit of extra estrogen in their bodies; this means fewer hot flashes during menopause and a lower risk of osteoporosis.

Weight reduction is also an issue for many women who are neither obese nor overweight. There are many women who diet to lose pounds for cosmetic reasons or because of feelings of inadequacy. In large part, this is due to the pressures of a society that idealizes thinness. Women who diet or exercise to an extreme could develop amenorrhea (loss of menstrual periods) and eating disorders, such as anorexia or bulimia, that could be fatal if not treated.

RECOMMENDED-WEIGHT CHARTS

The controversy about optimal body weight is long-standing. The first weight recommendations were based on charts created by insurance companies in the 1940s that analyzed which policyholders lived longest. These charts received criticism because they did not include a breakdown by age or bone structure, only height. In 1990 the "Age-Adapted Healthy Weight" chart was developed, breaking the information down by age group and height. However, critics say the data of the new charts, like that of previous ones, are based solely on statistics of people who are insured and present an incomplete—if not inaccurate—conclusion about optimal body weight.

The most recent studies on optimal weight reveal that even moderate weight gains (as little as 11 pounds after age 18), which are permissible according to the 1990 weight charts, can increase a woman's risk of early death.

RISKS OF BEING OVERWEIGHT

Many experts believe that the health risks of being overweight are not as dire as they may seem. They point out that studies often fail to account for the fact that overweight people are generally poorer than thin people—a demographic that includes other health risks. In addition, overweight people diet more than thin people, and constant dieting can often lead to increased health risks. Some experts also argue that overweight people may suffer stress-related health problems because of discrimination and prejudice. Other medical experts insist that it is healthier for people to gain weight as they age and that a little fat seems to help elderly people endure illness, an opinion reflected in current recommended-weight charts.

However, this advice is in direct conflict with that of most cardiologists and recent studies of heart disease. For example, researchers from the Harvard School of Public Health and Harvard School of Medicine conducted a 14-year study of nearly 116,000 women. They found that weight gains of even 11 to 18 pounds in adult life resulted in a 25 percent greater chance of suffering from or dying of a heart

BODY-MASS INDEX

Health risks are also measured by body-mass index, or BMI. While the current guidelines in the United States state that BMI should be between 21 and 27 for healthy men and women, current studies suggest that an index of 23 to 24 is more on target. To reduce the risk of diabetes, for example, a study reports that the BMI should be less than 24; to reduce heart disease, it should be less than 23.

BMI is computed by dividing your weight (in kilograms) into your height (in meters) squared. So, to determine your BMI, you first divide your weight by 2.2 to find the equivalent in kilograms. Then multiply your height in inches by .0245 to find your height in meters. Then multiply your height in meters by itself. Finally, divide your weight in kilograms by the square of your height in meters. The total equals your BMI.

attack compared with women who gained less than 11 pounds after the age of 18.

A similar study in the *Journal of the American Medical Association* reported that the risk of heart disease and cancer, especially breast, colon, and endometrial cancer, increases with a weight gain of 22 pounds or more after age 18. For women who are categorized as obese, the chances of an early death doubled, according to the study.

By these guidelines, a weight gain of 10 to 15 pounds in early adulthood should be a warning sign to monitor weight gain closely—even though the weight charts allow for moderate weight gain through the years. Experts also recommend that women stop smoking, a factor that greatly increases the risk of early death. The risk of any weight gain that occurs as a result of quitting smoking is much less than the risk of continuing to smoke.

Additionally, where a women carries her extra weight—whether she is apple-shaped and gains weight in the abdominal area or pear-shaped with extra pounds on her hips and thighs—also seems to matter. Most experts agree that being apple-shaped represents a greater health risk than being pear-shaped.

AGE-ADAPTED HEALTHY WEIGHTS FOR WOMEN

Height	Years				
	Age 20-29	Age 30-39	Age 40-49	Age 50-59	Age 60-69
4' 10"	84-111	92-119	99-127	107-135	115-142
4' 11"	87-115	95-123	103-131	111-139	119-147
5' 0"	90-119	98-127	106-135	114-143	123-152
5' 1"	93-123	101-131	110-140	118-148	127-157
5' 2"	96-127	105-136	113-144	122-153	131-163
5' 3"	99-131	108-140	117-149	126-158	135-168
5' 4"	102-135	112-145	121-154	130-163	140-173
5' 5"	106-140	115-149	125-159	134-168	144-179
5' 6"	109-144	119-154	129-164	138-174	148-184
5' 7"	112-148	122-159	133-169	143-179	153-190
5' 8"	116-153	126-163	137-174	147-184	158-196
5' 9"	119-157	130-168	141-179	151-190	162-201
5' 10"	122-162	134-173	145-184	156-195	167-207
5' 11"	126-167	137-178	149-190	160-201	172-213
6' 0"	129-171	141-183	153-195	165-207	177-219
6' 1"	133-176	145-188	157-200	169-213	182-225
6' 2"	137-181	149-194	162-206	174-219	187-232
6' 3"	141-186	153-199	166-212	179-225	192-238
6' 4"	144-191	157-205	171-218	184-231	197-244

Source: National Institutes of Health.

HELP YOURSELF

A schedule of well-balanced meals and exercise is the best way to reduce your weight and keep off pounds. Keep the following tips in mind:

■ Lose the "diet" mind-set. Stop dieting and choose to make a change in lifestyle. Make smart eating and exercise part of daily activities rather than viewing them as weight-reduction tools. By choosing to live healthier rather than concentrating on weight loss, you may find that the desired results are achieved more easily and last longer.

■ Be sure to drink at least eight glasses of water a day.

■ Eat more slowly. Experts say it takes 20 minutes after beginning to eat for the body to register that it is no longer hungry. If you eat too fast, you're more likely to overeat before you realize you're no longer hungry.

■ Try grazing. Have a selection of low-fat or nonfat foods, such as carrot and celery sticks, at your fingertips, and eat small snacks throughout the day to fight hunger.

However, watch your calories. The calories in nonfat desserts add up quickly and can sabotage a weight-reduction program.

■ Stay active. While exercise is an important part of weight reduction, keeping busy between workouts is also beneficial. Instead of watching TV or reading (two activities that promote snacking), try writing letters, cleaning the garage, or working in the garden.

■ Try not to snack before bedtime, when calories are least likely to be burned off.

■ Stay away from foods high in simple sugars, such as cake, candy, and ice cream.

■ Remember that not everyone loses weight at the same rate. Don't be discouraged if those around you drop pounds faster. Men, especially, lose weight faster with the same amount of exercise.

■ Stay in touch with your practitioner. This will ensure that you are losing weight in the healthiest, most efficient way possible. Practitioners are also good sources of encouragement and support.

This is because fat naturally deposits on the hips and thighs as the body's stores for pregnancy and childbirth: after birth, these stores are burned up by breast-feeding. However, fat that collects in the abdominal area is associated with obesity and increased risk of heart disease and other health problems.

DANGERS OF DIETING

While obesity may increase the risks of health problems, there are also dangers to constant

dieting. Crash diets, in particular, cause problems—and don't work. A severely reduced calorie intake (anything under 1,000 calories per day for a woman of average build) fails because the body is biologically conditioned to fight weight loss and starvation under those circumstances. Such diets also lead to fatigue, depression, sleep abnormalities, intolerance to cold, dry skin, dry hair, constipation, and dizziness. Women should also be aware that many well-known low-calorie commercial diets that encourage rapid weight loss have been linked to gallbladder disease. These programs often include prepackaged food and instant drinks.

Another reason semistarvation diets do not result in successful long-term weight loss and should be avoided is that most people have an urge to binge once they stop the diet. Not knowing when food will be available again, the body, which has just experienced a period of near starvation, instinctively overeats.

Constant dieting also encourages an obsession with body image, which may lead to serious eating disorders, such as anorexia nervosa and bulimia.

THE SAFE WAY TO LOSE WEIGHT

Before beginning any weight-reduction program, a woman should consult her practitioner.

The basic premise to weight reduction is to decrease calorie intake and increase calorie expenditure. The safest and most efficient way to do this is by eating 500 to 1,000 calories a day less than the body's energy requirements (recommended daily allowance charts are based on a 2,000-calorie-a-day diet). This should result in a weight loss of about 1 1/2 pounds per week. Women should expect a faster weight loss at the start of a diet, when the body's glycogen and fat stores are being depleted of water. Many recent studies suggest that cutting dietary fats may be more effective than counting calories in reducing weight. A practitioner or nutritionist should be able to provide information on specific food recommendations.

Exercise is an important part of a weight-reduction program. It not only burns calories and tones muscles, but aerobic exercise may also speed up the metabolism, making the body use energy more efficiently. Obese people should begin exercise programs gradually, with the goal of making it a daily habit to engage in more physical exertion.

Group therapy is another positive contributing factor to successful weight reduction. A number of weight-reduction organizations operate programs across the country. Weight Watchers and Overeaters Anonymous are the best known. People with similar problems appear to provide the emotional support and encouragement that many need when trying to lose weight.

SEE eating disorders; nutrition; physical fitness.

For more information on weight reduction, contact:

American Dietetic Association
Consumer Nutrition Hotline
216 W. Jackson Blvd., Suite 800
Chicago, IL 60606
800-366-1655
http://www.eatright.org

Overeaters Anonymous, Inc.
World Service Office
P.O. Box 44020
Rio Rancho, NM 87174-4020
505-891-2664

Take Off Pounds Sensibly (TOPS)
P.O. Box 07360
Milwaukee, WI 53207
800-932-8677

Weight Watchers International
175 Crossways Park W.
Woodbury, NJ 11797
516-390-1400

Yoga

Yoga is a science of life that originated in India and that espouses the uniting of body, mind, and spirit in order to achieve a higher self-realization; it has been practiced for some 6,000 years as a method for seeking self-discipline, concentration, and positive thinking. Yoga is a critical aspect of Ayur Veda, one of the most ancient systems of natural medicine. A person who practices yoga, follows its philosophy, or teaches yoga is a yogi. Yoga, a gentle alternative to more vigorous forms of exercise, is thought to benefit women by relieving premenstrual syndrome, dysmenorrhea (menstrual cramps), stress, postpartum depression, and other disorders. It is also sometimes used to prepare for childbirth.

The most common form of yoga in the United States is known as **hatha yoga.** It is deeply rooted in Eastern mysticism and the belief in a formless god who creates and arranges all matter. The yogi attempts to unite with this force and reach a state of consciousness and awareness in which harmony exists. But before reaching this state, the yogi must perform a series of exercises involving breathing, posture, and meditation.

Other forms of yoga are **mantra yoga,** in which a word or phrase is effortlessly repeated thousands of times to allow the mind to go beyond thoughts and feelings; **karma yoga,** which deals with good deeds producing good consequences and bad deeds producing bad consequences; and **raja yoga,** achieving the ultimate state of superconsciousness, or deep meditation, that yogis strive to attain.

For more information on all forms of yoga, contact:

Himalayan International Institute of Yoga
Science and Philosophy
R.R. 1, P.O. Box 400
Honesdale, PA 18431
800-822- 4547
717-253-5551

Samata Yoga and Health Institute
4150 Tivoli Ave.
Los Angeles, CA 90066
310-306-8845

APPENDICES

MEDICAL LANGUAGE

Medical practitioners use a precise language to communicate diagnosis and treatment. As a rule, these seemingly complex medical terms, which are derived from ancient Greek, are built from three blocks—the prefixes, roots, and suffixes. They can be easily deciphered if the meanings of the blocks are known.

The following list may help you translate the medical language you hear or read.

Prefixes are the blocks that sit at the front of words. They generally tell "where," "if," and "how much."

a, an = not, without
ab = away from
acid = sour
ad = near (*d* changes to *c, f, g, p, s,* or *t* when it precedes roots that begin with those letters)
alb = white
amphi(i) = both, twice as much
ante = before
anti = against
ap(o) = detached
brady = slow
contra = against, counter to
cry = cold
dia = through or passing through, going apart, between, across
dys = painful, difficult
e = out from
ecto = outside of, outer, exterior
endo = within
epi = upon, on, over
erythr = red
eso = inside
exo = outside of
hemi = half
hyper = increased, excessive, above
hypo = under, below, deficient
in = not (*n* changes to *l, m,* or *r* when it precedes roots that begin with those letters)
infra = below
inter = between
intra = within
leuco, leuko = white
macro = large
mal = bad, ill, wrongful, disordered

meta = after, beyond, changing
micro = small
para = beyond, beside
peri = around
poly = many, multiple
post = after
pre = before, in front of
pseud(o) = false
re = again
retro = backward, behind
sub = under, below
super = above, beyond, over
supra = above
syn, sy, syl, sym = with, together
tachy = fast

Roots are at the center of each word or at the beginning if there is no prefix. They usually indicate the affected body part.

abdomin = abdomen, stomach
adeno = gland
adip = fat
angi(o) = vessel (blood, lymph)
arteri(o) = artery
arthr(o) = joint
aur = ear
blephar = eyelid
brachi = arm
bronch = windpipe
cardi(o) = heart
cephal = head
cervic = neck
chole, cholo = bile, gall
cholecyst = gallbladder
chondr = cartilage
col(o) = colon
colpo = vagina
crani(o) = skull
cut = skin

cystido, cysto = bladder, sac, cyst
cyto = cell
dent = tooth
enter = intestine
fasci = face
gastr(o) = stomach
glyco = sugar
gnath = jaw
hema, hemato, hemo = blood
hepat(o) = liver
hyster(o) = uterus
ile, ili = intestines, lower abdomen
labi = lip
lact = milk
lapar = loin, flank, abdomen
laryng = windpipe
lipo = fat
lumbar = loin
mast = breast
meno = menstruation
ment = mind
myel = marrow
myelo = spinal cord
myo = muscle
nephro(o) = kidney
neur(o) = nerve
ocul = eye
odont = teeth
oophor = ovary
ophthalm = eye
orchii(o) = testicle
os = mouth, opening
oss, oste(o) = bone
ot(o) = ear
ov = egg
pharyng = throat
phleb = vein
pleur = rib
pneuma, pneumato, pneumo = air, gas, lung

pod = foot
procto = anus, rectum
pulmo = lung
ren = kidney
rhino = nose
salping = fallopian tube
sperm, spermato = semen
splen = spleen
staphyl = uvula
stear = fat
tact = touch
teno = tendon
thorac(o) = chest
thromb = clot, lump
tracheo = windpipe
ur = urine
ureter(o) = tube from kidney to bladder, carrying urine
urethra = tube from bladder to the exterior
vas = vessel, duct
veno = vein
vesic = bladder

Suffixes, the final block in the word, specify what has gone wrong with—or what will be done to—the part of the body designated by the prefix and root.

algia = pain
blast = a growth in its early stages
cele = tumor, hernia
cente = puncture
desis = fusion
dynia = pain
ectomy = excision of, surgical removal
hydr = water
itis = inflammation
lysis = freeing of
megaly = very large
oma = tumor, swelling
oscopy = looking at an organ or internal part
osis = disease, abnormal condition or process
ostomy = creation of an artificial opening

otomy = incision, cutting into
pathy = disease of, abnormality
pexy = fix, sew
plasty = reconstruct, formation of
pnea = breathing
ptosis = falling, drooping
rhage, rhagia, rrhage, rrhagis = bursting forth, bleeding
rhea, rrhea = flow, discharge
scler(osis) = hard, hardening
uria = urine (condition of, presence in)

Prefix, root, and suffix come together to form medical terms, such as "endocarditis." To decode the word, just consult the lists: prefix "endo" means "within"; "cardio" has to do with the heart; and "itis" means "inflammation." Therefore, "endocarditis" means "inflammation of the inside of the heart," a more or less accurate description of the condition.

APPENDIX B
MEDICAL TESTING

Medical tests can be divided into four categories. **Screening** is usually a simple test to determine if a particular problem is present in a person who appears healthy and has no complaints. **Diagnostic tests** confirm or deny a practitioner's impressions. **Prognostic tests** are conducted after a diagnosis has been made to gather additional information. **Monitoring** is done to evaluate medical treatment.

Medical tests can also be divided into two classification—**invasive** and **noninvasive.** A test that involves penetration of the body is an invasive test. Such tests normally pose greater risks than a noninvasive test, which is one that does not penetrate the body.

Amniocentesis. A sampling of the amniotic fluid that surrounds the fetus; used to detect certain birth defects and brain and blood disorders in the fetus.

Angiogram. An x-ray picture of a blood vessel made after injecting an opaque substance or dye through a thin tube (catheter) into blood vessels to make the vessels visible on x-ray film. An angiogram of the arteries is called *arteriogram;* of the veins, *venogram* or *phlebogram;* of the lymph vessels, *lymph angiogram;* of the heart's arteries, *coronary angiogram.*

Arthrogram. An x-ray picture of a joint; used to detect injury or damage.

Arthroscopy. An examination of a joint by means of a long, flexible viewing tube inserted into the joint; used to detect injury or damage.

Barium enema. X-ray pictures of the large intestine (colon) made after injecting barium sulfate into the rectum; used to locate abnormalities in the colon. Often called a lower gastrointestinal (GI) series.

Barium meal. X-ray pictures of the esophagus, stomach, and duodenum (first part of the small intestine) made after the patient swallows barium sulfate on an empty stomach; used to locate problems or abnormalities in the digestive tract. Often called an upper gastrointestinal (GI) series.

Biopsy. The removal of a small portion of body tissue for microscopic analysis; often used to check growths that might be cancerous.

Bronchoscopy. An examination of the bronchi (air passages) of the lungs with a flexible, fiberoptic viewing tube that has been inserted in the throat

Cardiac catheterization. The insertion of a thin, flexible tube (a catheter) through a vein or artery into the heart; used to collect information about the heart's structure and performance and to inject an opaque substance (dye) so that an x-ray can be made.

Carotid or **cerebral arteriogram.** An x-ray picture of the blood vessels of the brain; used in diagnosing stroke. See "Angiogram."

Cholesterol test. A sampling of the blood to determine the amount of cholesterol in the blood

Colonoscopy. An examination of the colon with a flexible, fiberoptic viewing tube

Complete blood cell count (CBC). An examination of blood samples to get a count of the number of red cells, white cells, and hemoglobin in the blood and to determine the percentage of red cells in the blood; used to check for infection or screen for blood disorders.

Computerized axial tomography scan (CAT scan). A highly detailed picture of internal body parts constructed by a computer from hundreds of x-rays; frequently used to locate disease, tumors, or abnormalities in the selected part of the body.

Coronary angiogram. An x-ray picture of the heart's arteries. Coronary angiography is a form of cardiac catheterization.

Cystogram. An x-ray picture of the bladder made by inserting a thin tube through the urethra into the bladder

Dilation and curettage (D&C). The removal of a layer of tissue from the wall of the uterus; as a diagnostic test, it is used to diagnose the cause of excessive vaginal bleeding or other problems with the reproductive system.

Echocardiogram. An ultrasound recording of the heart's internal structures; used to locate heart valve problems or heart deformities.

Electrocardiogram (ECG or EKG). A recording of the heart muscle's activity that is collected by electrodes placed on the body; used to detect heart damage, as after a heart attack, and to monitor the effect of certain drugs.

Electroencephalogram (EEG). A recording of the brain's electrical impulses and brain patterns that is collected by electrodes placed on the scalp; often used to detect brain damage, diagnose epilepsy, or confirm brain death.

Electromyogram (EMG). A recording of the electrical activity of resting and contracting muscles that is collected by an electrode and a thin needle attached to the skin; used to detect weakness, paralysis, or other problems in the muscle.

Endoscopy. The use of a hollow tube that contains a light source and a viewing lens to examine interior parts of the body. Some of the tubes are rigid for direct viewing, while others are flexible and can be "snaked" through various parts of the body. The newer flexible scopes owe their success in large part to the development and application of fiberoptics technology. Fiberoptic devices are thin, flexible tubes containing bundles of glass filaments that can transmit light around bends and curves to illuminate the inside of the body. In some cases forceps, scissors, or other tiny instruments can be threaded through channels in the scope to facilitate surgical procedures. In addition, the pictures taken by the lens of the scope can be fed to a television monitor for better viewing by practitioners. The more common endoscopes are:

Arthroscope: a fiberoptic instrument used to examine the interior of a joint, such as a knee or shoulder, by insertions through a small incision made above the joint

Bronchoscope: an instrument inserted through the mouth to examine the lungs and bronchial tree. A rigid bronchoscope is a straight, hollow tube that permits direct viewing of the airway passages. A flexible bronchoscope uses a fiberoptic system that permits an inspection of the full bronchial system.

Colonoscope: a flexible fiberoptic instrument inserted through the anus to examine the large intestine from the anus to the cecum (the first part of the large intestine)

Colposcope: a lighted instrument that looks like a pair of binoculars used to microscopically examine the vagina and the cervix and to target areas of suspicious tissue for biopsy

Culdoscope: a thin, lighted instrument that is inserted through an incision made in the vagina to view the uterus, fallopian tubes, and rectal wall

Cystoscope: a rigid or flexible instrument with a viewing lens and light source that is inserted through the urethra to view the urethra and bladder or to obtain urine and tissue samples

Gastroscope: a flexible fiberoptic instrument that is

413

inserted through the mouth or the nose to examine the upper portion of the digestive tract (esophagus, stomach, and duodenum)

Hysteroscope: a narrow instrument with a light source that is inserted through the vagina and cervix to examine the inside of the uterus

Laparoscope: a thin, lighted instrument that is inserted through a small incision in the abdomen, usually near the navel, and used to examine the liver, gallbladder, spleen, intestines, and, in women, the uterus, ovaries, and fallopian tubes

Laryngoscope: a thin fiberoptic instrument that is inserted through a nostril in order to view the base of the tongue, epiglottis, larynx, and vocal cords

Proctoscope: a short (about five or six inches), rigid or flexible tube that is inserted through the anus to examine the rectum

Sigmoidoscope: a rigid or flexible tube inserted through the anus to examine the sigmoid colon (the S-shaped portion of the colon just above the rectum). The rigid sigmoidoscope is a lighted tube about 12 inches long and one inch in diameter. The flexible sigmoidoscope employs fiberoptics and is about two feet long.

Hysterosalpingogram. An x-ray picture of the uterine cavity and the inside of the fallopian tubes

Lower gastrointestinal (GI) series. See "Barium enema."

Magnetic resonance imaging (MRI). A magnetic field process (instead of radiation) that produces detailed, computer-generated pictures of the body

Mammogram. An x-ray picture of the breast; used to diagnose certain conditions, including breast cancer.

Myelogram. An x-ray picture of the fluid-filled space around the spinal cord; used to locate tumors, nerve injuries, and slipped disks.

Pap test. A sampling of the tissue of the cervix; used to detect abnormal cells and cancer. Also called a cervical smear.

Positron emission tomography (PET). A technique for making computer-generated images of the brain or other body organs by injecting radioactive isotopes into the body; used to locate abnormal tissue.

Spinal tap. A sampling of cerebrospinal fluid removed by a long needle from the spinal canal; used to diagnose diseases of and injuries to the brain and spinal cord, especially in suspected cases of meningitis and stroke.

Thermogram. A photograph of the surfaces of the body made by a camera with heat-sensitive film; often used to detect varicose veins, breast tumors, inflammation, and decreased blood supply.

Ultrasound scan. A picture of organs and structures deep inside the body made by using high frequency sound waves; used to gather information about some part of the body; also used on pregnant women to gain information about the health or development of the fetus.

Upper gastrointestinal (GI) series. See "Barium meal" above.

Venogram. An x-ray picture of the interior of a vein. See "Angiogram."

X-ray. A picture of the body's internal structures made with electromagnetic rays with a short wavelength

APPENDIX C
SUGGESTED READING

Abortion

Chalker, Rebecca, and Carol Downer. *A Woman's Book of Choices: Abortion, Menstrual Extraction, and RU-486.* New York: Four Walls Eight Windows, 1992.

Adoption

Baldwin, Paul. *The 125 Most Asked Questions About Adoption (and the Answers).* New York: William Morrow, 1993.

Gilman, Lois. *The Adoption Resource Book.* New York: HarperCollins, 1992.

Johnston, Patricia A. *Adopting After Infertility.* Indianapolis, Ind.: Perspective Press, 1992.

Melina, Lois Ruskai, and Sharon Kaplan Roszia. *The Open Adoption Experience: A Complete Guide for Adoptive and Birth Parents—From Making the Decision Through the Child's Growing Years.* New York: HarperCollins, 1993.

Rappaport, Bruce. *The Open Adoption Book: A Guide to Adoption Without Tears.* New York: Macmillan, 1992.

Acupuncture

Bauer, Cathryn. *Acupressure for Everybody: Gentle, Effective Relief for More Than 100 Common Ailments.* New York: Holt and Company, 1991.

Aging

Doress-Worters, Paula B., and Diana Laskin Siegal. *The New Ourselves, Growing Older.* New York: Simon and Schuster, 1994.

AIDS/HIV

American Foundation for AIDS Research. *The AIDS/HIV Treatment Directory.* New York: The Foundation, 1995.

Ford, Michael Thomas. *100 Questions and Answers About AIDS: What You Need to Know Now.* New York: Beach Tree Books, 1993.

Greif, Judith, and Beth Ann Golden. *AIDS Care at Home: A Guide for Caregivers, Loved Ones, and People with AIDS.* New York: John Wiley and Sons, 1994.

Pinsky, Laura, and Paul Harding Douglas. *The Essential HIV Treatment Fact Book.* New York: Pocket Books, 1992.

Alternative Medicine

Bonk, Melinda, ed. *Alternative Medicine Yellow Pages.* Puyallup, Wash.: Future Medicine Publishing, 1994.

Burton Goldberg Group. *Alternative Medicine: The Definitive Guide.* Fife, Wash.: Future Medicine Publishing, 1994.

Westcott, Patsy, and Leyardia Black, N.D. *Alternative Health Care for Women: A Woman's Guide to Self-Help Treatments and Natural Therapies.* Rochester, Vt.: Healing Arts Press, 1988.

Alzheimer's Disease

Mace, Nancy L., M.A., and Peter V. Rabins, M.D., M.P.H. *The 36-Hour Day: A Family Guide to Caring for Persons with Alzheimer's Disease, Related Dementing Illnesses, and Memory Loss Later in Life.* Rev. ed. Baltimore, Md.: Johns Hopkins University Press, 1991.

Powell, Lenore S., Ed.D., and Katie Courtice. *Alzheimer's Disease: A Guide for Families.* Rev. ed. Reading, Mass.: Addison-Wesley, 1993.

Anemia

Beshore, George. *Sickle-Cell Anemia.* New York: F. Watts, 1994.

Larkin, Marylin. *What You Can Do About Anemia.* New York: Dell, 1993.

Arthritis

Childers, Norman F. *Arthritis—A Diet to Stop It: The Nightshades, Aging, and Ill Health.* Gainesville, Fla.: Horticultural Publications, 1986.

Pisetsky, David, M.D. *The Duke University Medical Center Book of Arthritis.* New York: Fawcett Columbine, 1991.

Sobel, Dava, and Arthur C. Klein. *Arthritis: What Works.* New York: St. Martin's Press, 1989.

Birth Defects

Gormley, Myra Vanderpool. *Family Diseases: Are You at Risk?* Baltimore: Genealogical Publishing Company, 1989.

Blood Pressure

Jones, Paul, M.D., and Angela Mitchell. *The Black Health Library Guide to Heart Disease and Hypertension.* New York: Henry Holt and Company, 1993.

Karpman, Harold L. *Preventing Silent Heart Disease: Detecting and Preventing America's Number 1 Killer.* New York: Crown, 1989.

Board Certification

Boyden, Karen, ed. *Medical and Health Information Directory, 1994-95.* 7th ed. Detroit: Gale Research Company, 1994

The Official ABMS Directory of Board Certified Medical Specialists, 1995. 27th ed. New Providence, N.H.: Marquis Who's Who, 1994.

Breast-Feeding

Huggins, Kathleen. *The Nursing Mother's Companion.* Boston: Harvard Common Press, 1991.

Jones, Carl. *Breastfeeding Your Baby: A Guide for the Contemporary Family.* New York: Macmillan, 1993.

La Leche League International. *The Womanly Art of Breastfeeding.* New York: New American Library, 1994.

Breast Health

Hirshaut, Yashar, and Peter I. Pressman. *Breast Cancer: The Complete Guide.* New York: Bantam, 1992.

Love, Susan M., M.D. *Dr. Susan Love's Breast Book.* Reading, Mass.: Addison-Wesley, 1991.

Simone, Charles B., M.D. *Breast Health: What You Need to Know About Disease Prevention, Diagnosis, Treatment, and Guidelines for Healthy Breast Care.* Garden City Park, N.Y.: Avery Publishing Group, 1995.

Breast Surgery

Bruning, Nancy. *Breast Implants: Everything You Need to Know.* Alameda, Calif.: Hunter House, 1992.

Wolfe, Sydney, and the Public Citizen Health Research Group with Rhonda Dolin Jones. *Women's Health Alert.* Reading, Mass.: Addison-Wesley, 1991.

Cancer

Altman, Roberta, and Michael J. Sarg, M.D. *The Cancer Dictionary.* New York: Facts on File, 1992.

Bruning, Nancy. *Coping with Chemotherapy.* New York: Ballantine, 1993.

Kemeny, Mary M., and Paula Dranov. *Beating the Odds Against Breast and Ovarian Cancer: Reducing Your Hereditary Risk.* Reading, Mass.: Addison-Wesley, 1992.

McGinn, Kerry, and Pamela Haylock. *Women's Cancers: How to Prevent Them, How to Treat Them, How to Beat Them.* Alameda, Calif.: Hunter House, 1993.

Montag, Thomas W. *A Woman's Cancer Book: A Complete Guide for Patients and Their Families.* Woodacre, Calif.: Penmarin Books, 1995.

Walters, Richard. Options: *The Alternative Cancer Therapy Book.* Garden City Park, N.Y.: Avery Publishing Group, 1993.

Williams, Wendy. *The Power Within: True Stories of Exceptional Patients Who Fought Back with Hope.* New York: Harper and Row, 1990.

Cancer, Breast

Fabian, Carol. *Recovering from Breast Cancer.* New York: HarperCollins, 1992.

LaTour, Kathy. *The Breast Cancer Companion.* New York: Avon, 1994.

Michnovicz, Jon J., and Diane S. Klein. *How to Reduce Your Risk of Breast Cancer.* New York: Warner Books, 1994.

Smith, Margaret D., Susie Henderson, and Monica Hashiguchi, eds. *Stealing the Dragon's Fire: A Personal Guide and Resource for Dealing with Breast Cancer.* Bothell, Wash.: Wilson Publishing, 1995.

Cesarean Section

Wolfe, Sydney, and the Public Citizen Health Research Group with Rhonda Dolin Jones. *Women's Health Alert.* Reading, Mass.: Addison-Wesley, 1991.

Childbirth

Curtis, Glade B., M.D., F.A.C.O.G. *Your Pregnancy, Questions and Answers.* Tucson, Ariz.: Fisher Books, 1995.

————, *Your Pregnancy Week-by-Week.* Tucson, Ariz.: Fisher Books, 1995.

Eisenberg, Arlene, Heidi E. Murkoff, and Sandee E. Hathaway, B.S.N. *What to Expect When You're Expecting.* New York: Workman, 1991.

Inch, Sally. *Birthrights: What Every Parent Should Know About Birth in Hospitals.* New York: Pantheon, 1984.

Kitzinger, Sheila. *Homebirth and Other Alternatives to Hospitals.* London: Dorling-Kindersley, 1991.

Korte, Diana, and Roberta Scaer. *A Good Birth, A Safe Birth: Choosing and Having the Childbirth Experience That You Want.* 3rd rev. ed. Boston: Harvard Common Press, 1992.

Lim, Robin. *After the Baby's Birth: A Woman's Way to Wellness.* Berkeley, Calif.: Celestial Arts Publishing Company, 1991.

Luke, Barbara. *Every Pregnant Woman's Guide to Preventing Premature Birth: A Program for Reducing the Sixty Proven Risks That Can Lead to Prematurity.* New York: Times Books, Random House, 1995.

Chronic Fatigue Syndrome

Bolles, Edmund Blair. *Learning to Live with Chronic Fatigue Syndrome.* New York: Dell, 1990.

Feiden, Karyn. *Hope and Help for the Chronic Fatigue Syndrome: The Official Book of the CFS/CFIDS Network.* New York: Prentice Hall, 1990.

Johnson, Hillary. *Osler's Web.* New York: Crown Publishing Group, 1996.

Contraception

Chalker, Rebecca. *The Complete Cervical Cap Guide.* New York: Harper and Row, 1987.

Hatcher, Robert. *Emergency Contraception: The Nation's Best Kept Secret.* Decatur, Ga.: Bridging the Gap Communications, 1995.

Hatcher, Robert, et al. *Contraceptive Technology.* New York: Irvington Publishers, 1994.

Juhn, Greg. *Understanding the Pill: A Consumer's Guide to Oral Contraceptives.* New York: Haworth Press, 1994.

Matteson, Peggy. *Advocating for Self: Women's Decisions Concerning Contraception.* Binghamton, N.Y.: Haworth Press, 1995.

Vecchio, Thomas J., M.D., F.A.C.P. *Birth Control by Injection—The Story of Depo-Provera.* New York: Vantage Press, 1993.

Weschler, Toni, M.P.H. *Taking Charge of Your Fertility—The Definitive Guide to Natural Birth Control and Pregnancy Achievement.* New York: HarperCollins, 1985.

Winikoff, Beverly, M.D., M.P.H., Suzanne Wymelenberg, and the editors of Consumer Reports Books. *The Contraceptive Handbook: A Guide to Safe and Effective Choices.* Yonkers, N.Y.: Consumer Reports Books, 1992.

Death and Dying

Cohen, B. D. *The Essential Guide to a Living Will: How to Protect Your Right to Refuse Medical Treatment.* Englewood Cliffs, N.J.: Prentice Hall, 1991.

Barnett, Terry J. *Living Wills and More: Everything You Need to Ensure That All Your Medical Wishes Are Followed.* New York: John Wiley and Sons, 1992.

Kubler-Ross, Elisabeth. *On Death and Dying: What the Dying Have to Teach Doctors, Nurses, Clergy, and Their Own Families.* New York: Macmillan, 1969.

Nuland, Sherwin B. *How We Die: Reflections on Life's Final Chapter.* New York: Alfred A. Knopf, 1994.

Taylor, Nick. *A Necessary End.* New York: Doubleday and Company, Inc., 1994.

Volkan, Vanik D., and Elizabeth Zintl. *Life After Loss: The Lessons of Grief.* New York: Scribner, 1994.

Depression

Braiker, Harriet B. *Getting Up When You're Feeling Down: A Woman's Guide to Overcoming and Preventing Depression.* New York: G. P. Putnam's Sons, 1988.

McGrath, Ellen. *When Feeling Bad Is Good.* New York: Holt, 1992.

————, ed. *Women and Depression.* Washington, D.C.: American Psychological Association, 1990.

Diabetes

Krall, Leo P., M.D., and Richard S. Beaser, M.D. *Joslin Diabetes Manual.* 12th ed. Philadelphia: Lea and Febiger, 1989.

Diethylstilbestrol

Cody, Nora, ed. *The DES Action Voice.* Oakland, Calif.: DES Action USA. Quarterly newsletter.

National Women's Health Network. *Diethylstilbestrol: Women's Health Resource Guide, No. 6.* Washington, D.C.: National Women's Health Network, 1980.

Domestic Violence

Berry, Dawn W. *Domestic Violence Sourcebook.* Los Angeles: Lowell House, 1995.

Lobel, Kerry. *Naming the Violence: Speaking Out About Lesbian Battering.* Seattle, Wash.: Seal Press, 1986.

McCue, Margaret. *Domestic Violence: A Reference Handbook.* Santa Barbara, Calif.: ABC-CLIO, 1995.

Renzetti, Claire M. *Violent Betrayal: Partner Abuse in Lesbian Relationships.* Thousand Oaks, Calif.: Sage, 1992.

Eating Disorders

Controlling Eating Disorders with Facts, Advice and Resources. Phoenix, Ariz.: Oryx Press, 1992.

Miller, Caroline. *My Name Is Caroline.* New York: Doubleday and Company, Inc., 1988.

Siegel, Michele, Judith Brisman, and Margot Weinshel. *Surviving an Eating Disorder.* New York: Harper and Row, 1988.

Zerbe, Kathryn J. *The Body Betrayed: Women, Eating Disorders, and Treatment.* Washington, D.C.: American Psychiatric Press, 1993.

Endometriosis

Carol, Ruth, ed. *Alternatives for Women with Endometriosis: A Guide by Women for Women.* Chicago: Third Side Press, 1994.

Herman, Phyllis, ed. *Natural Treatment of Fibroid Tumors and Endometriosis.* New Canaan, Conn.: Keats Publishing Company, 1995.

Lark, Susan. *Dr. Susan Lark's Fibroid Tumors and Endometriosis Self-Help Book.* Berkeley, Calif.: Celestial Arts Publishing Company, 1995.

Female Genital Mutilation

Porkenoo, Efua. *Cutting the Rose: Female Genital Mutilation: The Practice and Its Prevention.* Concord, Mass.: Paul and Company Publishers Consortium, 1995.

Walker, Alice, and Pratibha Parmar. *Warrior Marks: Female Genital Mutilation and the Sexual Binding of Women.* Orlando, Fla.: Harcourt Brace and Company, 1996.

Fibroids

Herman, Phyllis, ed. *Natural Treatment of Fibroid Tumors and Endometriosis.* New Canaan, Conn.: Keats Publishing Company, 1995.

Lark, Susan. *Dr. Susan Lark's Fibriod Tumors and Endometriosis Self-Help Book.* Berkeley, Calif.: Celestial Arts Publishing Company, 1995.

Fibromyalgia

Backstrom, Gayle. *When Muscle Pain Won't Go Away: The Relief Handbook for Fibromyalgia and Chronic Muscle Pain.* Dallas, Tex.: Taylor Publishing Company, 1992.

Gibson, Barbara A. *The Fibromyalgia Handbook.* 2nd ed. Clearwater, Fla.: Gemini Press, 1995.

Prudden, Bonnie. *Myotherapy: Bonnie Prudden's Complete Guide to Pain Free Living.* New York: Ballantine, 1985.

Heart Disease

Diethrich, Edward B., M.D., and Carol Cohan. *Women and Heart Disease: What You Can Do to Stop the #1 Killer of American Women.* New York: Random House, 1992.

Jones, Paul, M.D., and Angela Mitchell. *The Black Health Library Guide to Heart Disease and Hypertension.* New York: Henry Holt and Company, 1993.

Legato, Marianne J., M.D., and Carol Colman. *The Female Heart: The Truth About Women and Coronary Artery Disease.* New York: Simon and Schuster, 1991.

Ornish, Dean. *Dr. Dean Ornish's Program for Reversing Heart Disease.* New York: Random House, 1991.

Pashkow, Frederick, and Charlotte Libove. *The Woman's Heart Book: The Complete Guide to Keeping Your Heart Healthy and What to Do If Things Go Wrong.* New York: Dutton, 1993.

Herbal Medicine

Gladstar, Rosemary. *Herbal Healing for Women.* New York: Simon and Schuster, 1993.

McIntyre, Anne. *The Complete Woman's Herbal: A Manual of Healing Herbs and Nutrition for Personal Well-Being and Family Care.* New York: Henry Holt and Company, 1995.

Homeopathy

Handley, Rima. *Homeopathy for Women.* San Francisco: Thorsons, 1993.

Lockie, Andrew, and Nicola Geddes. *The Woman's Guide to Homeopathy.* New York: St. Martin's Press, 1994.

Moskowitz, Richard, M.D. *Homeopathic Medicines for Pregnancy and Childbirth.* Berkeley, Calif.: North Atlantic Books, 1992.

Hormone Replacement Therapy

Henkel, Gretchen. *Making the Estrogen Decision.* Los Angeles: Lowell House, 1992.

Ito, Dee. *Without Estrogen.* New York: Random House, 1994.

Kamen, Betty, Ph.D. *Hormone Replacement Therapy: Yes or No?* Novato, Calif.: Nutrition Encounter, 1993.

Lark, Susan M. *The Estrogen Decision: A Self-Help Program.* Los Altos, Calif.: Westchester Publishing, 1994.

Redmond, Geoffrey, M.D. *The Good News About Women's Hormones.* New York: Warner Books, 1995.

Rinzler, Carol Ann. *Estrogen and Breast Cancer: A Warning to Women.* New York: Macmillan, 1993.

Hysterectomy

Dennerstein, Lorraine, and Carol Wood. *Hysterectomy: Advances and New Options.* 2nd ed. New York: Oxford University Press, 1995.

Haas, Adelaide, and Susan L. Puretz. *The Woman's Guide to Hysterectomy: Expectations and Options.* Berkeley, Calif.: Celestial Arts Publishing Company, 1994.

Strausz, Ivan K. *You Don't Need a Hysterectomy: New and Effective Ways of Avoiding Major Surgery.* Reading, Mass.: Addison-Wesley, 1994.

West, Stanley, and Paula Dranov. *The Hysterectomy Hoax.* New York: Doubleday and Company, 1994.

Wolfe, Sydney, and the Public Citizen Health Research Group with Rhonda Dolin Jones. *Women's Health Alert.* Reading, Mass.: Addison-Wesley, 1991.

Incontinence

Chalker, Rebecca, and Kristine E. Whitmore. *Overcoming Bladder Diseases.* New York: Harper and Row, 1990.

Gartley, Cheryle B., ed. *Managing Incontinence: A Guide to Living with Loss of Bladder Control.* Ottawa, Ill.: Jameson Books, 1985.

Infertility

Andrews, Lori. *Between Strangers: Surrogate Mothers, Expectant Fathers and Brave New Babies.* New York: Harper and Row, 1989.

Glazer, Ellen S., and Susan L. Cooper. *Beyond Infertility: The New Paths to Parenthood.* New York: Simon and Schuster, 1994.

Harkness, Carla. *The Infertility Book: A Comprehensive Medical and Emotional Guide.* Berkeley, Calif.: Celestial Arts, 1992.

Johnson, Patricia Irvin. *Taking Charge of Infertility.* Indianapolis, Ind.: Perspective Press, 1994.

Scher, Geoffrey, M.D., and Virginia Marriage. *From Infertility to In Vitro Fertilization.* New York: McGraw-Hill, 1988.

Treiser, Susan, and Robin Levinson. *A Woman Doctor's Guide to Infertility: Essential Facts and Up-to-the-Minute Information on the Technology and Treatments to Achieve Pregnancy.* New York: Hyperion, 1994.

Insomnia

Ford, Norman O. *The Sleep Rx: 75 Proven Ways to Get a Good Night's Sleep.* Englewood Cliffs, N.J.: Prentice Hall, 1994.

Shapiro, Colin H., et al. *Conquering Insomnia: An Illustrated Guide to Understanding and Overcoming Sleep Disruption.* Chicago: Login Publishers Consortium, 1994.

Lesbian Health

Shernoff, Michael, ed. *Sourcebook on Lesbian/Gay Health Care.* Washington, D.C.: National Lesbian/Gay Health Foundation, 1988.

Stern, Phyllis M., ed. *Lesbian Health: What Are the Issues?* Bristol, Pa.: Hemisphere Publishing Company, 1993.

Long-Term Care

Inlander, Charles B., et al. *Long-Term Care and Its Alternatives.* Allentown, Pa.: People's Medical Society, 1996.

Lupus

Blau, Sheldon Paul. *Living with Lupus: All the Knowledge You Need to Help Yourself.* Reading, Mass.: Addison-Wesley, 1993.

Dibner, Robin, M.D., and Carol Colman. *The Lupus Handbook for Women: Up-to-Date Information on Understanding and Managing the Disease Which Affects 1 in 500 Women.* New York: Simon and Schuster, 1994.

Wallace, Daniel. *The Lupus Book: A Guide for Patients and Their Families.* New York: Oxford University Press, 1995.

Massage Therapy

DePaoli, Carlo. *The Healing Touch of Massage.* New York: Sterling Publishing Company, 1995.

LaCroix, Nitya. *Erotic Massage: Simple, Sensuous Techniques for Enhancing Sexual Pleasure.* San Francisco: Harper San Francisco, 1994.

McGilvery, Carole. *Step by Step Massage: A Guide to Massage Techniques for Health, Relaxation, and Vitality.* New York: Smithmark Publications, 1994.

Waters, Bette L. *Massage During Pregnancy.* Fuquay Varina, N.C.: Research Triangle Publications, 1995.

Medical Rights

Inlander, Charles B., and Eugene I. Pavalon. *Your Medical Rights: How to Become an Empowered Consumer.* Allentown, Pa.: People's Medical Society, 1990.

Medications

Long, James W., M.D., and James J. Rybacki, Pharm.D. *The Essential Guide to Prescription Drugs.* New York: HarperCollins, 1994.

The Physician's Desk Reference. Montvale, N.J.: Medical Economic Data, 1996.

The PDR Guide to Women's Health and Prescription Drugs. Montvale, N.J.: Medical Economic Data, 1994.

Menopause

Barbach, Lonnie, Ph.D. *The Pause—Positive Approaches to Menopause.* New York: Penguin Books, 1993.

Cherry, Sheldon H., M.D., and Carolyn D. Runowicz, M.D. *The Menopause Book: A Guide to Health and Well Being for Women After Forty.* New York: Macmillan, 1994.

Cobb, Janine O'Leary. *Understanding Menopause: Answers and Advice for Women in the Prime of Life.* New York: Penguin Books, 1993.

———, ed. *A Friend Indeed: For Women in the Prime of Life.* Montreal, Quebec: A Friend Indeed Publications. Monthly newsletter.

Greer, Germaine. *The Change: Women, Aging and the Menopause.* New York: Alfred A. Knopf, 1992.

Jacobowitz, Ruth S., and Wulf H. Utian. *Managing Your Menopause.* New York: Prentice Hall, 1990.

Landau, Carol, Ph.D., Michele G. Cry, M.D., and Anne W. Moulton, M.S. *The Complete Book of Menopause.* New York: Perigee Books, 1994.

Notelovitz, Morris, M.D., Ph.D., and Diana Tonnessen. *Menopause and Midlife Health.* New York: St. Martin's Press, 1993.

Porcini, Jane, ed. *Hot Flash: Newsletter for Midlife and Older Women.* Stony Brook, N.Y.: National Action Forum for Mid-Life and Older Women. Newsletter.

Sand, Gayle. *Is It Hot in Here or Is It Me? A Personal Look at the Facts, Fallacies, and Feelings of Menopause.* New York: HarperCollins, 1993.

Sheehy, Gail. *Silent Passage.* New York: Random House, 1992.

Wolfe, Honora Lee. *Menopause, A Second Spring: Making a Smooth Transition with Traditional Chinese Medicine.* Boulder, Colo.: Blue Poppy Press, 1995.

Menstruation

Taylor, Dena. *Red Flower: Rethinking Menstruation.* Freedom, Calif.: The Crossing Press, 1988.

Migraine Headache

American Council for Headache Education. *Migraine: The Complete Guide.* New York: Dell Publishing Company, 1994.

Burks, Susan L. *Managing Your Migraine: A Migraine Sufferer's Practical Guide.* Totowa, N.J.: Humana Press, 1994.

Rapoport, Alan M., M.D., and Fred D. Sheftell, M.D. *Headache Relief.* New York: Simon and Schuster, 1990.

Miscarriage

Allen, Marie, and Shelly Marks. *Miscarriage: Women Sharing from the Heart.* New York: John Wiley and Sons, 1993.

Friedman, Rochelle, and Bonnie Gradstein. *Surviving Pregnancy Loss: A Complete Sourcebook for Women and Their Families.* New York: Little, Brown and Company, 1992.

Semchyshyn, Stefan. *How to Prevent Miscarriages and Other Crises of Pregnancy.* New York: Macmillan, 1989.

Nutrition

Brown, Judith E. *Everywoman's Guide to Nutrition.* Minneapolis: University of Minnesota Press, 1990.

Garrison, Robert H., Jr., M.A., R.Ph., and Elizabeth Somer, M.A., R.D. *The Nutrition Desk Reference.* New Canaan, Conn.: Keats Publishing Company, 1990.

Gittleman, Ann Louise, and J. Lynne Dodson. *Supernutrition for Women: A Foodwise Guide for Health, Beauty, and Immunity.* New York: Bantam Books, 1991.

Osteoporosis

Bonnick, Sydney L. *The Osteoporosis Handbook: Every Woman's Guide to Prevention and Treatment.* Dallas, Tex.: Taylor Publishing Company, 1994.

Gaby, Alan R. *Preventing and Reversing Osteoporosis: Every Woman's Essential Guide.* Rocklin, Calif.: Prima, 1994.

Jacobowitz, Ruth S. *150 Most Asked Questions About Osteoporosis: What Women Really Want to Know.* New York: Hearst Books, 1993.

Pap Test

Wilson, Margaret. *What an Abnormal Pap Smear Means.* Cincinnati, Ohio: Seven Hills Book Distribution, 1995.

Physical Fitness

Butler, Joan M. *Fit and Pregnant: The Pregnant Woman's Guide to Exercise.* Waverly, N.Y.: Acorn Publishing, 1995.

Harris, Raymond, et al., eds. *Physical Activity, Aging, and Sports Series.* 4 vols. Albany, N.Y.: Center for the Study of the Aging, 1994.

Melopomene Institute for Women's Health Research. *The Bodywise Woman: Reliable Information on Physical Activity and Health.* New York: Prentice Hall, 1990.

Shangold, Mona, and Gabe Mirkin. *The Complete Sports Medicine Book for Women: Revised for the '90s.* New York: Simon and Schuster, 1992.

Plastic Surgery

Davis, Kathy. *Reshaping the Female Body: The Dilemma of Cosmetic Surgery.* New York: Routledge, 1994.

McCoy, Betsy. *Cosmetic Plastic Surgery.* Sacramento, Calif.: Paradise Publications, 1993.

Practitioners, How to Choose

Boyden, Karen, ed. *Medical and Health Information Directory, 1994–5.* 7th ed. Detroit: Gale Research Company, 1994.

The Official ABMS Directory of Board Certified Medical Specialists, 1996. 28th ed. New Providence, N.H.: Marquis Who's Who, 1995.

Pregnancy

See "Childbirth."

Premenstrual Syndrome

Dalton, Katharina, M.D. *Once a Month: The Original Premenstrual Syndrome Handbook.* Alameda, Calif.: Hunter House, 1990.

Lark, Susan. *Dr. Susan Lark's the Menstrual Cramps Self-Help Book: Effective Solutions for Pain and Discomfort Due to Menstrual Cramps and PMS.* Berkeley, Calif.: Celestial Arts Publishing Company, 1995.

Moe, Barbara. *Everything You Need to Know About PMS.* New York: Rosen Publishing Group, 1995.

Repetitive Motion Injuries

Tannenhous, Norra. *Relief from Carpal Tunnel Syndrome and Other Repetitive Motion Disorders.* New York: Dell, 1991.

Sexual Assault

Bohmer, Carol, and Andrea Parrot. *Sexual Assault on Campus: The Problem and the Solution.* New York: The Free Press, 1993.

Brave, Ellen, and Ellen Cassedy. *The 9 to 5 Guide to Combatting Sexual Harassment.* New York: John Wiley and Sons, 1992.

Los Angeles Commission on Assaults Against Women. *Surviving Sexual Assault*. Chicago: Congdon and Weed, 1992.

Martin, Laura. *Life Without Fear: A Guide to Preventing Sexual Assault*. Nashville, Tenn.: Rutledge Hill Press, 1992.

Warshaw, Robin. *I Never Called It Rape: The Ms. Report on Recognizing, Fighting, and Surviving Date and Acquaintance Rape*. New York: Harper and Row, 1988.

Sexuality

Comfort, Alex, M.D., D.Sc. *The New Joy of Sex*. New York: Crown Publishers, 1991.

Davis, Elizabeth. *Women, Sex and Desire—Understanding Your Sexuality at Every Stage of Life*. Alameda, Calif.: Hunter House, 1995.

DeCotiis, Sue. *A Woman's Guide to Sexual Health*. New York: Pocket Books, 1989.

Ogden, Gina, Ph.D. *Women Who Love Sex*. New York: Pocket Books, 1994.

Reiss, Ira L., Ph.D. *An End to Shame: Shaping Our Next Sexual Revolution*. Buffalo, N.Y.: Prometheus Books, 1990.

Steinberg, Ruth, M.D., and Linda Robinson, R.N., C.N.M. *Women's Sexual Health: An Up-to Date, Comprehensive Guide to Female Sexuality and Health*. New York: Primus, 1995.

Sexually Transmitted Infections

Ebel, Charles. *Managing Herpes—How to Live and Cope with a Chronic STD*. Research Triangle Park, N.C.: American Social Health Association, 1994.

Hager, David, and Don Joy. *Women at Risk*. Anderson, Ind.: Bristol House, Ltd., 1993.

Novotny, Pamela P. *What Every Woman Should Know About Chronic Infection and Sexually Transmitted Diseases*. New York: Dell, 1991.

Smoking

Delany, Sue F. *Women Smokers Can Quit*. Evanston, Ill.: Women's Healthcare Press, 1989.

Stress

Powell, J. Robin, and Holly George-Warren. *The Working Woman's Guide to Managing Stress*. Englewood Cliffs, N.J.: Prentice Hall, 1994.

Witkin-Lanoil, Georgia. *The Female Stress Syndrome: How to Become Stress-Wise in the '90s*. New York: Newmarket Press, 1991.

Stroke

Caplan, Louis R., M.D., Mark L. Dyken, M.D., and J. Donald Easton, M.D. *The American Heart Association Family Guide to Stroke Treatment, Recovery and Prevention*. New York: Times Books, 1994.

Frye-Pierson, Janice, R.N., B.S.N., C.N.R.N., and James F. Toole, M.D. *Stroke: A Guide for Patient and Family*. New York: Raven Press, 1987.

Urinary Tract Infections

Gillespie, Larrian. *You Don't Have to Live with Cystitis! How to Avoid It, What to Do About It*. New York: Avon, 1988.

Schrotenboer, Kathryn. *The Woman Doctor's Guide to Overcoming Cystitis*. New York: New American Library, 1987.

Vaginitis

Bumslag, Naomi, and Dia L. Michaels. *A Woman's Guide to Yeast Infections*. New York: Pocket Books, 1992.

Crook, William G. *The Yeast Connection and the Woman*. Jackson, Tenn.: Professional Books, 1995.

Varicose Veins

Baron, Howard C., and Barbara A. Rose. *Varicose Veins: A Guide to Prevention and Treatment*. New York: Facts on File, 1995.

Navarro, Luis, et al. *No More Varicose Veins*. New York: Bantam, 1988.

Women's Health

Ammer, Christine. *A to Z of Women's Health: A Concise Encyclopedia*. New York: Facts on File, 1995.

Boston Women's Health Collective. *The New Our Bodies, Ourselves*. New York: Simon and Schuster, 1992.

DiMona, Lisa, and Constance Herndon, eds. *The 1995 Information Please Women's Sourcebook: Resources and Information to Use Every Day*. Boston: Houghton Mifflin Company, 1994.

Doress-Worters, Paula B., and Diana Laskin Siegal. *The New Ourselves, Growing Older*. New York: Simon and Schuster, 1994.

Hoffman, Eileen, M.D. *Our Health, Our Lives: A Revolutionary Approach to Total Health Care for Women*. New York: Pocket Books, 1995.

Korte, Diana. *Every Woman's Body*. New York: Fawcett Columbine, 1994.

Selmer, Tracy Chutorian. *All About Eve: The Complete Guide to Women's Health and Well Being*. New York: HarperCollins, 1995.

Thompson, D. S., M.D., ed. *EveryWoman's Health*. New York: Simon and Schuster, 1993.

Villarosa, Linda, ed. *Body and Soul: The Black Women's Guide to Physical Health and Emotional Well-Being*. New York: HarperCollins, 1994.

White, Evelyn C., ed. *The Black Women's Health Book: Speaking for Ourselves*. Seattle: Seal Press, 1994.

Yoga

Jordan, Sandra. *Yoga for Pregnancy: Ninety-Two Safe, Gentle Stretches Appropriate for Pregnant Women and New Mothers*. New York: St. Martin's Press, 1988.

O'Brien, Paddy. *A Gentler Strength: The Yoga Book for Women*. San Francisco: Thorsons, 1992.

PLANNED PARENTHOOD FEDERATION OF AMERICA PUBLICATIONS

The national office of Planned Parenthood Federation of America publishes a series of sexual and reproductive health pamphlets. More than 1.5 million are sold and distributed every year. Current titles on the following subjects include:

Birth Control

All About Tubal Sterilization
All About Vasectomy
The Condom
Diaphragms and Cervical Caps
Facts About Birth Control
Is Depo-Provera for You?
Norplant and You
Understanding IUDs
You and the Pill
Your Contraceptive Choices

Family Communication

How to Be a Good Parent
How to Talk with Your Child About Sexuality:
    A Parent's Guide
How to Talk with Your Teen about the Facts of Life
Kids and AIDS: A Guide for Parents
Talking About Sex: A Guide for Families (animated
    video, parent's guide, and children's activity book)

Sexuality Education

Feeling Good About Growing Up
Human Sexuality: What Children Should Know and
    When They Should Know It
A Man's Guide to Sexuality
TeenSex? It's OK to Say No Way!
A Woman's Guide to Sexuality

Sexual Health Care

AIDS and HIV: Questions and Answers
Chlamydia: Questions and Answers
Herpes: Questions and Answers
HPV & Genital Warts: Questions and Answers
Sex—Safer and Satisfying
Sexually Transmitted Infections: The Facts

Women's Health Care

Abortion: Questions and Answers
Having Your Period
Infertility: Questions and Answers
Menopause: Another Change in Life
Vaginitis: Commonly Asked Questions
Ways to Chart Your Fertility Pattern
What If I'm Pregnant?
Your Key to Good Health: The Gynecological Exam

For information about purchasing Planned Parenthood publications, call 800-669-0156, or write:

    Marketing Group
    Planned Parenthood Federation of America, Inc.
    810 Seventh Avenue
    New York, NY 10019
    212-541-7800

For the Planned Parenthood health center nearest you, call:

    800-230-PLAN
    http://www.ppfa.org/ppfa

INDEX